CHEMOTHERAPY

Volume 3
Special Problems in Chemotherapy

Edited by
J.D. Williams
The London Hospital Medical College
London, U.K.

and
A.M. Geddes
East Birmingham Hospital
Birmingham, U.K.

AF793578

Plenum Press · New York and London

Library of Congress Cataloging in Publication Data

International Congress of Chemotherapy, 9th, London, 1975.
Special problems in chemotherapy.

(Chemotherapy; v. 3)
1. Chemotherapy – Congresses. 2. Antitubercular agents – Congresses. 3. Genito-urinary organs – Diseases – Chemotherapy – Congresses. 4. Drugs resistance in micro-organisms – Congresses. 5. Antiseptic medication – Congresses. I. Williams, John David, M.D. II. Geddes, Alexander McIntosh. III. Title. IV. Series.
RM260.2.G45 vol. 3 615'.58s [615'.58] 76-1947
ISBN 978-1-4684-3122-3 ISBN 978-1-4684-3120-9 (eBook)
DOI 10.1007/978-1-4684-3120-9

Proceedings of the Ninth International Congress of Chemotherapy
held in London, July, 1975 will be published in eight volumes,
of which this is volume three.

©1976 Plenum Press, New York
Softcover reprint of the hardcover 1st edition 1976
A Division of Plenum Publishing Corporation
227 West 17th Street, New York, N.Y. 10011

United Kingdom edition published by Plenum Press, London
A Division of Plenum Publishing Company, Ltd.
Davis House (4th Floor), 8 Scrubs Lane, Harlesden, London, MW10 6SE, England

All rights reserved

No part of this book may be reproduced, stored in a retrieval system, or transmitted,
in any form or by any means, electronic, mechanical, photocopying, microfilming,
recording, or otherwise, without written permission from the Publisher

CHEMOTHERAPY

Volume 3
Special Problems in Chemotherapy

CHEMOTHERAPY

Volume 1 **Clinical Aspects of Infections**
Prophylaxis; life-threatening infections; infection in leukaemia; surgical infection; anaerobic infection; respiratory and urinary tract infections; amikacin.

Volume 2 **Laboratory Aspects of Infections**
Sensitivity testing; assay methods; animal models of infection; sisomycin; tobramycin.

Volume 3 **Special Problems in Chemotherapy**
Tuberculosis; genital tract infections; antibiotic resistance and mode of action; topical chemotherapy and antisepsis.

Volume 4 **Pharmacology of Antibiotics**
Tissue concentrations; pharmacokinetics; untoward effects of antibiotics.

Volume 5 **Penicillins and Cephalosporins**
Penicillins and cephalosporins; betalactamases; new agents.

Volume 6 **Parasites, Fungi, and Viruses**
Parasitic infections; fungal infections; chemotherapy of viruses; co-trimoxazole.

Volume 7 **Cancer Chemotherapy I**
Symposia – new drugs and approaches; cell and pharmacokinetics; potentiators of radiotherapy; in vitro screening systems; immunological aspects.

Volume 8 **Cancer Chemotherapy II**
Free papers – new drugs and approaches; cell and pharmacokinetics; mechanisms of action; new analogues; cancer chemotherapy of specific organs.

CHEMOTHERAPY

Proceedings of the
9th International Congress of Chemotherapy
held in London, July, 1975

Editorial Committee

K. Hellmann, *Chairman* (Anticancer)
Imperial Cancer Research Fund, London.

A. M. Geddes (Antimicrobial)
East Birmingham Hospital.

J. D. Williams (Antimicrobial)
The London Hospital Medical College.

Congress Organising Committee

W. Brumfitt	I. Phillips	H.P. Lambert
K. Hellmann	M.R.W. Brown	P. Turner
K.D. Bagshawe	D.G. James	A.M. Geddes
H. Smith	C. Stuart-Harris	D. Armitage
E.J. Stokes	R.G. Jacomb	D. Crowther
F. Wrigley	D.T.D. Hughes	D.S. Reeves
J.D. Williams	T. Connors	R.E.O. Williams

International Society
of Chemotherapy Executive - to July 1975

P. Malek	H.P. Kuemmerle	H. Ericsson
C. Grassi	Z. Modr	G.M. Savage
G.H. Werner	K.H. Spitzy	H. Umezawa
	P. Rentchnick	

Preface

The International Society of Chemotherapy meets every two years to review progress in chemotherapy of infections and of malignant disease. Each meeting gets larger to encompass the extension of chemotherapy into new areas. In some instances, expansion has been rapid, for example in cephalosporins, penicillins and combination chemotherapy of cancer - in others slow, as in the field of parasitology. New problems of resistance and untoward effects arise; reduction of host toxicity without loss of antitumour activity by new substances occupies wide attention. The improved results with cancer chemotherapy, especially in leukaemias, are leading to a greater prevalence of severe infection in patients so treated, pharmacokinetics of drugs in normal and diseased subjects is receiving increasing attention along with related problems of bioavailability and interactions between drugs. Meanwhile the attack on some of the major bacterial infections, such as gonorrhoea and tuberculosis, which were among the first infections to feel the impact of chemotherapy, still continue to be major world problems and are now under attack with new agents and new methods.

From this wide field and the 1,000 papers read at the Congress we have produced Proceedings which reflect the variety and vigour of research in this important field of medicine. It was not possible to include all of the papers presented at the Congress but we have attempted to include most aspects of current progress in chemotherapy.

We thank the authors of these communications for their cooperation in enabling the Proceedings to be available at the earliest possible date. The method of preparation does not allow for uniformity of typefaces and presentation of the material and we hope that the blemishes of language and typographical errors do not detract from the understanding of the reader and the importance of the Proceedings.

K. HELLMANN, Imperial Cancer Research Fund
A. M. GEDDES, East Birmingham Hospital
J. D. WILLIAMS, The London Hospital Medical College

Contents

SINGAPORE STUDY OF INTERMITTENT RIFAMPICIN PLUS ISONIAZID FOR PULMONARY TUBERCULOSIS

S C Poh

Tan Tock Seng Hospital
Moulmein Road, Singapore 11

SUMMARY

In Singapore, 481 adult patients with newly diagnosed pulmonary tuberculosis were allocated at random to four regimens of intermittent rifampicin plus isoniazid. All patients received an initial two weeks of daily chemotherapy with streptomycin plus isoniazid plus rifampicin in standard daily dosages, followed by isoniazid 15 mg/kg body weight plus rifampicin 900 mg, both drugs twice a week (HR2 regimen) or once a week (HR1 regimen), or by isoniazid 15 mg/kg plus rifampicin 600 mg, both drugs twice a week (LR2 regimen) or once a week (LR1 regimen). All patients in addition received a supplementary daily capsule containing at random either rifampicin 25 mg or a matched placebo, to see if the daily supplement would reduce the incidence of adverse reactions to rifampicin.

The first 334 patients with fully drug-sensitive strains pretreatment were currently available for assessment at 12 months. Every single patient on the 2 twice-weekly regimens had a favourable bacteriological status at 12 months, as had 96% of the HR1 and 92% of the LR1 patients. Adverse reactions to intermittent rifampicin occurred in 26% of the HR1 patients, but on the other three regimens their incidence was low. In contrast, the incidence of rifampicin-dependent antibodies ranged from 21% (LR2) to 54% (HR1). The incidence of adverse reactions and antibodies was unaffected by the rifampicin supplement.

INTRODUCTION

At the time this study was planned, animal and in vitro experimental evidence suggested that in man both isoniazid and rifampicin should be suitable for intermittent chemotherapy (Dickinson et al. 1968; Grumbach et al. 1969; Verbist 1969; Dickinson and Mitchison 1970). In clinical practice, however, rifampicin in dosages of 900 to 1800 mg once a week and twice a week although effective, induced a high incidence of adverse reactions (Girling and Fox 1971; Poole et al. 1971; Aquinas et al. 1972; Hong Kong Tuberculosis Treatment Services/Brompton Hospital/British Medical Research Council 1974; Hong Kong Tuberculosis Treatment Services/ British Medical Research Council 1974). The commonest of these was the 'flu' syndrome, a febrile reaction which came on one to two hours after a dose, lasted for several hours and was often associated with circulating rifampicin-dependent antibodies. It occurred more frequently during once weekly rifampicin treatment then during twice weekly treatment with the same dose size and it could sometimes be stopped simply by reducing the intermittent dose size. It did not occur during daily chemotherapy and was thought to be immunological in origin. Therefore, it was envisaged that a small daily dose of rifampicin given as a supplement to an intermittent regimen might prevent or reduce the incidence of adverse reactions and the development of rifampicin-dependent antibodies.

The present study was, therefore, designed to find out, first, whether intermittent rifampicin in lower dosages would be both therapeutically effective and of low toxicity when given with high dosage isoniazid, and secondly, whether adverse reactions and the development of antibodies could be reduced or avoided by giving a very small dose of rifampicin i.e. 25 mg daily in addition to the intermittent doses.

CRITERIA OF ELIGIBILITY

Patients were admitted to the study if they had pulmonary tuberculosis, were aged 15 years or more, had received no previous antituberculosis chemotherapy and had sputum positive for tubercle bacilli on direct smear examination.

REGIMENS STUDIED

All patients received an initial two weeks of daily chemotherapy with streptomycin plus isoniazid plus rifampicin in standard daily dosages. They were allocated at random to one of four intermittent continuation regimens as follows:

1. Rifampicin 900 mg twice weekly (HR2 regimen)

2. Rifampicin 900 mg once weekly (HR1 regimen)

3. Rifampicin 600 mg twice weekly (LR2 regimen)

4. Rifampicin 600 mg once weekly (LR1 regimen)

All patients on all four regimens received the same dose size of isoniazid, i.e. 15 mg per kg body weight per dose. In addition, all patients received a supplementary capsule every morning containing at random either rifampicin 25 mg or a matched placebo, so that this part of the study was conducted double blind.

Of the 481 patients admitted, the first 371 have been under observation in the study for 12 months or longer. Of these, 13 patients were excluded for pretreatment reasons which were bacteriological in all except two. Another 24 were excluded for reasons encountered during treatment, the majority because of alteration to chemotherapy for drug toxicity (9 patients) or intercurrent disease (7 patients), leaving 334 patients with fully drug-sensitive strains pretreatment in the main bacteriological comparison. These patients have all completed a year under study and the findings at one year are presented.

PRETREATMENT COMPARISONS

The four regimens were similar in the pretreatment distribution of a number of factors including the following:

race (81% Chinese), age (average 43 years), sex (74% male), body weight (average 45 kg), radiological extent of disease (69% had moderate to gross disease), cavitation (55% had cavitation on a postero-anterior chest radiograph) and isoniazid inactivation rate (72% were rapid acetylators).

THERAPEUTIC RESPONSE

Patients with Fully Sensitive Strains Pretreatment

The single monthly culture results based on patients with fully drug sensitive strains pretreatment showed that the LR1 regimen lagged behind the other three regimens in the rate at which it produced sputum negativity in the early months of chemotherapy. At 12 months, all the HR2 patients had negative cultures, as did 90% of the HR1, 97% of the LR2 and 91% of the LR1 patients.

The bacteriological status at 12 months based on a total of 8 cultures at 10, 11 and 12 months is shown in Table 1. A favourable status was defined as all cultures negative or no more than 1 culture with a growth of 5 or more colonies. All patients on the two twice weekly regimens had a favourable status as did 96% of the HR1 and 92% of the LR1 patients. The therapeutic response on the twice-weekly regimens was significantly better than that on the once-weekly regimens (P = 0.005), but the dose size had no significant effect.

Table 1

BACTERIOLOGICAL STATUS AT 12 MONTHS

(based on 8 cultures at 10, 11 and 12 months)

	HR2		HR1		LR2		LR1	
	No.	%	No.	%	No.	%	No.	%
Patients assessed	85		78		87		84	
Favourable status	85	100	75	96	87	100	77	97

Ten patients (3 HR1, 7 LR1) had an unfavourable status. All 10 were excreting drug-resistant strains. Three of them developed isoniazid resistance followed by rifampicin resistance, 1 rifampicin resistance and then isoniazid resistance and another developed resistance to the two drugs at the same time. The remaining 5 developed resistance to isoniazid alone. All 10 were rapid acetylators of isoniazid.

Patients with Drug-Resistant Strains Pretreatment

The incidence of initial resistance to isoniazid was low. Of 7 patients with pretreatment strains resistant to isoniazid who were available for assessment at 12 months, only one had an unfavourable bacteriological status at 12 months.

ADVERSE REACTIONS

The analysis of the incidence of adverse reactions is based on the 359 patients who were followed up for 6 months or longer and is concerned with reactions to rifampicin in the intermittent phase (Table 2). Adverse reactions occurred in 26% of the HR1 patients but on the other regimens their incidence was low. The commonest was the 'flu' syndrome. The majority of the reactions were mild. Thus, of the 49 patients with reactions, 32 (65%) had no change to their chemotherapy or no more than a temporary dose reduction. A further 9 patients had their rifampicin dosage reduced or interrupted, while 4 were changed to a daily rhythm of chemotherapy. The only patients who had their rifampicin terminated were 4 with thrombocytopenia, and in these 4 the platelet count returned to normal within 48 hours.

Table 2

INCIDENCE OF ADVERSE REACTIONS IN 12 MONTHS

Adverse reaction	HR2		HR1		LR2		LR1	
	No.	%	No.	%	No.	%	No.	%
Any type	11	12	23	26	5	5	10	11
'Flu' syndrome	7	8	20	23	4	4	7	8
Thrombocytopenia	2	2	1	1	1	1	0	0
Patients assessed	89		88		94		88	

RIFAMPICIN-DEPENDENT ANTIBODIES

Rifampicin-dependent antibodies were detected in 48% of 89 HR2 patients, 54% of 88 HR1, 21% of 94 LR2 and 36% of 88 LR1 patients, an incidence on all 4 regimens considerably higher than that of adverse reactions. The effect of dosage on the incidence was highly significant but the effect of the interval between doses was not significant.

DAILY RIFAMPICIN SUPPLEMENT

The daily rifampicin 25 mg supplement had no significant effect on the bacteriological results, on the incidence of adverse reactions, or on the incidence of rifampicin-dependent antibodies.

CONCLUSIONS

In conclusion, this study has shown that high-dosage isoniazid plus rifampicin 900 mg or 600 mg twice a week or once a week (preceded by an initial two weeks of daily chemotherapy) achieved good therapeutic results at 12 months, particularly the two twice weekly regimens.

Adverse reactions were infrequent (except on the 900 mg once a week regimen) and were in general mild but there was still a small risk from thrombocytopenia even on the lower dosage twice weekly regimen.

A daily rifampicin 25 mg supplement had no effect on the incidence of adverse reactions or on the development of rifampicin-dependent antibodies.

(Paper presented on behalf of the Singapore Tuberculosis Research Committee and the MRC Tuberculosis and Chest Disease Unit, London).

REFERENCES

Aquinas, M., Allan, W.G.L., Horsfall, P.A.L., Jenkins, P.K., Wong, Hung-Yan, Girling, D., Tall, R. & Fox, W. (1972). British Medical Journal 1, 765.

Dickinson, J.M., Ellard, G.A. & Mitchinson, D.A. (1968). Tubercle, 49, 351.

Dickinson, J.M. & Mitchison, D.A. (1970). Tubercle,51,82.

Girling, D.J. & Fox, W. (1971). British Medical Journal, 4, 231.

Grumbach, F., Canetti, G.& Le Lirzin, M. (1969). Tubercle, 50, 280.

Hong Kong Tuberculosis Treatment Services/British Medical Research Council (1974). Clinical Allergy, 4, 59.

Hong Kong Tuberculosis Treatment Services/Brompton Hospital/British Medical Research Council (1974). Tubercle, 55, 1.

Poole, G., Stradling P. & Worlledge, S. (1971). British Medical Journal, 3, 343.

Verbist, L. (1969). Acta Tuberculosea et Preumologica Belgica, 60, 397.

ADVERSE REACTIONS TO INTERMITTENT RIFAMPICIN

D J Girling

MRC Tuberculosis and Chest Diseases Unit

Brompton Hospital, London SW3 6HP

SUMMARY

Adverse reactions to the commonly used dosage schedules of rifampicin are more frequent during intermittent than during daily chemotherapy, the commonest being a febrile reaction called the 'flu' syndrome which rarely occurs during daily treatment. During intermittent chemotherapy, the syndrome is less common with lower dosage schedules, less common during twice-weekly than during once-weekly treatment with the same dose size, less common when intermittent treatment is preceded by a daily phase and less common when small daily doses of rifampicin are given in addition to the larger intermittent doses. It is associated with circulating rifampicin-dependent antibodies and occurs during the period of high serum rifampicin concentration and reduced antibody concentration after an intermittent dose of the drug. It probably has an immunological origin.

INTRODUCTION

Intermittent antituberculosis regimens have the advantages over daily regimens of being fully supervisable in outpatients and usually less toxic. However, rifampicin is an exception, and a major problem with intermittent rifampicin in the dosages currently used is the high incidence of adverse reactions. In contrast, adverse reactions to daily rifampicin are infrequent. The types of reaction to intermittent rifampicin have been fully described by Aquinas and others (1972) from a study in Hong Kong (Hong Kong Tuberculosis Treatment Services/Brompton Hospital/ British Medical Research Council, 1974 and 1975).

TYPES OF REACTION TO INTERMITTENT RIFAMPICIN

There are 6 main types of adverse reaction to intermittent rifampicin.

1. Cutaneous reactions - mild episodes of flushing and itching, with or without a rash, affecting particularly the face and scalp and sometimes including redness and watering of the eyes.

2. Abdominal reactions - mild episodes of abdominal pain and nausea, occasionally with vomiting and diarrhoea.

3. 'Flu' syndrome - fever, chills and malaise, sometimes with headache, dizziness or bone pain.

4. Respiratory syndrome - shortness of breath, sometimes with wheezing and rhonchi, sometimes with shock.

5. Hepatic reactions - usually no more than transient increases in the serum transaminase concentration without symptoms, but jaundice does occur.

6. Purpura - thrombocytopenic in type. The platelet count rapidly returns to normal once rifampicin has been terminated.

   Cutaneous, abdominal, 'flu' and respiratory reactions typically come on 1 to 2 hours after a morning dose and are gone by the evening of the same day.

The adverse reactions to daily rifampicin are generalised hypersensitivity reactions, cutaneous reactions, transient increases in serum transaminase concentrations, jaundice, and rarely purpura.

Rarely, acute renal failure occurs during intermittent rifampicin or when daily rifampicin is resumed after an interval. It sometimes follows a severe clinical episode such as shock or actue haemolysis, but can also occur without any such precipitating crisis.

The size of the problem of adverse reactions to rifampicin is well illustrated by the Hong Kong study (Hong Kong Tuberculosis Treatment Services/Brompton Hospital/British Medical Research Council 1974 and 1975). Chinese patients whose primary chemotherapy had failed were allocated at random to daily or intermittent re-treatment regimens of rifampicin plus ethambutol. The rifampicin plus ethambutol combination was given daily (ER7 regimen), twice-weekly (ER2 regimen), once-weekly (ER1 regimen) and daily for 2 months and then once-weekly (ER7ER1 regimen). The daily rifampicin dosage was 450 mg, and the intermittent dosages were 900, 1050 and 1200 mg according to body weight in both the once-weekly and twice-weekly regimens.

INCIDENCE OF ADVERSE REACTIONS

During 18 months of chemotherapy, adverse reactions occurred in only 5 (11%) of 47 ER7 patients, but in 22 (32%) of 68 ER2, 44 (61%) of 72 ER1 and 37 (48%) of 77 ER7ER1 patients. The 'flu' syndrome was by far the commonest reaction to intermittent rifampicin and the one which most frequently led to modifications to the regimen. At 12 months its incidence was significantly lower on the ER2 and ER7ER1 regimens that on the ER1 regimen ($P < 0.001$ and 0.02 respectively).

By 18 months the syndrome had occurred in 40% of the ER7ER1 patients and 50% of the ER1 patients, compared with 22% of the ER2 patients. Although the difference between the ER2 and ER1 regimens was still statistically significant at 18 months ($P < 0.001$), the difference between the two once-weekly regimens was not ($P = 0.3$). The uniformly higher incidence of the syndrome on the ER1 than on the ER2 regimen demonstrates the importance of the rhythm of rifampicin administration in producing the syndrome. The individual dose size of rifampicin was the same on these two regimens. On the ER7ER1 regimen, the effect of the initial 2 months of daily chemotherapy was to delay the onset of the 'flu' syndrome during subsequent once-weekly chemotherapy.

MANAGEMENT OF ADVERSE REACTIONS

During the course of the study it was found that adverse reactions to intermittent rifampicin were comparatively easy to manage clinically. If purpura occurred rifampicin was terminated immediately and not given again. Some reactions required no more than simple symptomatic treatment, while others could be stopped simply by reducing the intermittent rifampicin dosage. If these measures failed, the rhythm of rifampicin administration was changed from intermittent to daily, and the ethambutol was then also given in standard daily dosage. Changing to daily administration was almost always successful, and only if this failed was the rifampicin terminated.

MECHANISM OF THE 'FLU' SYNDROME

Serological tests for rifampicin-dependent antibodies were introduced a year after the intake to the study had begun, using an indirect antiglobulin method (Worlledge, 1973). Antibodies were detected in only 1 of 47 patients on daily rifampicin (ER7), on a single occasion only during 18 months. In contrast, 45% of 40 ER2 patients had developed antibodies by 18 months, as had 55% of 47 ER1 and 41% of 51 ER7ER1 patients, and on all threee intermittent regimens there was a statistically significant association between the production of antibodies and the occurrence of the 'flu' syndrome ($P < 0.001$), strongly suggesting that it had an immunological origin.

The investigation of the nature, incidence and management of adverse reactions and of the incidence of antibodies was supplemented by detailed studies of a few patients by Gabriel and Chew in Hong Kong (Gabriel and Chew, 1973). They studied 12 patients who were having episodes of the 'flu' syndrome. During the 24 hours after a dose of intermittent rifampicin they recorded the serum rifampicin concentration, the nature and duration of symptoms of the 'flu' syndrome and the serum antibody score, a semiquantitative measure of antibody concentration based upon the degree of agglutination in the antiglobulin reaction. In a typical response, the serum rifampicin concentration reached a maximum 2 to 4 hours after a dose and had reached the predose level by 24 hours. The symptoms of the 'flu' syndrome coincided with the period of maximum serum rifampicin concentration and during the same period, the antibody score fell.

METHODS OF REDUCING THE INCIDENCE OF ADVERSE REACTIONS

Episodes of the 'flu' syndrome can sometimes be stopped simply by reducing the dose-size of intermittent rifampicin. It was therefore important to find out whether rifampicin in lower dosages once a week or twice a week would be therapeutically effective and of low toxicity. The study in Singapore, the results of which have just been presented (Poh Soo-Chuan, above) has shown that rifampicin in dosages of only 900 mg and 600 mg twice a week and once a week is therapeutically effective and carries a low risk of adverse reactions, and that reactions when they do occur are in general mild and easy to manage.

Nevertheless, even at these low dosages of intermittent rifampicin, there is still a small risk from thrombocytopenic purpura. However, the risk to the patient is small in fully-supervised chemotherapy for two reasons. First, the platelet count rapidly returns to normal once rifampicin treatment has been terminated and secondly, purpura need never occur more than once since the rifampicin can be terminated as soon as the patient reports symptoms, and the supervising staff can question the patient about purpura after the last dose before administering the next supervised dose on each occasion.

The 'flu' syndrome hardly ever occurs during daily rifampicin administration. It was therefore argued that it might be possible to prevent it during intermittent chemotherapy by giving a small daily supplement of the drug in addition to larger intermittent therapeutic doses. A daily supplement of 25 mg rifampicin had no effect on the incidence of adverse reactions to 600 or 900 mg of rifampicin once a week or twice a week in the Singapore study, but a little more success was achieved with larger rifampicin dosages and a 75 mg supplement in Hong Kong (Hong Kong Tuberculosis Treatment Services/British Medical Research Council, 1974).

In the Hong Kong study, all patients were receiving once-weekly rifampicin 900, 1050 or 1200 mg according to body weight, and were allocated at random to receive a daily capsule of rifampicin 75 mg or a matched placebo. By 12 months, 45% of 58 patients on rifampicin supplement had developed adverse reactions, compared with 60% of 58 on placebo, and 34% of the patients on the rifampicin supplement had developed the 'flu' syndrome compared with 55% on placebo ($P = 0.04$). Thus, the rifampicin 75 mg supplement had a definite effect, but one not large enough to have practical application.

CONCLUSIONS

1. The 'flu' syndrome is less common during twice-weekly than during once-weekly treatment with the same dose size of rifampicin. It is not therefore a simple toxic reaction (patients on the twice-weekly regimen receiving twice the total weekly amount of rifampicin), but is probably immunological in origin since in immunological reactions the interval between successive exposures to antigen is known to be important.

2. The incidence of the 'flu' syndrome depends not only upon the interval between doses of rifampicin but also on the dose size, being less common with smaller dosages.

3. The syndrome is less common during once-weekly rifampicin when this is preceded by a daily phase. It is possible that rifampicin is weakly immunogenic *in vivo* so that daily administration produces specific immune tolerance, whereas intermittent administration favours sensitisation.

4. The syndrome is less common during moderate-dosage intermittent rifampicin when a small daily 75 mg supplement of the drug is given, but a daily supplement of only 25 mg has no effect on the incidence of reactions to lower intermittent dosages. The small daily 75 mg doses may have served to "mop up" circulating antibody by providing an excess of antigen in the serum.

5. The occurrence of the 'flu' syndrome is significantly associated with the detection of circulating rifampicin antibodies. Whether these antibodies are responsible for the syndrome is not known. Other antibodies, complement or rifampicin complexes may be involved.

6. Symptoms of the 'flu' syndrome coincide with the period of maximum serum rifampicin concentration and reduced antibody concentration. This observation suggests that a rifampicin-antibody complex is being formed.

7. The recurrence of episodes of the 'flu' syndrome can be prevented by reducing the dose size of rifampicin or by changing to a daily rhythm of

treatment. The proportion of antigen to antibody is known to be important in the production of immunological reactions, and this could be an example of this effect.

REFERENCES

Aquinas, M., Allan, W.G.L., Horsfall, P.A.L., Jenkins, P.K., Wong, H.Y., Girling, D., Tall, R., & Fox, W. (1972). British Medical Journal 1, 765.

Gabriel, O'M.M., & Chew, W.K. (1973). Clinical Allergy, 3, 353.

Hong Kong Tuberculosis Treatment Services /British Medical Research Council (1974). Tubercle, 55, 193.

Hong Kong Tuberculosis Treatment Services /Brompton Hospital /British Medical Research Council (1974). Tubercle, 55, 1.

Hong Kong Tuberculosis Treatment Services /Brompton Hospital /British Medical Research Council (1975). Tubercle, in press.

Worlledge, S. (1973). Scandinavian Journal of Respiratory Diseases, Supplementum 84, 60.

CHOICE OF DRUGS FOR SHORT COURSE CHEMOTHERAPY

D.A. Mitchison

British Medical Research Council, Unit for Laboratory
Studies of Tuberculosis
Royal Postgraduate Medical School, Ducane Road
London W12 OHS

The concept that the duration of chemotherapy for tuberculosis might be drastically shortened has arisen from a considerable body of experimental evidence. I am going to review this evidence, describe how it leads to a choice of regimens for clinical studies in man and also discuss why some of the drugs are particularly effective.

EXPERIMENTAL TUBERCULOSIS IN THE MOUSE AND GUINEA PIG

The findings which are of the greatest immediate importance in designing short course regimens come from work on the chemotherapy of experimental tuberculosis of the mouse, particularly the early studies at Cornell University (McCune *et al*., 1966) and more recently at the Pasteur Institute, Paris (Grumbach *et al*., 1969, Le Lirzin, 1972). In these experiments, mice were infected by the intravenous route with *Mycobacterium tuberculosis*, strain H37Rv, and were then treated for periods of several months. Counts of the number of surviving bacilli in the lungs and spleen were done during and at the end of treatment.

Sterilizing Drugs

The results of some of the more important experiment done at Cornell University are summarized in Table I. Treatment with isoniazid (INH), streptomycin (SM) or PAS or with any combination of these drugs resulted in an initial fall in the viable counts which then levelled off, leaving a large (2+) viable population of "persisters", particularly in the spleen. Only when pyrazinamide

Table I. STERILIZING ACTIVITY OF DRUG COMBINATIONS IN MURINE TUBERCULOSIS

Drugs	Months of treatment	Lung/spleen culture		Relapse	Place of study
INH + SM + PAS	3	2+		-	
SM + PZA	3	0	1/8*	-	Cornell
INH + PZA	3	0	0/77*	2+	University
INH + PZA	6	0		0	
INH + SM	4 - 6	2+		-	Pasteur
INH + RMP	6	0	0/20†	1+	Institute
SM + RMP	4	1+	2/8†	-	

*spleen †lung PZA = pyrazinamide RMP = rifampicin

(PZA) was given did the counts continue to fall. This sterilizing effect was greatest when PZA was given with INH, since cultures from the organs were always negative after treatment for three months. A lesser sterilizing effect was obtained when PZA was given with other drugs including SM. If animals treated with PZA + INH were allowed to survive for three months, cultures of the organs from about two-thirds of mice became positive, indicating a relapse. Relapse could apparently be prevented by prolonging the treatment period from three to six months. Table I also shows experiments done at the Pasteur Institute which demonstrate that rifampicin (RMP) is, like PZA, a sterilizing drug. The sterilizing action was again most effective when INH was given with RMP, but the number of surviving organisms was far less if any of several drugs tested was combined with RMP rather than with INH.

These experiments show that PZA and RMP are unique in their ability to prolong the initial bactericidal activity of a drug regimen by killing or rendering non-viable for prolonged periods persisting sensitive bacilli. In this sense they are sterilizing drugs and the sterilizing effect is best demonstrated when they are given with INH. We should note that in the mouse experiments all three drugs were given in dosages, expressed as mg/kg body weight, considerably above the dosage used in man.

Table II. STREPTOMYCIN AND ETHAMBUTOL IN MURINE TUBERCULOSIS

Treatment		Per cent culture negative			
		End of treatment		4 months later	
		Lungs	Spleen	Lungs	Spleen
RMP + INH	5 months	100	100	80	70
RMP + INH + SM	daily	100	100	92	77
RMP + INH	5 months	50	50	71	36
RMP + INH + SM	twice-weekly	50	50	56	19
RMP + EMB	6 months	75	87		
INH + EMB	daily	9	0		

RMP 25 mg/kg INH 25 mg/kg SM 200 mg/kg

Companion Drugs

In addition to INH, PZA and RMP, additional drugs, usually SM or ethambutol (EMB), are often prescribed in short course regimens in man, in part because they may prevent a failure due to the emergence of drug resistance if the strain has initial resistance to INH and in part because they might contribute to the bactericidal activity of the regimen. The extent to which they increase the bactericidal activity in the murine model is shown in Table II, taken from work at the Pasteur Institute. The addition of SM to a regimen of INH + RMP, given daily or twice weekly, did not increase the proportion of negative organ cultures at the end of treatment nor the proportion of negative cultures in mice examined four months after chemotherapy had been stopped. Similar experiments with EMB have not been done in the mouse, but the lower part of Table II shows that INH + EMB had very low bactericidal activity.

Fig.1 summarizes an experiment done with Dr. Jean Dickinson in the guinea pig. Animals with established disease following intramuscular infection were given no treatment or were treated with EMB. Other groups received INH, INH plus EMB, INH plus RMP and INH plus RMP plus EMB. Treatment was given for five days every week for a total of 11 weeks. Groups of 5-7 guinea pigs were killed at the end of the treatment period and at intervals thereafter. The amount of disease visible naked eye in the organs was scored out of a total of 100 and viable counts were set up on the spleens. The scores shown in Fig.1 indicate that EMB alone had little or no antibacterial action. Addition of EMB to a regimen

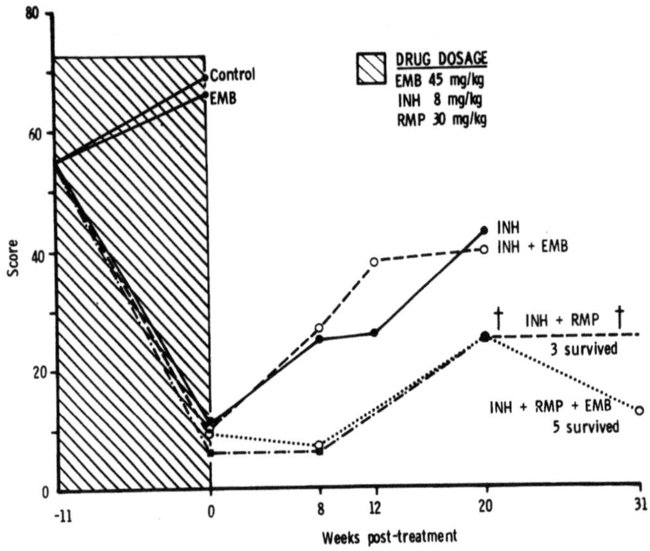

Fig. 1. POST-MORTEM SCORES IN GUINEA PIGS TREATED FOR ELEVEN WEEKS

of INH did not influence the results. Inclusion of RMP in the regimen considerably prolonged the period before relapse occurred, but the addition of EMB again failed to influence the relapse rates. The results of spleen viable counts (not illustrated here) confirmed the conclusions drawn from the scores.

DESIGN OF SHORT COURSE REGIMENS

The animal experiments show us that effective short course regimens depend on the use of RMP and PZA and that their sterilizing activity is greatest when they are given with INH. Thus these 3 drugs are the basis of current short course regimens. SM and EMB do not increase or decrease the bactericidal activity of regimens containing RMP, but they may be of value in the prevention of failure due to the emergence of drug-resistant strains of tubercle bacilli. For reasons discussed elsewhere (Fox and Mitchison, 1975), bacilli may be in a more alkaline environment in human than in mouse lesions so that PZA may be less effective and SM more effective in man than in mouse.

Table III. BACTERICIDAL ACTIVITY IN VITRO AND IN VIVO OF ANTITUBERCULOSIS DRUGS ALONE OR IN COMBINATION

	Bactericidal Activity	
	In vitro Kill at 7 days*	In vivo Mouse lungs
SM 2 μg/ml	3.05, 3.18	
RMP 0.33 μg/ml	1.64, 2.43	
INH 1 μg/ml	1.07, 1.86	
EMB 4 μg/ml	-0.77	
INH + SM	>5.11	2+
RMP + SM	3.80	3+
EMB + INH	2.52	1+
RMP + INH	2.47	4+

*Difference in $\log_{10}$ cfu/ml between drug-containing and drug-free Tween-albumin cultures.

MODE OF ACTION OF STERILIZING DRUGS

A simple explanation for the special sterilizing activity of PZA and RMP might be that they are, when given alone or in combination with other drugs, more bactericidal in vitro than, say, INH or SM and that the sterilizing activity is simply an expression of their high innate bactericidal activity. Experiments were done with Dr. Jean Dickinson to test this possibility. To log phase cultures of M.tuberculosis, strains H37Rv, in 7H9 Tween-albumin liquid medium with an initial viable count of $\log_{10}$ 6.1 - 7.1 cfu/ml was added RMP, INH, SM, or EMB, alone and in combination. The fall in viable counts that occurred during a 7-day exposure period is shown in Table III. When cultures were exposed to a single drug, SM was much the most bactericidal even though its concentration was only about 4 times higher than the MIC in this medium. Of the drug combinations, INH + SM was the most bactericidal and RMP + INH the least bactericidal, indicating a lack of correlation between in vitro bactericidal activity and sterilizing activity in the mouse, and probably in man also. Thus the simple hypothesis that a good sterilizing regimen has greater bactericidal activity in vitro does not appear to be true.

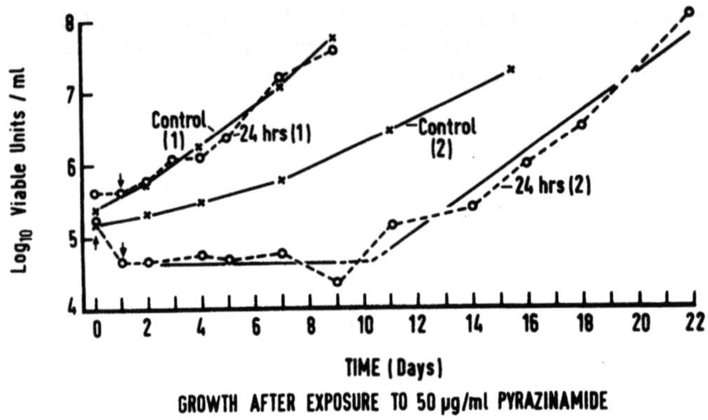

Fig. 2. VIABLE COUNTS AFTER EXPOSURE TO 50 µg/ml PYRAZINAMIDE FOR 24 HOURS

Arrows indicate addition and removal of pyrazinamide

Pyrazinamide

In vitro experiments have shown that PZA is only active in acid medium. When sufficiently acid, the growth of drug-free control cultures was slow and an exposure to 50 µg/ml PZA was bactericidal and was followed, as with other bactericidal drugs, by a lag period of several days before growth restarted (Dickinson and Mitchison, 1970b) (Fig.2). The more acid the medium and the slower the rate of growth, the shorter was the exposure to PZA necessary to produce a lag period and the longer was the lag period itself, which could extend to more than 76 days (Table IV). These findings suggest that pyrazinamide may be effective as a sterilizing drug because it can kill or at least inhibit for long periods bacilli that are almost completely inhibited by their acid environment. These bacilli may well be intracellular and may not be killed by other drugs because of their slow growth or their intracellular site.

Table IV. LAG PERIOD AFTER PULSED EXPOSURE TO 50 µg/ml PYRAZINAMIDE RELATED TO pH

pH	Rate of growth	Lag (days) after exposure for: 6 hr.	96 hr.
6.2	0.36	0	9
5.8	0.27	0	72
5.6	0.14	40	> 76

Rifampicin

It is less easy to suggest why RMP is so much more effective than INH as a sterilizing drug. RMP is no more bactericidal than INH and like INH does not kill dormant bacilli. However, the onset of its bactericidal action is rapid being demonstrable in exposures of 6 hours or less whereas INH was only bactericidal after exposures of 24 hours or more (Dickinson and Mitchison, 1970a). Thus organisms showing a temporary spurt of growth might be killed by RMP but not by INH. Since RMP and PZA may well be effective sterilizing drugs for different reasons and may therefore kill different members of the persisting bacterial population, strong bactericidal synergism between them is to be expected. Thus, there are good reasons for exploring regimens containing both PZA and RMP in man.

References

Dickinson, J.M., and Mitchison, D.A., Tubercle, 1970a, 51, 82.

Dickinson, J.M., and Mitchison, D.A., Tubercle, 1970b, 51, 389.

Fox, W., and Mitchison, D.A., Amer. Rev. Resp. Dis., 1975, 111, 325

Grumbach, F., Canetti, G., and Le Lirzin, M., Tubercle, 1969, 50, 280.

Le Lirzin, M., Ciba Foundation Symposium: Rifampicin and current policies in antituberculosis chemotherapy, Ciba Laboratories, 1972, p.7.

McCune, R.M., Feldmann, F.M., Lambert, H.P., and McDermott, W., J. exp. Med., 1966, 123, 445.

SHORT-COURSE CHEMOTHERAPY IN PULMONARY TUBERCULOSIS

J.H. Angel

British Thoracic & Tuberculosis Association

Harefield, U.K.

Chemotherapeutic agents for the treatment of pulmonary tuberculosis have been with us now for nearly thirty years but only comparatively slowly have we learnt how best to deploy them. As a result of a mixture of clinical experience and well-planned controlled clinical trials, we learnt that the use of any single agent alone would lead to a substantial proportion of treatment failures due to the development of bacteriological resistance. This problem was virtually overcome when two or more drugs were used in combination but gradually it became clear that the duration of chemotherapy would have to be prolonged way beyond that employed for most other bacterial infections, failing which a substantial proportion of patients would relapse, with re-emergence of tubercle bacilli in their sputum. This is exemplified by the results of the controlled clinical trial initiated by the British Medical Research Council in 1956 in which different durations of therapy with a combination of PAS plus isoniazid, supplemented in some instances by an initial course of streptomycin, were compared in patients with chronic cavitated tuberculosis. (see Table 1).

TABLE 1 : RELAPSE RATES AFTER DIFFERENT DURATIONS OF CHEMOTHERAPY

M.R.C. Trial (1962)

Comparison	Duration of Chemotherapy			
	Six Months	One Year	Two Years	Three Years
6/12/24 Month	62%	14%	0%	-
1/2/3 Year	-	22%	4%	3%

It will be seen that in the smaller section of the trial, in which comparisons of 6 months, 1 year and 2 years were made, as many as 62% of the patients relapsed after stopping chemotherapy at 6 months and even after a one year's duration of therapy, 14% relapsed. Gradually it became accepted that, for those countries whose health services could meet the cost, the standard chemotherapeutic regimen should be PAS plus isoniazid, with an initial two to three months' supplement of streptomycin and the total duration of therapy should be between eighteen months and two years. The widespread use of this regimen over the past fifteen to twenty years has led to the virtual elimination of relapse, provided that the patient is co-operative and takes his drugs regularly. In the past few years there has been a move towards replacing the unpalatable PAS by ethambutol or rifampicin but the total duration of chemotherapy has remained unchanged.

Such prolonged chemotherapy has considerable disadvantages - the inconvenience to the patient, the tendency of patients not to take their drugs and the need for treatment services to continue close monitoring for long periods of time. Further, both PAS and streptomycin have a high incidence of adverse effects.

The advent of rifampicin, a powerful bactericidal anti-tuberculosis drug, and the demonstration that its combination with isoniazid formed a highly potent regimen, suggested that it might be possible to reduce the duration of chemotherapy. The British Thoracic and Tuberculosis Association accordingly initiated a study in October 1972, the aims of which were as follows: (see Table 2) The design of the study is set out in Table 3.

TABLE 2

A Controlled Trial by the British Thoracic and Tuberculosis Assoc.	
Primary Objective	: To compare the efficacy of different durations of rifampicin plus isoniazid (supplemented initially by a third drug)
Secondary Objective	: To compare the efficacy of ethambutol and streptomycin as the third drug.

TABLE 3

SHORT-COURSE CHEMOTHERAPY IN NEWLY DIAGNOSED PULMONARY TUBERCULOSIS

Cavity Size	Regimen: RMP + INH	Third Drug (for initial 8 weeks)
$<$2 cms or none	6 or 12 months	$<$60 - EMB or SM $>$60 - EMB
$>$2 cms	9 or 18 months	$<$60 - EMB or SM $>$60 - EMB

Patients were divided into two groups according to the physician's reading of their pre-treatment radiograph. Those with little or no cavitation, i.e. with no single cavity of diameter greater than 2 cms. were allocated at random to 6 or 12 months' chemotherapy; those with any cavity larger than 2 cms. were allocated 9 or 18 months' chemotherapy. All patients were given a supplementary third drug for the first 8 weeks of therapy; those under the age of 60 received either ethambutol or streptomycin by random allocation all those above the age of 60 automatically received ethambutol. The physician was left free to treat the patient either at home or in hospital according to his usual practice. All patients received isoniazid 300 mgm. plus rifampicin in a dose depending on their weight - 600 mgm. if over 50 kg., 450 mgm. if under 50 kg. During the first eight weeks, they received in addition either streptomycin 0.75 g. on 6 days per week, or ethambutol daily in a dose of 25mgm/kg.

Bacteriological surveillance of the patients included the examination of two sputum specimens before treatment, followed by that of a monthly specimen during the course of chemotherapy; at each of the last three months of chemotherapy two specimens were examined. In the first year after the cessation of chemotherapy, two specimens were examined at two-monthly intervals; subsequently, two specimens were examined at three-monthly intervals.

111 were excluded because they did not satisfy the protocol; in a few, the diagnosis of tuberculosis was mistaken but the most common reasons were bacteriological i.e. negative pre-treatment cultures, disease due to opportunistic mycobacteria and pre-treatment isoniazid resistance. A further 106 patients did not complete their allocated duration of therapy for the reasons shown in Table 4, thus 695 patients remain for analysis.

TABLE 4

Submitted		913
Excluded		111
Did not complete allocated treatment:-		
Lack of co-operation	37	
Toxicity (RMP and/or INH)	29	
Death	19	
Withdrawn by physician	15	
Emigrated	6	106
Remaining for analysis		696

Before giving the results, I should like to define the terms we have used:

> FAILURE OF CHEMOTHERAPY : The presence of two or more positive cultures at different months during the last three months of chemotherapy.
>
> RELAPSE AFTER CHEMOTHERAPY : The presence of two or more positive cultures in any period of 4 months in specimens taken at least two weeks apart. (This last proviso has been inserted to exclude those patients who may, over a brief period of time, cough up a small residual nidus of caseous material).

The period of intake was from October 1972 to May 1973. The results presented today relate to the period up to the end of May 1975. In other words, all patients have had a period of follow-up of 24 months and some up to 32 months from the start of chemotherapy.

RESULTS

On Table 5 are the results in those patients allocated 6 or 12 months' chemotherapy, i.e. those with little or no cavitation. Of the 174 patients who received 6 months' chemotherapy, only one was regarded as a failure of chemotherapy, having produced positive cultures at 5 and 6 months after having satisfactorily converted earlier. 5 patients relapsed between 7 and 18 months i.e. in the twelve months following the end of chemotherapy and 3 more patients have relapsed in the subsequent period of follow-up, giving a total of 8 in all. In the 12 months group only 1 patient has relapsed. There was no difference in the relapse rates between those patients given streptomycin and those given ethambutol as the initial supplement. The failure of chemotherapy patient and all nine relapses, relapsed with organisms sensitive to the drugs used in the study, suggesting that the duration of chemotherapy had been inadequate to kill of all sensitive bacilli. All of them have responded to further chemotherapy.

Table 6 shows the results in those patients allocated 9 or 18 months' chemotherapy, ie. those with cavities larger than 2 cms. in diameter. It will be seen that there were no failures of chemotherapy and no patient has as yet relapsed since the cessation of chemotherapy.

We have looked critically at the characteristics of those patients who did relapse to determine whether there were any adverse prognostic factors. They did not appear to be any liable to have positive direct smears or to have heavier growths on culture than did the 6 and 12 months groups as a whole. As far as the appearances of the chest radiograph were concerned, there was a slightly higher incidence of moderate and extensive disease and of a moderate degree of cavitation, when compared with the 6 and 12 months groups as a whole but with such small numbers the differences do not achieve statistical significance.

TABLE 5 : FAILURE OF CHEMOTHERAPY AND RELAPSES

Patients without cavities or no cavity >2 cm
(6 or 12 months chemotherapy)

Age	Regimen	Total	Failure of chemotherapy 1-6 months	Relapse 7-18mo.	After 18 mth	Total Relapses
<60	EHR 6	68	0	2	2	3
<60	SHR 6	64	0	1	1	2
<60	SHR 6/EHR 6	12	0	1	0	1
>60	EHR 6	30	1	1	0	1
	TOTAL	174	1	5	3	8

Age	Regimen	Total	Failure of Chemotherapy 1-12 months	Relapse 13-18 mo.	After 18mth	Total Relapses
<60	EHR 12	71	0	0	0	0
<60	SHR 12	68	0	0	1	1
<60	SHR 12/EHR 12	10	0	0	0	0
>60	EHR 12	30	0	0	0	0
	TOTAL	177	0	0	1	1

TABLE 6 : RELAPSES OF PATIENTS WITH CAVITIES >2 CM
(9 or 18 months' chemotherapy)

Regimens	Total	Failure of Chemotherapy	Relapses
EHR 9 and SHR 9	151	0	0
EHR 18 and SHR 18	155	0	0

TABLE 7: CHARACTERISTICS OF PATIENTS WITH RELAPSE

SPUTUM	DIRECT SMEAR	Positive 5 Negative 4
	GROWTH ON CULTURE	Heavy 5 Moderate 2, Slight 2.
CHEST RADIOGRAPH	EXTENT OF DISEASE	Slight 1, Limited 4, Moderate 3, Extensive 1.
	EXTENT OF CAVITATION	Nil 5, Slight 1, Moderate 3.

As has been reported in other studies, other bacteriological phenomena have occurred since the end of chemotherapy. 16 patients in all produced sputun which was positive on direct smear but negative on culture, and a further 5 patients produced isolated positive cultures. Three patients produced sputum containing opportunistic mycobacteria. By definition, none of these have been regarded as constituting a bacteriological relapse. It is however, of interest that one of the patients with an isolated positive culture did later have a true bacteriological relapse, having produced subsequent negative cultures in the meantime.

TABLE 8: BACTERIOLOGICAL FINDINGS AFTER CHEMOTHERAPY IN PATIENTS WHO DID NOT RELAPSE

	6-month groups	9-month groups	12-month groups	Total Patients
Positive smears with negative cultures	7	5	4	16*
Isolated positive cultures	3**	2	3	8**
Opportunistic mycobacteria	2 (M.Intracellulare) (M.Xeonopii)	1 (M.Terrae)	-	3

* 4 patients produced such results on two separate occasions

** 1 patient had subsequent negative cultures before having a true bacteriological relapse.

COMPARISON OF ETHAMBUTOL AND STREPTOMYCIN

We now turn to the comparison of ethambutol and streptomycin given as an initial 8 weeks' supplement. It will be seen that the rate of sputum conversion was similar in the ethambutol and the streptomycin groups, both in those with little or no cavitation,

TABLE 9 : SPUTUM CONVERSION DURING CHEMOTHERAPY

Patients without cavities or no cavity > 2 cm (6 or 12 months chemotherapy)

Regimen	Total	% culture negative (monthly) 1	2	3	4	5	6
EHR 6) EHR 12)	150	39	69	95	97	98	100
SHR 6) SHR 12)	141	45	77	92	97	99	100

or in those with more extensive cavitation,

TABLE 10 : SPUTUM CONVERSION DURING CHEMOTHERAPY

Patients with any cavity > 2 cm (9 or 18 months chemotherapy)

Regimen	Total	% culture negative (monthly) 1	2	3	4	5	6	7	8	9
EHR 9) EHR 18)	131	18	53	85	97	99	100	100	100	100
SHR 9) SHR 18)	126	25	60	87	98	98	100	100	100	100

although the rate of conversion is slower by about a month in those with the more extensive disease. There were no advers effects in any of the patients receiving ethambutol whereas 8% of those receiving streptomycin experienced adverse effects which required discontinuation of the drug and substitution of ethambutol; 10 of them had hypersensitivity reactions, 11 had vestibular symptoms and 2 patients refused injections.

TABLE 11 : ADVERSE EFFECTS OF ETHAMBUTOL COMPARED WITH STREPTOMYCIN

Third Drug	Number Eligible	Adverse Effects
Ethambutol	286	0 (0%)
Streptomycin	298	23 (8%)

TABLE 12 : RIFAMPICIN/ISONIAZID TOXICITY IN 802 PATIENTS

Nature of Adverse Effect	Isoniazid	Rifampicin	Rifampicin + Isoniazid
Rash and/or Fever	3	3	2
Peripheral Neuropathy	3	-	-
Psychosis	2	-	-
Abnormal liver function tests			
Raised Transaminases only	-	6	-
Raised Transaminases + Jaundice	-	8	-
Gastrointestinal upset	-	2	-
TOTAL	8(1%)	19(2.4%)	2(0.2%)

Adverse effects caused by rifampicin and/or isoniazid which were severe enough to require discontinuation of treatment occurred in 29 of the 802 patients in the study (3.6%). All but 2 of those attributed to rifampicin occurred in the first month of therapy. 8 patients developed jaundice with a serum bilirubin range between 2 and 5.5mg/100ml. and 6 patients had persistently raised serum transaminase levels without evidence of jaundice; all but one of these patients achieved normal serum enzymes afer rifampicin was stopped. The 5 patients who had developed rashes, pyrexia or gastro-intestinal upsets on rifampicin recovered on stopping the drug.

SUMMARY

The results of this study have yielded a relapse rate of 5% over an 18-26 month period following 6 months' chemotherapy with rifampicin plus isoniazid in patients with newly diagnosed sputum positive pulmonary tuberculosis, infected with sensitive bacilli. In patients with a similar extend of disease and cavitation allocated 12 months' chemotherapy, only 1 relapse occurred.

Patients with more extensive disease and cavitation allocated 9 months' chemotherapy have produced no relapses in a 15-23 month post-chemotherapy follow-up, nor have any relapses occurred in patients with similar disease given 18 months' chemotherapy.

There was no difference in the rate of sputum conversion during chemotherapy in those patients given an initial supplement of ethambutol compared with those given initial streptomycin. Similarly there was no difference in the relapse rates between these two groups. A higher incidence of adverse effects was reported with streptomycin than with ethambutol.

There was no undue incidence of toxicity with the rifampicin/isoniazid regimen. There was a low incidence of patients producing sputum specimens which were positive on smear and negative on culture and an even lower incidence os isolated positive cultures. In only one instance was either of these phenomena a precursor of true bacteriological relapse.

On the present evidence we would conclude that 6 months' chemotherapy with rifampicin plus isoniazid is not quite sufficient to achieve 100% success, whereas 9 months' chemotherapy may prove sufficient, both in cavitated and non-cavitated disease. The limited period of follow-up makes this conslusion only tentative. However, most studies of short-course chemotherapy have shown that the majority of relapses occur during the first few months after stopping chemotherapy and we anticipate that the relapse rate in the 9-months group can now only be minimal.

SUMMARY

1. In 174 patients receiving six months' chemotherapy, the relapse rate, in an 18-26 month follow-up period was 5%.

2. In 483 patients receiving 9,12 or 18 months' chemotherapy, the relapse rate, over slightly shorter period of follow-up was 0.2%.

3. No difference between ethambutol and streptomycin supplements in:
   (a) Rate of sputum conversion to negative
   (b) Incidence of relapse.

4. Ethambutol produced fewer adverse effects than streptomycin (o% vs 8%).

5. Comparatively low incidence of side-effects to rifampicin/isoniazid (3.6%)

5. Low incidence of smear positive/culture negative results after chemotherapy (16/657).

7. Even lower incidence of isolated positive cultures after chemotherapy (8/657).

HONG KONG STUDY OF 6-AND 9- MONTH REGIMENS OF DAILY AND INTERMITTENT STREPTOMYCIN, ISONIAZID AND PYRAZINAMIDE FOR PULMONARY TUBERCULOSIS

Sister Mary Gabriel

Ruttonjee Sanatorium

Wanchai, Hong Kong

SUMMARY

A comparison has been made between 6-and 9-month regimens of streptomycin, isoniazid and pyrazinamide given daily, 3 times a week or twice a week from the start of chemotherapy, in the treatment of newly-diagnosed, smear positive pulmonary tuberculosis in Chinese patients.

At 6 months the twice weekly regimen was marginally inferior to the two other regimens in that 5 (4%) of 126 patients with drug-sensitive strains pretreatment had an unfavourable bacteriological status compared with only 2 (1%) of 141 on the 3 times weekly and none of 137 on the daily regimen. Of a total of 211 patients treated for 9 months, only 1 of 74 on the twice weekly regimen relapsed bacteriologically between 6 and 9 months.

The bacteriological relapse rates in the first 9 months of follow up after 6 months' chemotherapy were 17% on the daily, 21% on the three times weekly and 18% on the twice weekly regimen, and after 9 months' chemotherapy they were 5%, 5% and 4% respectively. All the relapses were with strains sensitive to isoniazid and streptomycin, and 63% occurred in the first 3 months after the end of chemotherapy.

The patients with drug-resistant strains pretreatment fared less well. One third of them had an unfavourable bacteriological status at 6 months. However, the relapse rates after the end of chemotherapy were similar to those for patients with sensitive strains pretreatment.

INTRODUCTION

A study in East Africa showed that regimens of streptomycin plus isoniazid plus rifampicin, and of streptomycin plus isoniazid plus pyrazinamide given daily for 6 months were highly effective, caused little toxicity and were followed by low relapse rates (East African/British Medical Research Councils, 1972). These findings, and previous experience from Madras that daily, twice weekly or once weekly regimens of streptomycin and isoniazid eliminated sensitive tubercle bacilli from the sputum equally rapidly in the early months of treatment (Tuberculosis Chemotherapy Centre Madras, 1970) led our group to predict that short course regimens intermittent from the start would be effective. The treatment services in Hong Kong are based on fully supervised outpatient treatment, so there was a special interest in short course regimens intermittent from the start of treatment.

Intermittent rifampicin is associated with immunological toxicity, the incidence depending on the dose size and the interval between doses. For this reason and because of the high cost of rifampicin it was decided to study regimens containing streptomycin, isoniazid and pyrazinamide given daily, three times weekly and twice weekly. Because in the East African study, streptomycin plus isoniazid plus pyrazinamide given for 6 months was followed by a relapse rate of 8%,in the present study it was decided to investigate 2 durations of chemotherapy, 6 and 9 months.

PLAN AND CONDUCT OF THE STUDY

Patients Admitted to the Study

Chinese patients with pulmonary tuberculosis were eligible if they were aged 15 years or more, had received no previous antituberculosis chemotherapy and were producing sputum positive for tubercle bacilli on direct smear examination. Patients with non-tuberculous disease which contraindicated the use of any of the drugs under study were ineligible, as were pregnant women and drug addicts. A total of 620 patients was admitted to the stuay between June 1, 1972 and July 1973.

REGIMENS OF CHEMOTHERAPY

Patients were allocated at random to 1 of 3 regimens of streptomycin, isoniazid and pyrazinamide given daily (SHZ regimen), 3 times a week ($S_3H_3Z_3$ regimen) or twice a week ($S_2H_2Z_2$ regimen), and to a total duration of chemotherapy of either 6 or 9 months.

The drug dosages were as follows:

Streptomycin	1 g for patients less than 40 years old; 0.75 g for older patients, in all 3 regimens.
Isoniazid	300 mg daily; and 15 mg/kg body weight per dose in both intermittent regimens.
Pyrazinamide	SHZ regimen 1.5 g for patients weighing less than 50 kg; 2 g for heavier patients. $S_3H_3Z_3$ and $S_2H_2Z_2$ regimens 2 g and 3 g respectively for patients weighing less than 45 kg; 2.5 g and 3.5 g respectively for heavier patients.

All 3 drugs were given at the same time in a single dose under the direct supervision of the staff, except that outpatients on daily chemotherapy (SHZ) were given no streptomycin on Sundays or public holidays and were handed their oral drugs for these days to take at home. After the end of chemotherapy, all patients were given monthly supplies of placebo (calcium gluconate), 1 tablet to be taken each day, to encourage their continued clinic attendance.

POPULATION STUDIED

Of the total 620 patients 106 were excluded from the main bacteriological analysis for various reasons which did not introduce bias. There remained 404 patients (137 SHZ, 141 $S_3H_3Z_3$, 126 $S_2H_2Z_2$) with fully sensitive strains pretreatment, and 110 (33 SHZ, 41 $S_3H_3Z_3$, 36 $S_2H_2Z_2$) with pretreatment strains resistant to isoniazid, to streptomycin or to both drugs. The bacteriological results for these 2 groups are presented separately.

PATIENTS WITH SENSITIVE STRAINS PRETREATMENT

Culture Results in First 6 Months

In the rate at which they produced culture negativity, the twice weekly regimen lagged a little behind the other two regimens which were very similar. Thus, at 3 months, 93% of the SHZ and 94% of the $S_3H_3Z_3$ patients were culture negative compared with 86% of the $S_2H_2Z_2$ patients. At 6 months the corresponding negativity rates were 96%, 96% and 93%. This lag of the twice weekly regimen in the early months of chemotherapy was associated with the emergence of isoniazid resistance.

Bacteriological Status During Chemotherapy

The bacteriological status at 6 months was based on 6 cultures at 4, 5 and 6 months. An unfavourable status was defined as 4 or more positive cultures, or 3 positive cultures at least 1 of which grew 5 colonies or more. Bacteriological status at 9 months was based on 4 cultures at 7, 8 and 9 months. An unfavourable status was defined as 2 or more positive cultures. Patients were assessed at the end of 6 months, whether they had been allocated to 6 or to 9 months of chemotherapy.

At 6 months (table 1) none of the 137 SHZ patients had an unfavourable bacteriological status. Of 141 $S_3H_3Z_3$ patients, 2 had an unfavourable status, but one of these had a favourable status at 9 months and so was, in fact, a late converter to culture negativity. In contrast 5 (4%) of 126 $S_2H_2Z_2$ patients had an unfavourable status. Of 70 SHZ, 67 $S_3H_3Z_3$ and 74 $S_2H_2Z_2$ patients who continued chemotherapy to 9 months, only 1 ($S_2H_2Z_2$) relapsed between 6 and 9 months. In all the patients whose chemotherapy failed, failure was associated with the emergence of isoniazid resistance.

Thus the daily and three times weekly regimens produced an excellent and equally good therapeutic response during chemotherapy. The twice weekly regimen was marginally less effective in its partial inability to prevent bacteriological failure during chemotherapy - a failure associated with the emergence of isoniazid resistance.

Table 1

BACTERIOLOGICAL STATUS DURING CHEMOTHERAPY

	Patients assessed at end of:						
	6 months' chemotherapy			9 months' chemotherapy			
	Total	Unfavourable at 6 months No.	%	Favourable at 6 months	Relapse in months 7-9 No.	%
SHZ	137	0	0	70	0	0
$S_3H_3Z_3$	141	2*	1	67	0	0
$S_2H_2Z_2$	126	5	4	74	1	1

* One had a favourable status at 9 months.

Relapses in the First 9 Months After Stopping Chemotherapy

In the first 9 months after stopping chemotherapy (table 2) the relapse rates for all 3 6-month regimens were high; 17% for SHZ patients, 21% for $S_3H_3Z_3$ and 18% for $S_2H_2Z_2$ patients, that is 19% for all 3 regimens combined.

After the 9-month regimens the relapse rates were much lower, only 5%, 5% and 4%, that is 4% for all 3 regimens combined.

Relapses in both 6- and 9-month groups occurred early after the end of chemotherapy (63% of them in the first 3 months after stopping chemotherapy and 90% in the first 6). All relapses were with strains fully sensitive to isoniazid and streptomycin.

PATIENTS WITH RESISTANT STRAINS PRETREATMENT

Bacteriological Status During Chemotherapy

Table 3 shows the bacteriological status during chemotherapy of patients with strains resistant to isoniazid and/or streptomycin pretreatment. Approximately one third of the patients had an unfavourable status at 6 months on all 3 regimens, but of the 36 patients who continued chemotherapy to 9 months, only 3 relapsed between 6 and 9 months.

Table 2

BACTERIOLOGICAL RELAPSE IN FIRST 9 MONTHS AFTER STOPPING CHEMOTHERAPY

Duration of chemotherapy	Regimen	Favourable at end of chemotherapy	Relapses: Total* No.	%		Months after stopping chemotherapy 1-3	4-6	7-9
	SHZ	63	11	17		5	4	2
6 months	$S_3H_3Z_3$	68	14	21	19	9	4	1
	$S_2H_2Z_2$	39	7	18		6	1	0
	SHZ	64	3	5		2	0	1
9 months	$S_3H_3Z_3$	66	3	5	4	2	1	0
	$S_2H_2Z_2$	54	2	4		1	1	0

*All with strains sensitive to isoniazid and streptomycin.

Table 3

BACTERIOLOGICAL STATUS DURING CHEMOTHERAPY OF PATIENTS WITH STRAINS RESISTANT TO ISONIAZID AND/OR STREPTOMYCIN

	Patients assessed at end of: 6 months' chemotherapy: Total	Unfavourable at 6 months No.	%	9 months' chemotherapy: Favourable at 6 months	Relapse in months 7-9 No.	%
SHZ	33	10	30	14	0	(0)
$S_3H_3Z_3$	41	15	37	11	1	(9)
$S_2H_2Z_2$	36	14	39	11	2	(18)

Relapses in First 9 Months After Stopping Chemotherapy

The relapse rates in the first 9 months after stopping chemotherapy (table 4), although based on relatively few patients, are of special interest because the rates were similar to those for patients with fully sensitive strains pretreatment, namely 17% for the 6-month regimens and 4% for the 9-month regimens.

Table 4

BACTERIOLOGICAL RELAPSES IN FIRST 9 MONTHS AFTER STOPPING CHEMOTHERAPY IN PATIENTS WITH STRAINS RESISTANT TO ISONIAZID AND/OR STREPTOMYCIN

Duration of chemotherapy	Regimen	Favourable at end of chemotherapy	Relapses No.	%	
	SHZ	7	2	(29)	
6 months	$S_3H_3Z_3$	13	1	(8)	17
	$S_2H_2Z_2$	9	2	(22)	
	SHZ	10	0	(0)	
9 months	$S_3H_3Z_3$	9	0	(0)	4
	$S_2H_2Z_2$	7	1	(14)	

DRUG TOXICITY

Drug toxicity was not a major problem. Only 7% of the SHZ patients, 3% of the $S_3H_3Z_3$ and 5% of the $S_2H_2Z_2$ patients had one or more drugs terminated for adverse reactions. Reactions to streptomycin were mainly vestibular.

Reactions to isoniazid alone were uncommon. The commonest reaction to pyrazinamide was arthralgia, which was less common on the intermittent than on the daily regimen. Only one patient ($S_3H_3Z_3$) developed jaundice.

CONCLUSIONS

In conclusion:

1. The 9-month daily and three times weekly regimens are effective for patients with drug-sensitive strains pretreatment.

2. They also produce a measure of therapeutic success in patients with resistant strains.

3. The incidence of adverse reactions is acceptable.

4. Intermittent regimens can constitute effective short-course chemotherapy.

REFERENCES

East African/British Medical Research Councils (1972). Lancet, 1, 1079.

Tuberculosis Chemotherapy Centre Madras (1970). Bulletin of the World Health Organization, 43, 143.

STRUCTURE-ACTIVITY STUDY ON THE KASUGAMYCIN FAMILY

Makoto Hori, Kayoko Suzukake, Yoshimasa Uehara &
Hamao Umezawa
Institute of Microbial Chemistry

Kamiosaki 3-14-23, Shinagawa-ku, Tokyo, Japan

Minosaminomycin (MSM), which is structurally related to kasugamycin (KSM), is active against mycobacteria but not against Gram negative bacteria. In vivo studies showed that MSM inhibits protein synthesis in mycobacteria. MSM, at $2x10^{-7}$M, also inhibits f_2 RNA-directed protein synthesis in an E. coli cell-free system by 50%. This inhibition is 100 times stronger than that caused by KSM in the same system. Like KSM, MSM preferentially inhibits the initiation process of protein synthesis. No increase in miscoding is observed in the presence of MSM. KG-8, a chemical derivative of KSM, is 10 times more inhibitory to the growth of E. coli than KSM. However, in the in vitro protein synthesizing system, KG-8 is not as inhibitory as KSM. These discrepancies between in vivo and in vitro activities may be ascribed to a difference in permeability, since E. coli cells with modified permeability show altered sensitivity to MSM. There is no indication that MSM is inactivated in E. coli cells. Based on these findings, the structure essential for binding to ribosomes and for permeation are discussed.

KSM is an antibiotic active against Piricularia oryzae. At high concentrations, it also inhibits the growth of E. coli. The mode of action of KSM has been extensively studied with cell-free protein synthesizing systems of E. coli and it is known that KSM primarily inhibits the formation of the 30S-initiation complex. To obtain some KSM derivatives active against Gram-negative bacteria, chemical modification has been attempted. KG-8 is the most promising derivative so far obtained, inhibiting the growth of E. coli about 10 times more strongly than KSM. However this derivative was not as active as KSM in cell-free protein synthesizing systems of E. coli. MSM was isolated as an inhibitor of the growth of mycobacteria (Hamada et al., 1974). This antibiotic is slightly active against *E. coli*. Based on the structural similarity of MSM to KSM, an analogous mode of action was presumed. We have found that this antibiotic also inhibits the initiation of protein synthesis in cell-free systems of *E. coli*, being 100 times as active as KSM on a molar concentration basis. These discrepancies between the *in vivo* and *in vitro* activities prompted us to reveal essential structures of the KSM family for attacking the ribosomes and for permeation. This paper deals with these problems.

With exponentially growing mycobacteria, MSM at $3x10^{-4}M$ preferentially inhibited protein synthesis without significantly affecting cell wall and nucleic acid syntheses. Plasmolysed cells of *E. coli*, permeability being modified (Gros et al., 1967), became susceptible to MSM: 50 µg/ml of MSM inhibited protein synthesis by 50% with these cells. Thus, it was suggested that the ineffectiveness of MSM on *E. coli* is due to a permeability barrier. The effect of MSM on cell-free protein synthesizing systems of *E. coli* was determined. MSM inhibited the poly-U directed incorporation of ^{14}C-phe into polypeptide chains by 91%, 81% and 35% at $10^{-4}M$, $10^{-5}M$ and $10^{-6}M$, respectively. This inhibition was more than 100 times that of KSM and KG-8. MSM did not stimulate the poly-U directed incorporation of ^{14}C-ile into peptide chains, or miscoding, at a concentration of $2x10^{-4}M$. Protein synthesis can be divided into 3 distinct steps: initiation, elongation and termination. On which step MSM acts was determined. To a cell-free protein synthesizing system directed by RNA of phage f_2, $2x10^{-4}M$ MSM was added at 3 minutes of incubation, and the amounts of ribosome-bound peptides and of released peptides at 3, 10 and 20 minutes of incubation were determined. After the addition of MSM, the amount of ribosome-bound peptide decreased rapidly, while that of released peptide increased at a comparable rate with that of a control run by 10 minutes of incubation. This result indicated that MSM primarily inhibited initiation, but not or to a lesser extent, elongation and termination. MSM at a concentration of $10^{-6}M$ inhibited the binding reaction of ^{14}C-fmet-tRNA with ribosomes by 70 to 90% depending on the initiator codon, any of AUG, poly GU and RNA of phage f_2. This inhibition was also more than 100 times that of KSM and KG-8. Considering the similarity in the mode of action, we presumed that the ribosomes from a KSM resistant strain (ksg C) of *E. coli* (Okuyama et al., 1974) should be insensitive to MSM and KG-8, as were insensitive to KSM. However, these ribosomes were still sensitive to MSM and KG-8. The minute structural differences of these compounds could be recognized by ribosomes, although these compounds should share a common binding locus on a ribosome, leading to the same mode of action.

With a cell-free protein synthesizing system, various members and derivatives of this family were tested for the direct effect on ribosomes. A reaction mixture of the assay contained in 100 µl; 50 mM Tris·HCl, pH 7.8, 3 mM ATP, 0.2 mM GTP, 160 mM NH_4Cl, 2 mM

Table I

Structures of kasugamycin family antibiotics and their effects on f2 RNA directed protein synthesis

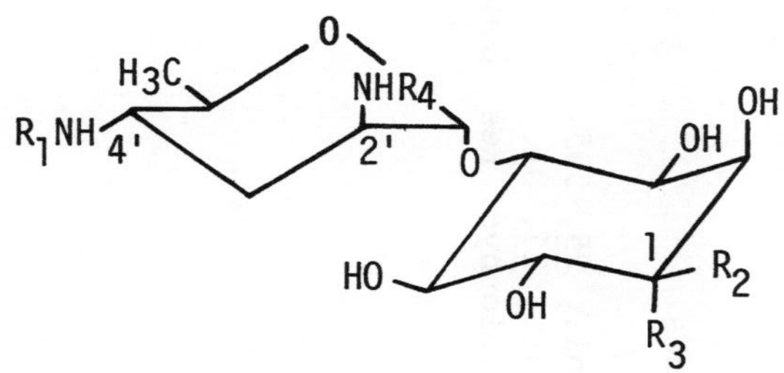

*

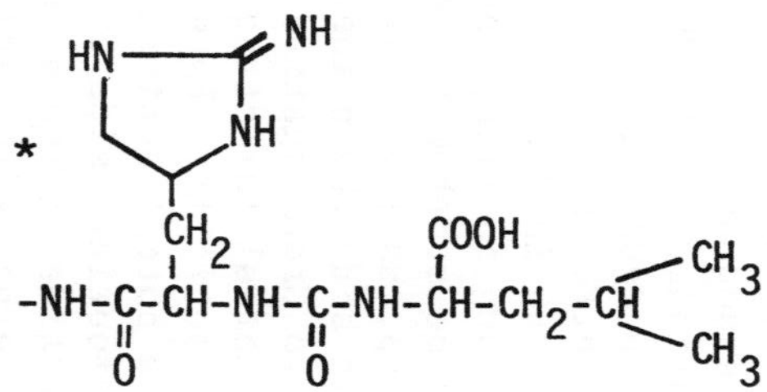

	R_1	R_2	R_3	R_4	% inhibition at $2x10^{-4}M$ or ($1x10^{-6}M$)
Minosaminomycin	-H	*	-H	-H	89 (90)
Minobiosamine	-H	$-NH_2$	-H	-H	6
Kasugamycin	-C(=NH)-COOH	-H	-OH	-H	81 (0)
Kasuganobiosamine	-H	-H	-OH	-H	0
Kasugamycinic acid	-C(=O)-COOH	-H	-OH	-H	31
Kasugamycin KG-8	$-C(=NH)-NH-CH_2-CH_2-NH_2$	-H	-OH	-H	65 (0)
TK-27	-C(=NH)-COOH	-H	-OH	$-CH_2-$ 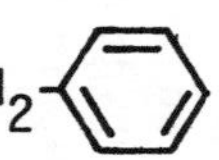	50

phosphoenol pyruvate, 5 mg of pyruvate kinase, 2 mM dithiothreitol, 18 μM of ^{14}C-Val (233 mCi/m mole), 20 μM each of 19 amino acids, 10 mM $Mg(OAc)_2$, 0.6 A_{260} u. of uncharged tRNA, 0.2 mg protein equivalent of S-30, a desired amount of a test compound, 1.7 A_{260} u. of phage f_2 RNA and water. After incubation at 37°C for 20 minutes, acid insoluble radioactivity was measured. The results are summarized in Table I. The effect is expressed as % inhibition exerted by each compound at indicated concentrations. Since MSM was a much stronger inhibitor than KSM in vitro, the equatorial N-blocked amino group on C-1, as in MSM, seems to be a better structure than the axial hydroxyl group on the same carbon, as in KSM. Since minobiosamine, in which the equatorial amino group is free, was only slightly active, the amino group should be somehow blocked. About the structure on C-4', a free amino group, as in MSM, was sufficient for in vitro activity. However, a basic side chain there, as in KG-8, should increase the permeability to Gram-negative bacteria. The free amino group on C-2' is not essential for attacking ribosomes, since TK-27 showed some in vitro activity. Based on these observations, we hopefully expect that a potent antimicrobial agent will be obtained by introduction of appropriate side chains on minobiosamine. Function of presumptive side chains on the C-4' and C-2' amino groups will primarily be concerned with permeation while that on the amino group at the C-1 position will be concerned with both direct effect on ribosomes and permeation.

References

Gros, F. et al. (1967), J. Mol. Biol., 25, 555.
Hamada, M. et al. (1974), J. Antibiot., 27, 81.
Okuyama, A. et al. (1974), Biochem. Biophys. Res. Comm., 60, 1163.

EXPERIMENTAL DATA ON THE ANTIMYCOBACTERIAL ACTIVITY OF ISOPRODIAN[(R)]

Richard Urbanczik

Saarstickstoff Fatol Ltd.
Schwarzwald-Sanatorium
D-7542 Schoemberg

Until today, it is not common to discuss the chemotherapy of "mycobacterioses" as a single topic. Treatment of tuberculosis, leprosy etc. is considered more or less separately, in spite of the obvious advantage of a common approach recognized e.g. by Mayer (1964) or possibly even earlier. Prothionamide (PTH) and/or diaphenylsulphone (DDS) were claimed to increase the antimycobacterial activity of rifampicin (RMP, Freerksen and Rosenfeld, 1972) or of isoniazid (INH, Freerksen, 1973). Also, it has been reported by Middlebrook and Yegian (1946) that no resistance to streptomycin (SM) occured in mycobacteria exposed in vitro simultaneously to SM and DDS. According to Shepard (1972), B-663 (LAMPRENE), ethionamide (ETH) and DDS were reported to give mutually additive results with their combinations against M.leprae; longer bacterial growth delay was observed in M.leprae by Matsuo (1974) with RMP+DDS than with RMP alone. The rationale for combined chemotherapy in tuberculosis has been for years that the development of mycobacterial resistance to each drug alone may be prevented. Obviously, if this were the only advantage of combined chemotherapy, then all drugs of the combination should be given in "full" daily dosage, as claimed e.g. by Radenbach (1973); consequently, some drugs were in fact eliminated from use on the large scale because of side-effects or cost problems. Nevertheless, at least under experimental conditions, even sub-inhibitory concentrations of drugs were reported to exert some effect on bacteria, as shown e.g. by Hobby and Lenert (1972) for RMP or by Urbanczik (1974a) for cycloserine (CS); Awaness and Mitchison (1973) demonstrated that the effect of daily small exposures of M.tuberculosis to INH was cumulative and was related more to the total period over which contact was maintained than to the time-concentration product. Numerous differences in opinion regarding this subject may be due, at least in part, to the known difficulties of evaluating combined antibiotic activity, as discussed thoroughly by Garrett (1958). For all these reasons it appeared interesting to investigate the compound ISOPRODIAN, a chemotherapeutic unit consisting of INH+PTH+DDS, because of its suggested activity in both tuberculosis and leprosy, and perhaps in other mycobacterial diseases too.

Bacteriological studies, in part already published as preliminary communication (Urbanczik, 1974b), were based on the effect, single or in combination, of subinhibitory concentrations of INH, PTH and/or DDS on the growth of several mycobacteria in liquid medium monitored by nephelometry and/or by viable units counts. Also, pulse experiments with higher drug concentrations were performed in M.tuberculosis, basically according to the technique of Jenne and Beggs (1973), however without aeration. The overall results may be summarized as follows:

INH+PTH+DDS (i.e. the components of ISOPRODIAN) provoked in M.tuberculosis H37Rv and M.parafortuitum 16009 (kindly supplied by Dr.Tsukamura, TABLE 1) considerable extension of lag time; also, the logarithmic growth rate coefficients (TABLE 1) with INH alone, INH+PTH or PTH+DDS were different (P lower than 0,05) from those seen with INH+PTH+DDS. Similar results were observed also in 7 recently isolated strains of M.tuberculosis, the effect of ISOPRODIAN was, however, considerably impaired in INH-resistant strains of M.tuberculosis;

the enhanced activity of INH+PTH+DDS compared to that of individual components was also observed in M.kansasii (2 strains), M.marinum (kindly supplied by Dr.Schroeder, Borstel), M.smegmatis ATCC 607 and, to a lesser degree, in a strain of the M.avium - M.intracellulare complex;

DDS seems to be essential for this effect, though it exerted alone, except with M.marinum, hardly any growth inhibition under the conditions of this study. Preliminary investigations with M.parafortuitum 16009 revealed that DDS also increased the activity of RMP, SM, LAMPRENE, but not of CS, ethambutol, polymyxin B and PTH.

TABLE 1

Logarithmic growth rate coefficients in M.parafortuitum 16009 with subinhibitory concentrations of INH,PTH and/or DDS[a]

Group	Growth rate coefficient [b]		Statistical significance [c]
Control	(5)	0,1653	P = > 0,1
DDS 2,5 mcg/ml	(4)	0,1592	
INH 1,37 mcg/ml	(4)	0,0453	P = < 0,05
INH + DDS	(4)	0,0136	
PTH 0,9 mcg/ml	(5)	0,0588	P = > 0,1
PTH + DDS	(4)	0,0501	
INH + PTH	(4)	0,0250	P = < 0,05 [d]
INH + PTH + DDS	(5)	0,0031	P = < 0,05 [e]

[a] The experiments were performed in Dubos liquid medium (Difco) without ADC enrichment and without aeration. The growth rate coefficient was calculated according to the formula $k = 2{,}303/t.(\log E_1 - \log E_2)$ where $t = 4$ days beginning from the time when log of extinction or viable units plotted against time showed the start of a straight line (the 2nd day in these experiments with inocula around 10^5 viable mycobacterial units, and where E_1 and E_2 are nephelometric data or viable units.

[b] Number in parenthesis indicate the individual experiments from which the mean value of the growth rate coefficient was calculated.

[c] Calculated with use of the Wilcoxon test.

[d] Compared to INH or PTH alone.

[e] Compared to INH + PTH.

INH+PTH+DDS appear to increase the bacteriostatic effect, not the killing rate. Pulse studies (INH 1,37 mcg/ml, PTH 0,9 or 1,8 mcg/ml and DDS 0,5 mcg/ml) showed in 2 strains of M.tuberculosis a decrease in number of viable units after 48 hours of contact with INH+DDS or INH+PTH+DDS (about 10 and 1 per cent, respectively, of the values seen with INH alone), but almost no effect was observed after 2 hours of contact.

Pharmacologic experiments were performed in cross - over studies on 12 healthy volunteers (6 men and 6 women) selected so that both rapid and slow INH-inactivators were present. With the single dose peroral administration following results were obtained (Franz et al., 1974):

serum PTH levels are significantly higher in women than in men;

after the administration of PTH 350 mg as part of ISOPRODIAN significantly higher serum levels of free PTH and "areas under the curve" about 70 per cent greater have been observed, compared to the values obtained after the same dosage of PTH administered alone. In fact, PTH 350 mg given as part of ISOPRODIAN resulted in in PTH serum levels approaching those seen after the administration of PTH 750 mg alone. Preliminary studies in 2 persons suggest the conclusion that INH is responsible for this effect.

In order to verify whether drug accumulation occurs during long term treatment, 6 healthy volunteers were given ISOPRODIAN once daily over six days (this investigation was organized and evaluated by Prof.H.M.von Hattingberg, Gießen, Germany). The following results were obtained (TABLE 2):

INH and PTH concentrations were not found to be higher on the 6th day as compared to the 1st day (intraindividual comparison);

as the concentrations of DDS rose significantly during the test period, a pharmacokinetic analysis was perfomed; using a Bateman-type model (Dost, 1968), all data points were fitted simultaneously under the conditions of multiple dosing. The relative volume of distribution ranged from 0,8 to 1,2 (1/kg), the rate constant of elimination from 0,029 to 0,043 (1/h) with half-time values from 16 to 24 hours. The goodness of fit is documented by correlation coefficients ranging from 0,898 to 0,972. The peak concentrations (Y_{max}), theoretically

TABLE 2

Pharmacologic analysis of data observed after DDS administration (as part of ISOPRODIAN) once daily over six days in 3 male and 3 female volunteers

Person	Dose (mg/kg)	V/kg [a]	k_1 [b]	k_2 [c]	Y_{max} (mcg/ml)	Y_{max}/Y_{min}	$s.d._{res}$	r [d]
BU,m,78kg	1,28	1,09	0,681	0,0428	1,57	2,24	0,14	0,962
HE,m,74kg	1,35	1,19	1,056	0,0385	1,69	2,18	0,14	0,937
BR,m,76kg	1,32	1,08	0,873	0,0414	1,70	2,26	0,14	0,972
CE,f,55kg	1,82	1,05	1,000	0,0288	3,20	1,78	0,23	0,937
TH,f,61kg	1,64	0,91	0,552	0,0354	2,70	1,88	0,14	0,972
GI,f,70kg	1,43	0,79	0,202	0,0422	2,11	1,64	0,21	0,898

Samples were taken five times during the first day, immediately before each following dose and up to nine times after cessation of the medication.

(a) Relative volume of distribution in kg^{-1}.

(b) Rate constant of invasion in $hours^{-1}$.

(c) Rate constant of elimination in $hours^{-1}$.

(d) Correlation coefficient.

never to be exceeded during long term therapy, were calculated from the parameters: they cover a range of 1,57 to 3,2 mcg/ml DDS and they are reached within 6 days. From this point of view, there is no particular need to recommend one therapy-free day weekly.

References

Awaness, A.M. and Mitchison, D.A., (1973), Tubercle, 54, 153

Dost, F.H., (1968), Grundlagen der Pharmakokinetik, Georg Thieme, Stuttgart

Franz, H., Urbanczik, R., Stoll, K. and Müller, U., (1974), Praxis der Pneumologie, 28, 605

Freerksen, E., and Rosenfeld, M., (1972), Arzneimittel-Forschung (Drug Research), 22, 1235

Freerksen, E., (1973), Lecture presented during the 13th Meeting of the North German Association for Tuberculosis and Pulmonary Diseases, Celle (Germany), October 19 - 21

Garrett, E.R., (1958), Antibiotics and Chemotherapy, 8, 8

Hobby, G.L. and Lenert, T.F., (1972), American Review of Respiratory Diseases, 105, 292

Jenne, J.W. and Beggs, W.H., (1973), American Review of Respiratory Diseases, 107, 1013

Matsuo, Y., (1974), Japanese Journal of Microbiology, 18, 15

Mayer, R.L., (1964), Advances in Tuberculosis Research (S.Karger, Basel/New York) 13, 219

Middlebrook, G. and Yegian, D., (1946), American Review of Tuberculosis, 54, 553

Radenbach, K.L., (1973), Internist, 14, 100

Shepard, C.C., (1972), International Journal of Leprosy, 40, 33

Urbanczik, R., (1974a), Arzneimittel-Forschung (Drug Research), 24, 723

Urbanczik, R., (1974b), Infection, 2, 80

PRELIMINARY EXPERIENCES WITH ISOPRODIAN(R) IN THE TREATMENT OF PULMONARY TUBERCULOSIS

H. Blaha and W.Müller

Zentralkrankenhaus, D - 8035 Gauting

Federal Republic of Germany

The WHO Committee on Tuberculosis emphasized in its last report (1974) the importance to secure adequate chemotherapy to every patient with infectious pulmonary tuberculosis. Such treatment should combine effectivity and acceptable toxicity, should be convenient both to dispense and for the patient to take and, last but not least, its cost should also be "adequate", which certainly does not apply only to so called developing countries.

In the last years, there has been a progressive crystallization of two general trends concerning the future of tuberculosis chemotherapy, which in fact are very much related each to the other: the first, short-course chemotherapy usually with isoniazid (INH) and rifampicin was recently reviewed by Fox and Mitchison (1975) and we do not intend to discuss it here. The other one is the simplified chemotherapy directed to (a) intermittent administration of suitable, not necessarily less expensive or less toxic drugs, or to (b) regimens where the acceptability by the patient and the low cost are predominant factors. The possibly first representative of the last type was INH monotherapy extensively studied in particular by the Madras Chemotherapy Center; today, the best known among them is INH + thiacetazone (TH, e.g. Fox, 1964). However, other combinations have been tried too: so, in 1952, INH + diaphenylsulphone (DDS, East African/British Medical Research Council), or later INH + ethionamide (Lees, 1965; Chicou <u>et al</u>., 1968).

Based on this motivation and on the experimental work of Freerksen (1973), we started the clinical trial with ISOPRODIAN which contains in 1 coated tablet 175 mg INH, 175 mg prothionamide (PTH) and 50 mg DDS and which was administered usually in a single dose of 2 tablets daily. A limited number of previously untreated persons with cavernous pulmonary tuberculosis were chosen for the study. The standard type of controlled clinical trial i.e. randomized allocation of patients to a "known" and to an "investigational" chemotherapeutic regimen groups was not employed; at the Gauting hospital, a center for chest diseases in Southern Germany, sputum conversion rates achieved with currently employed regimens are well known - usually between 90 to 95 per cent - and we dispose of sufficient data to be able to recognize whether a given regimen is better, approx. equal or worse than our standard therapy (Blaha and Rottach, 1974, TABLE 1).

The condition of patients on admission to the ISOPRODIAN trial is presented in TABLE 2; from 30 persons available for evaluation so far, 12 were treated 2 months or less, 18 received ISOPRODIAN 4 months or more (TABLE 3).

TABLE 1

Overall sputum conversion rates (Gauting 1972)[a]

Type of therapy	Conversion after 3 months	Conversion after 6months	Mean conversion time in months
First treatment	92%	95%	1,4
Re-treatment	85%	92%	1,5

[a] Sputum conversion on culture.

Bacteriologic results are summarized in TABLE 4. Sputum conversion on smear was achieved in all 23 persons available for evaluation at the 3 months, 69 per cent of them already after 1 month of ISOPRODIAN therapy. Sputum conversion on culture was achieved in 18 from 19 persons available for evaluation; one of them, however, suffered a bacteriologic relapse with a typical "fall and rise" phenomenon. One person continued to

TABLE 2

Condition of the patients on admission to trial

All patients admitted to treatment	32	
male		22
female		10
Extent of disease (ATS classification)		
I		0
II		20
III		12
Bacteriological status		
positive on smear & culture		30
positive on culture only		2
Exclusion for pretreatment factors (drug resistance of M.tuberculosis)		2
Total patients remaining for evaluation	30	

discharge bacilli on culture after 3 months of ISOPRODIAN administration. Comparing these results e.g. to sputum conversion rates achieved with INH + streptomycin + PAS for 3 months followed by INH + PAS (British Medical Research Council, 1973) which amounted to 79 per cent on

TABLE 3

Duration of treatment[(a)]

Less than 1 month	4
1 month	4
2 months	4
3 months	0
4 months	6
5 months	4
6 months	1
7 months	7

(a) June 1975.

smear and to 57 per cent on culture at 3 months, then ISOPRODIAN certainly appears worth while of further investigation, as far as early results are concerned. On the other hand, there is no need to stress that regimens containing rifampicin will undoubtedly achieve better results more rapidly. Radiological development is shown in TABLE 5.

TABLE 4

Sputum conversion

Smear:			
Total patients evaluated (June '75)		23	
negative after	1 month of therapy	16	(69 %)
	2 months of therapy	6	
	3 months of therapy	1	
Culture:			
Total patients evaluated (June '75)		19	
negative after	1 month of therapy	3	
	2 months of therapy	8	(a)
	3 months of therapy	7	(b)
positive after	3 months of therapy	1	

(a) 1 patient in this group relapsed with sputum positive on culture (5th month) and on smear (6th month); results of susceptibility determination are not yet available.

(b) Since only early results can be evaluated, the 3 months' interval was arbitrarily chosen as the limit.

Following laboratory parameters were monitored at regular intervals using the SMA-12 apparatus for SGOT, SGPT, creatinine, alkaline phosphatase, LDH, serum bilirubin, serum urea nitrogen and serum uric acid, the SMA-6 apparatus for glucose, serum chloride, potassium, calcium and sodium values, and the Coulter counter for white and red (RBC) blood counts, hemoglobin (Hb), hematocrit, MCV and MCHC value determinations. Also, in specific cases reticulocytes and serum iron values were determined. The overall results are shown in TABLE 6 stressing exclusively the negative observations. At the present time and in comparable groups of patients, we are observing around 25 per cent of side-effects. It is, of course, rather difficult to compare percentages because of the low numbers in the ISOPRODIAN group; RBC and Hb changes might be considered worth of further investigation, though we saw similar effects also in patients treated by other regimens.

TABLE 5

X-ray development

Total patients with cavity on admission	30	
Total patients evaluated (June '75)	22	
Cavity closed		10
Cavity decreased in size		12

TABLE 6

Side effects and change of chemotherapy

Side effects:	
Decrease of RBC and Hb values	9
Decrease of RBC and Hb values followed by their increase, with eventual repetition	11 (a)
Chemotherapy changed:	
Considerable decrease of RBC and Hb values accompanied by increase of reticulocytes and bilirubin	3
Excessive vomiting	1
Considerable increase in SGOT and SGPT values	2
Hemoptoe	2

(a) without interrupting ISOPRODIAN administration.

Summarizing our results, we consider it worth while to continue this trial and we think that, regarding the acceptance by the patients, technology of administration and the price, ISOPRODIAN could be an advantage in extending our chemotherapeutic possibilities in mycobacterial diseases.

Literature

Blaha H. and Rottach H. (1974), Praxis der Pneumologie 28, 930
British Medical Research Council Co-operative Study (1973), Tubercle, 54, 99
Chicou, F.J., et al. (1968), Bulletin of the World Health Organization, 39, 731
East African/British Medical Research Council Sulphone Investigation (1959), Tubercle 40, 1
Fox, W. (1964), British Medical Journal, 1, 135
Fox, W. and Mitchison, D.A. (1975), American Review of Respiratory Diseases, 111, 325
Freerksen, E. (1973), Lecture presented during the 13th Meeting of the North German Association for Tuberculosis and Respiratory Diseases, Celle, Germany, October 19 - 21
Lees, A.W., (1965), 18th Conference of the International Union Against Tuberculosis, Munich, Excerpta Medica, International Congress Series No. 96, 112
WHO Expert Committee on Tuberculosis (1974), 9th Report, World Health Organization Technical Report Series No. 552, 17

COMPARATIVE STUDY OF THE INACTIVATION OF ISONIAZID IN AFRICANS AND EUROPEANS

E. Bergogne-Berezin and J. Modai

Bichat and Claude Bernard Hospitals

Paris, France

The determination of concentrations of free isoniazid (INH) in the blood of patients treated for tuberculosis has not yet become part of routine examination procedures; for the last 15 years, this test has nevertheless greatly helped to gain a deeper knowledge of the 2 classes of slow and rapid inactivators of isoniazid into which humans are divided, the distribution of these types of inactivators into various ethnical groups studied since 1960 by various authors (Armstrong, Harris, Jeanes, etc.), the genetic determinism of the phenotypes of inactivation determined by Evans.

These studies have found immediate therapeutic application since the doses of INH can now be adjusted to each individual patient according to his type of inactivation, in order to make sure that the drug is therapeutically effective and avoid untoward toxic reactions which might result from overdosage.

While numerous reports on the pharmacokinetics of isoniazid in caucasian Europeans are available, the number of publications dealing with the fate of the drug in negroid Africans is scarce. The recrudescence of tuberculosis in black people, as well as the frequency of tuberculosis recurrences or relapses that these people are subject to, raise the question as to whether rapid inactivators are prevalent in this ethnic group. Harris, Sunamara and Armstrong determined high percentages of rapid inactivators among Japanese (90%), Eskimos (nearly 100%) and American Indians (70%). As far as negroid patients are concerned, Harris concluded after a study on 15 patients, that the distribution of the types of inactivation was very heterogenous, with rapid inactivators amounting to only 45%. The small number of reports published on this subject, together with the difficulties of interpretation related to the choice of one or several criteria for discrimination, have led us to make another study on the frequency of occurrence of rapid inactivators in a sample of negroid African population, as compared with an equivalent sample from caucasian Europeans studied simultaneously.

MATERIALS AND METHODS

The tubercular patients who participated in this study were hospitalized at the Claude Bernard Hospital, Paris. The sample from negroid African population consisted in a group of 58 patients free from any liver or renal impairment liable to modify INH acetylation or excretion processes. A group of 55 caucasian Europeans served as controls. Single doses of 4 mg/kg INH were administered orally to patients fasting for 24 hours. Blood samples were collected 1, 3, and 6 hours later. The vertical diffusion technique advocated by Schmiedel, and revised by Canetti and Grosset in France, was used.

In the present study, we had recourse to a "Serum isoniazid quick assay method," using as the test strain the Pasteur Institute atypical Mycobacterium aurum REB strain with rapid growth. Inhibition heights of the reference standard series of tubes were measured in mm, and data were plotted on scale paper to give the reference curve of inhibition heights versus INH concentrations. The inhibition height values for each serum permitted direct measurement of corresponding concentrations of INH. In order to improve the precision of inhibition height conversions, especially with regard to the lower concentrations of INH, we transformed the curves by plotting data on semilog paper.

INTERPRETATION OF RESULTS

Choice of a Criterion of Discrimination for Types of Inactivation

The numerous criteria that have been put forward since 1960 show how difficult it is to find a strict classification.

(a) The Armstrong test (1960) based on the residual level of INH at the 6th hour has long been the recognized criterion of discrimination: according to this test, isoniazid serum levels of 0.6 mcg/ml or lower at hour 6 are said to belong to "rapid inactivators" and those amounting to at least 0.8 mcg/ml are said to belong to "slow inactivators."

(b) Vivien shows that the distribution of third hour concentrations is bimodal, and confirmed the existence of two categories of inactivators (slow and rapid inactivators amounted to 59% and 41% respectively in 134 patients from a caucasian population).

(c) Measurement of the half-life of INH in the serum is a third criterion for discrimination between the 2 metabolism types. However, the figures reported vary. INH serum half-life ranges from 60 minutes to 150 minutes according to Ritschel and from 30 minutes to 6 hours with a wide scatter of values according to Vivien. More recently, Tiitinen put forward that the only boundary to be set to the 2 metabolism types was an INH serum half-life value of 110 minutes.

Overall Comparison of the Two Groups Studied in Our Report

Comparison of curves of inactivation shows that the slopes of elimination of both groups do not seem different. For greater precision, statistical analysis was applied to compare the means and slopes.

Comparison of means at hours 1, 3, and 6 reached statistical significance.

Comparison of slopes of the 2 groups between hours 1 and 3, 3 and 6, and 1 and 6 were not statistically significant either.

Comparison of half-lives did not show great differences: the mean half-lives measured in the samples studied were found to be equally long in both groups, 190 minutes for white people and 170 minutes for black people. According to most authors, such values as these belong to slow inactivators.

The histograms of the data obtained at hours 1, 3, and 6 were compared with Vivien bimodal curve for hour 3 (the same experimental procedure was used). This comparison allowed neither a bimodal distribution of INH serum levels to be brought out clearly, nor any differentiation between slow and rapid inactivators to be made in the black and white populations.

A new criterion of discrimination, the multidimensional factor analysis applied to technical comparisons, has been introduced in our study with the collaboration of Prof. Gremy's team. Graphical representation of the patients were determined from the analysis of the principal component with data gathered at hours 1, 3, and 6 standing for variables. They showed first that the most important contribution is that of INH serum levels at hour 3 and, secondly, that the differentiation between 2 categories of inactivators, the slow and the rapid ones, is rather good. This suggested the possibility of calculating a discriminating linear function which might allow patients to be classified fairly accurately into one of these categories, depending on the INH levels determined at hours 1, 3, and 6. The complex formula is as follows:

$$Y = 3.38 + 0.009 X_1 + 0.002 X_2 + 0.010 X_3$$

in which X_1, X_2, and X_3 represent INH serum levels at hours 1, 3, and 6.

The first results were not steady, probably because of the small size of our samples.

Distribution of Types of Inactivation in Each of the Groups Studied

As the overall comparison of INH inactivation rate in the two groups studied failed to show statistical significance, the respective proportions of slow and rapid inactivators in each group were determined using Armstrong criteria. Calculation was based on the data gathered at hour 6 (which represent the residual INH serum levels).

With this simple criterion of discrimination, it was possible to bring out a significant difference between the proportions of slow and rapid inactivators among caucasian Europeans and negroid Africans the percentage of rapid inactivators being of 62% in the black population versus 43.6% in controls. The comparison of the two percentages observed (62 and 43.6% of 58 and 55 patients respectively) was based on the chi-square test. The difference was significant at the 5% level of probability, X_2 being equal to 3.841, we reached here the limit of significance.

CONCLUSION

A critical study has been presented. Few reports on the differences liable to exist between caucasian and negroid populations as far as the frequency of occurrence of rapid inactivators is concerned are yet available. A number of parameters serving as criteria of discrimination between the two phenotypes covering INH inactivation rate (slow and rapid inactivators) were used in this study. Only one of them, which takes into account the residual serum level of INH at hour 6 was retained. It allowed a significant difference between the respective percentages of rapid inactivators among caucasian Europeans and negroid Africans to be evidenced; this difference was significant at the 5% level of probability and the limit of significance was reached ($X_2 = 3.841$).

A new parameter based on the multi-dimensional analysis was put forward in this study; a discriminating linear function was used but discrimination within the 2 groups could not be made owing to the small size of the samples.

BIOAVAILABILITY OF RIMACTAZID

R.L. PARSONS[1], G.M. HOSSACK[1], P.F.G. BOON[2], &
D.M. BURLEY[2]

Department of Clinical Pharmacology[1]

Guy's Hospital Medical School. London. SE1.9RT

Ciba Laboratories, Ltd.[2] Horsham. Sussex

Introduction Rifampicin has now got an established place as a first line agent in the management of tuberculosis. Its advantages include proven efficacy(1), nausea is relatively infrequent (2), a low incidence of bacterial drug resistance (3) and the possibility of shortening the normally prolonged course of antituberculous chemotherapy.

The availability of Rimactazid, (a combined preparation of rifampicin & isoniazid) now means that effective treatment can be given with less risk of patient default resulting from the unpleasant upper gastrointestinal side effects associated with PAS. In view of the known interactions previously described between a number of antituberculous agents (4-6), it is important to establish whether this combination provides therapeutically effective plasma concentrations of both its components.

Subjects & methods 8 normal subjects (6 male, 2 female) weight (52.2 - 65.9 kg.) participated in a double blind cross over study. Each subject received either 2 capsules of Rimactazid (each capsule contained 300 mg. of rifampicin & 150 mg. of isoniazid) or 2 x 300 mg. capsules of rifampicin with 3 x 100 mg. tablets of isoniazid. The participants had not previously been exposed to rifampicin prior to this study. They were studied following an overnight fast and performed their normal working activities throughout the study.

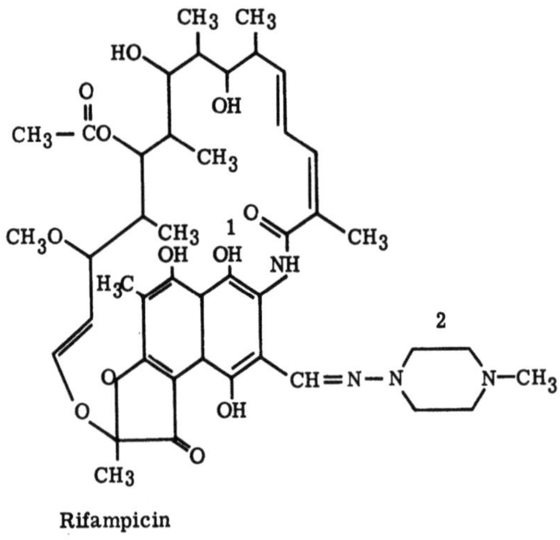

FIGURE 1: Structural Formulae of Rifampicin

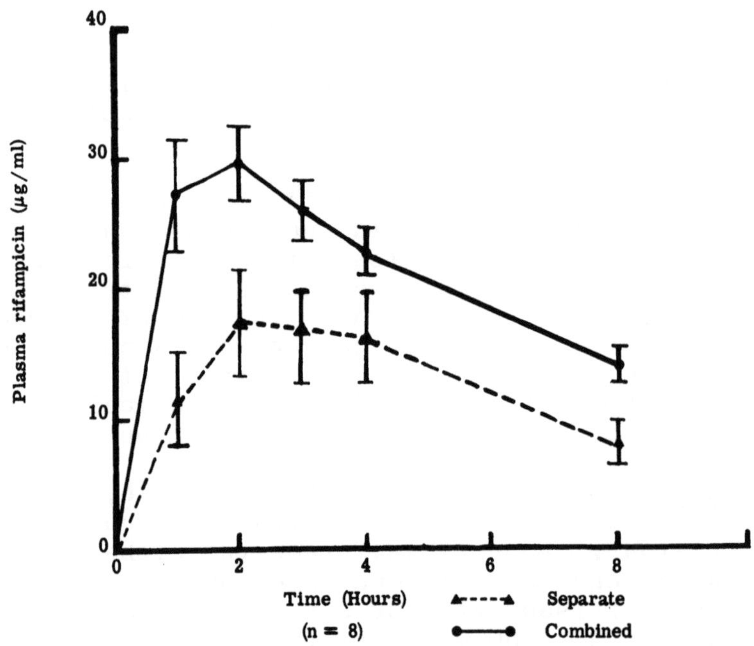

FIGURE 2: Mean ± SEM plasma Rifampicin in normal subjects after separate (Rifampicin 300 mg. X 2 + isoniazid 100 mg. X 3) & combined (Rimactazid) preparations. Assay organism. Sarcina lutea.

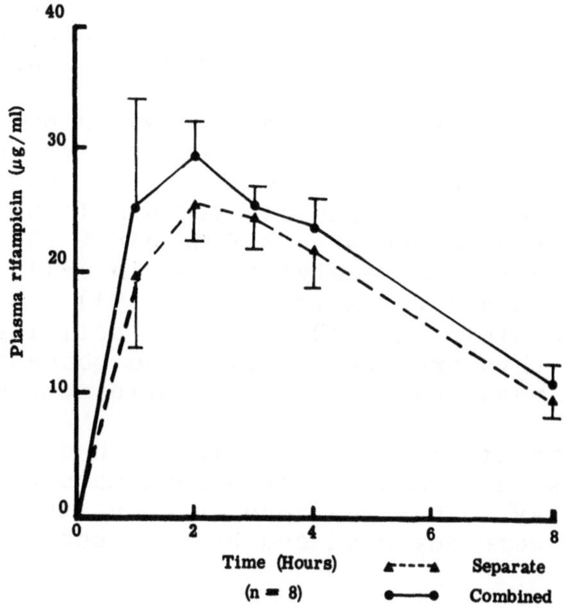

FIGURE 3: Mean ± SEM plasma Rifampicin in normal subjects after separate (Rifampicin 300 mg. X 2 + isoniazid 100 mg. X 3) & combined (Rimactazid) preparations. Assay organism. Bacillus Brevis.

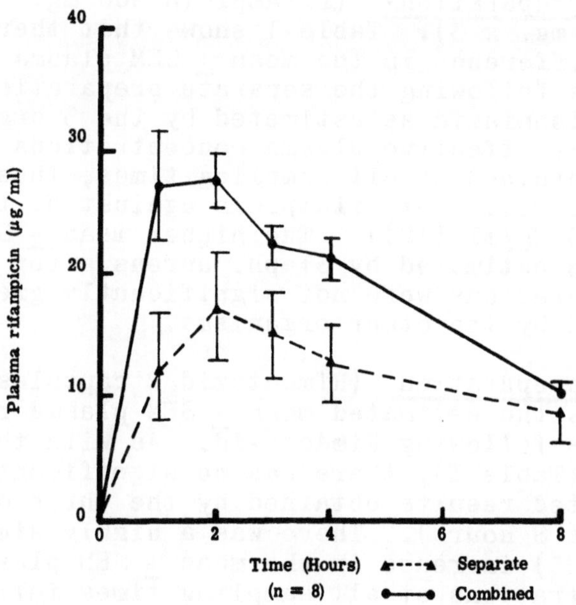

FIGURE 4: Mean ± SEM plasma rifampicin in normal subjects after separate (rifampicin 300 mg. X 2 + isoniazid 100 mg. X 3) and combined (Rimactazid) preparations. Assay organism. Staph. aureus.

Blood samples were collected prior to dosing, and at 1, 2, 3, 4 & 8 hours afterwards. The subjects were given breakfast after collection of the 1 hour sample.

Plasma from these blood samples was stored at $-20^{o}C$ until analysed by small plate microbiological assay for rifampicin by a method based on that of Grove & Randall (1955) (7). Each sample was assayed simultaneously with Sarcina lutea (which measures rifampicin & the biologically active metabolite desacetylrifampicin (8)), Bacillus brevis (which assays rifampicin alone (9)) & S aph. aureus (desacetylrifampicin has 1/25th of the activity of rifampicin against this organism (10)). The concentration of isoniazid was measured by a colorimetric method (11).

Known concentrations of isoniazid in solution were assayed against all three assay organisms used for the rifampicin assay. This was done to check that the zones of inhibition were not produced by the isoniazid in the combination.

Results

Plasma rifampicin

(a) Separate preparations (rifampicin 300 mg. x 2 + isoniazid 100 mg. x 3). Table I shows that there was no significant difference in the mean ± SEM plasma rifampicin concentrations following the separate preparations of rifampicin & isoniazid as estimated by the 3 organisms. Therapeutically effective plasma concentrations of rifampicin were obtained at all sampling times, these being well above the M.I.C. of rifampicin against M. tuberculosis (0.1 - 0.5 µg/ml (12)). The higher mean ± SEM plasma concentrations estimated by Staph. aureus after the separate preparations were not significantly greater than those obtained by the other organisms.

(b) Combined preparation (Rimactazid 2 capsules) Table II shows the estimated mean ± SEM plasma rifampicin concentrations following Rimactazid. As with the separate preparations (Table I), there was no significant difference in the estimated results obtained by the three organisms. (apart from at 8 hours). There was a highly significant ($P<0.01 - 0.025$) increase in the mean ± SEM plasma rifampicin concentrations at all sampling times following Rimactazid (S. lutea. Table III) and similar differences were found with B. brevis. There was no significant difference between the results of the separate & combined preparations when using Staph. aureus as the assay organism.

Table I: Mean ± SEM plasma rifampicin after separate preparations of rifampicin & isoniazid

Assay organism	Sarcina lutea	Bacillus brevis		Staph.aureus	
Timing	μg/ml	μg/ml		μg/ml	
1 hour	11.24±3.51	12.41±4.31	NS	19.88±5.59	NS
2 hours	17.25±3.85	16.40±4.10	NS	25.46±2.47	NS
3 hours	16.12±3.28	14.87±3.11	NS	24.45±1.93	NS
4 hours	16.01±3.21	12.95±2.65	NS	21.58±2.62	NS
8 hours	7.93±1.46	8.74±2.36	NS	9.65±0.97	NS

Table II: Mean ± SEM plasma rifampicin after combined preparation of rifampicin & isoniazid

Assay organism	Sarcina lutea	Bacillus brevis		Staph.aureus	
Timing	μg/ml	μg/ml		μg/ml	
1 hour	27.24±4.49	27.16±4.24	NS	25.36±8.24	NS
2 hours	29.76±2.61	27.71±1.75	NS	29.63±2.85	NS
3 hours	25.99±2.09	22.54±1.20	NS	25.30±1.87	NS
4 hours	22.84±1.69	21.02±1.35	NS	23.94±2.06	NS
8 hours	13.68±1.21	10.21±0.87	<0.02	11.09±1.44	NS

TABLE III: Mean Plasma Levels of Rifampicin & Isoniazid (μg/ml ± SEM) after 600 mg. Rifampicin & 300 mg. Isoniazid Given Separately & as a Combined Capsule (Rimactazid).

PLASMA RIFAMPICIN & DESACETYL RIFAMPICIN				PLASMA RIFAMPICIN & DESACETYL RIFAMPICIN		
Assay Organism: Sarcina lutea				Bacillus brevis		
Timing	Separate preparations	Combined preparation		Separate preparations	Combined preparation	
1 hr.	11.24 ± 3.51	27.24 ± 4.49	< 0.01	12.41 ± 4.31	27.16 ± 4.24	< 0.025
2 hr.	17.25 ± 3.85	29.76 ± 2.61	< 0.01	16.40 ± 4.10	27.71 ± 1.75	< 0.0125
3 hr.	16.12 ± 3.28	25.99 ± 2.09	< 0.01	14.87 ± 3.11	22.54 ± 1.20	< 0.025
4 hr.	16.01 ± 3.21	22.84 ± 1.69	< 0.025	12.95 ± 2.65	21.02 ± 1.35	< 0.025
8 hr.	7.93 ± 1.46	13.68 ± 1.21	< 0.005	8.74 ± 2.36	10.21 ± 0.87	NS
PLASMA RIFAMPICIN & DESACETYL RIFAMPICIN				PLASMA ISONIAZID		
Assay Organism: Staph. aureus						
Timing	Separate preparations	Combined preparation		Separate preparations	Combined preparation	
1 hr.	19.88 ± 5.59	25.36 ± 8.24	NS	7.73 ± 0.56	8.43 ± 0.41	NS
2 hr.	25.46 ± 2.47	29.63 ± 2.85	NS	6.49 ± 0.34	6.39 ± 0.24	NS
3 hr.	24.45 ± 1.93	25.30 ± 1.87	NS	4.95 ± 0.26	4.98 ± 0.12	NS
4 hr.	21.58 ± 2.62	23.94 ± 2.06	NS	4.17 ± 0.22	3.99 ± 0.20	NS
8 hr.	9.65 ± 0.97	11.09 ± 1.44	NS	1.74 ± 0.16	1.70 ± 0.17	NS

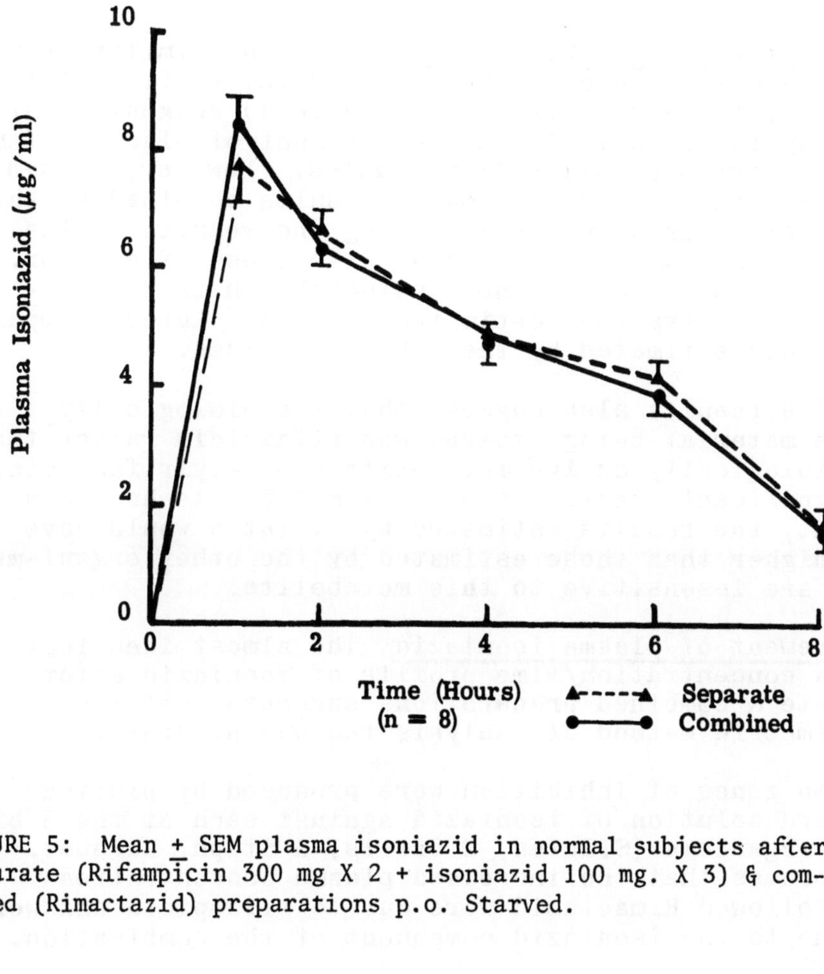

FIGURE 5: Mean ± SEM plasma isoniazid in normal subjects after separate (Rifampicin 300 mg X 2 + isoniazid 100 mg. X 3) & combined (Rimactazid) preparations p.o. Starved.

Plasma isoniazid (Fig. 5). The plasma concentration/time profile after 300 mg. of isoniazid followed an almost identical pattern after both the separate & combined preparations. The levels obtained were all well in excess of the M.I.C. of isoniazid against sensitive strains of M. tuberculosis (12) (0.05 - 0.2 μg/ml).

Discussion

Reliability of microbiological assay The similar results obtained with each organism after administration of rifampicin and tablets of isoniazid (Table I) suggests that bioassay is reliable in the measurement of plasma rifampicin during bioavailability studies. However, consider able variation in the estimated results obtained by the assay method is shown by comparing the results of the samples assayed by one organism with those of another. This is illustrated by the considerably higher mean ± SEM plasma concentrations estimated by Staph. aureus compared with those estimated by the other organisms.

The results also suggest that the biologically active material being assayed was rifampicin rather than its biologically active metabolite desacetylrifampicin. If significant quantities of this metabolite had been present, the results estimated by S. lutea would have been higher than those estimated by the other organisms, which are insensitive to this metabolite.

Measurement of plasma isoniazid The almost identical plasma concentration/time profile of isoniazid after separate & combined preparations suggests that the colorimetric method of analysis too was accurate.

No zones of inhibition were produced by plating standard solution of isoniazid against each of the 3 bio assay organisms (S.lutea, B.brevis, & Staph. aureus). This proves that the increased plasma concentrations that followed Rimactazid were due to rifampicin and were not due to the isoniazid component of the combination.

Clinical significance of these results The bioavailability of rifampicin following Rimactazid was considerably greater than that after rifampicin and isoniazid given separately. This was largely due to low plasma rifampicin concentrations in two subjects after the separate preparations. Whilst small numbers were studied, occasional erratic oral absorption of this potent antituberculous drug is of considerable practical importance, since it might lead to therapeutically ineffective levels in some patients. This would also increase the risk of bacterial drug resistance. These findings remain to be confirmed in patients on permanent treatment with Rimactazid. On these results it would appear that the combined preparation of rifampicin and isoniazid has several advantages over separate preparations.

Problems resulting from interactions such as have occurred with PAS have not so far occurred with Rimactazid Thus there appears to be no risk of increased isoniazid toxicity resulting from its combination with rifampicin.

Conclusions

1). There was no change in the plasma concentrations of isoniazid as a result of combining this antibiotic with rifanpicin in a single capsule.

2). In-vitro pharmaceutical interactions between the constituents of Rimactazid do not seem to occur.

3). The gastrointestinal side effects associated with combined preparations of PAS & isoniazid do not appear to be a serious problem.

4). The bioavailability of rifampicin following Rimactazid is better than that after rifampicin alone.

5). The risk of bacterial drug resistance is reduced by using combinations such as Rimactazid in the treatment of Tuberculosis.

References

(1) Neuman, R., Doster, B., Murray, F.J. & Ferebee, (1971) Rifampicin in initial treatment of pulmonary tuberculosis. Amer. Rev. resp. Dis. 103, 461 - 476.

(2) Mattson, K., (1972) Rifampicin induced side effects. Symposium on Rifampicin & current policies in antituberculous chemotherapy. Ciba Foundation, London.

(3) Grumbach, F. & Rist, N. (1967) Experimental antituberculous activity of rifampicin, derivative of rifamycin SV. Rev. Tuberc. Pneumol. (Paris) 31, 749.

(4) Boman, G. Borga, O., Hanngren, A. et. al. (1970) Pharmacokinetic interactions between the tuberculostatics rifampicin, para-aminosalicylic acid and isoniazid. Acta. Pharmac. Toxicol. 28, Suppl. 1, 15.

(5) Acocella, G. (1971)
A metabolic & kinetic study on the association rifampicin-isoniazid. Respiration, 28, Suppl. 1-6.
(6) Burley, D.M. (1972)
Rifampicin, isoniazid & hepatotoxicity. Proceedings of the 258th meeting of the Danish Pneumological society. p. 25.
(7) Grove, D.C. & Randall, W.A. (1955)
Assay methods of antibiotics. A laboratory manual. Medical Encyclopedia. Inc., New York.
(8) Burley, D.M. Personal communication.
(9) Porven, G. & Canetti, G. (1968)
Revue Tuberc. 32 (5) 707 - 716.
(10) Gialdroni-Grassi, G. (1969) Some aspects of the antimycobacterial activity of rifampicin. Simposi Scientifici Lepetit 20, 51 - 57.
(11) Ellard, G.A., Gammon, G.T. & Wallace, S.M. (1972)
The determination of isoniazid and its metabolites acetylisoniazid, isonicotinic acid and isonicotinylglycine in serum and urine. Biochem. J. 126, 449 - 458.
(12) Pallanza, R., Arioli, V., Furesz, S. et al. (1967)
Rifampicin: a new rifamycin II. Laboratory studies on the antituberculous activity & preliminary clinical observations. Arzneimittel-Forsh, 17. 529 - 534.

RATE OF STERILIZATION OF SPUTUM FROM PATIENTS WITH PULMONARY TUBERCULOSIS

Gladys L. Hobby, Ph.D.[1], H. William Harris, M.D.[2], Charles Felton, M.D.[3], and John Edsall, M.D.[3]
Veterans Administration Hospital, East Orange, New Jersey[1], and the Bellevue[2] and Harlem[3] Hospitals, New York, New York

In 1973 , as part of a study to evaluate the usefulness of a procedure developed by us for precise microscopic enumeration of acid-fast bacilli in the sputum of patients with pulmonary tuberculosis, the number of culturable mycobacterial cell units per ml. of sputum was determined in 28 patients before and during chemotherapy. The data obtained clearly showed, perhaps for the first time, that there is a very significant decrease in the acid-fast burden, at least in some patients, during the first two weeks of treatment. The data further suggested that quantitation of the culturable mycobacterial burden might well provide a useful mechanism for comparison of chemotherapeutic drug regimens. The present study was prompted by these observations.

The present study was designed to evaluate, in a controlled trial, the rates of sterilization of sputum from tuberculous patients, effected by rifampin plus isoniazid as compared with rifampin plus isoniazid plus pyrazinamide, a three-drug combination which we believed to be potentially the most active available.

All patients included in the study had moderately or far advanced tuberculosis, no previous antituberculosis chemotherapy, and pretreatment sputum microscopically positive for acid-fast bacilli. Individuals in whom the number of <u>microscopically</u> detectable mycobacteria per ml. of sputum was less than 1×10^5 prior to or at the time of institution of chemotherapy in most instances were eliminated from the study.

Patients with no evidence of acute or chronic hepatic disease, based on medical history and physical examination, were randomized between the two regimens: (1) isoniazid 300 mg. daily plus rifampin 600 mg. daily, each drug administered in a single daily dose, and (2) isoniazid 300 mg. daily plus rifampin 600 mg. daily plus pyrazinamide 1.5 grams daily. Patients with hepatic abnormality were not randomized; rather, they were treated with isoniazid and rifampin only.

Sputum was collected from each patient prior to the start of chemotherapy, and, insofar as was feasible, at 7-day intervals thereafter. Sputum was concentrated by the N-acetyl-L-cysteine method, and the number of culturable mycobacterial cell units per ml. of each specimen was determined by the conventional microbial population count technique of Fenner, Martin, and Pierce. All patients were infected with strains of M. tuberculosis fully susceptible to isoniazid, rifampin, and other antituberculosis drugs.

The present report concerns only the effect of chemotherapy on the numbers of culturable mycobacterial cell units per ml. of sputum in patients with previously untreated pulmonary tuberculosis.

In 19 patients treated with isoniazid plus rifampin, the initial number of culturable cell units per ml. ranged from 2.0×10^4 to 5.6×10^9 (mean 3.7×10^8). A 99.9 per cent decrease in the number of cell units occurred within 4.6 to 42.4 days (mean time, 23.5 days). All patients from whom sufficient specimens were obtained to permit evaluation showed fewer than 1×10^1 culturable cell units per ml. of sputum in less than 9 weeks after start of chemotherapy (mean time, 46.7 days). There was no apparent relation between the size of the initial microbial burden and the rate of decrease in the number of culturable cell units after institution of chemotherapy. In 13 patients treated with the three drugs, isoniazid, rifampin, and pyrazinamide, the initial number of culturable cell units ranged from 5.0×10^4 to 1.3×10^{10} (mean, 9.5×10^8); the number decreased by 99.9 per cent within 5.5 to 43.8 days (mean time, 18.6 days); and the mean time to apparent sterilization (i.e., to $< 1 \times 10^1$ cell units per ml. of sputum) was 44.8 days. On both regimens, there was considerable variation from patient to patient in the rate of decrease in number of culturable cell units.

In conclusion, (1) apparent sterilization was achieved in all patients in less than 9 weeks after start of chemotherapy with either rifampin plus isoniazid, or rifampin plus isoniazid plus pyrazinamide; (2) inclusion of pyrazinamide in the regimen used did not speed the rate of sterilization; (3) the rate at which sterilization was achieved seemed unrelated to the size of the initial mycobacterial burden; (4) following apparently effective chemotherapy, persisting culturable mycobacteria were detected with equal frequency in the sputum of tuberculous patients treated with rifampin plus isoniazid, or with rifampin plus isoniazid plus pyrazinamide.

RE-TREATMENT OF CHRONIC PULMONARY TUBERCULOSIS WITH LOW AND HIGH DOSAGES RIFAMPICIN REGIMENS IN THE CONTINUATION INTERMITTENT PHASE (A controlled comparison study)

M. Zierski*, E. Bek*, J. Marcinia+, B. Szelagowicz+

*Department of Respiratory Diseases and Tuberculosis
National Institute for Research of Tuberculosis Study Centre, Lodz, Poland
+District Chest Dispensary, Poznan, Poland

The great value of rifampicin as a suitable anti-tuberculous agent for intermittent therapy has been confirmed in several experimental and clinical studies. Unfortunately our actual knowledge of which size of doses should be chosen for rifampicin in the intermittent therapy after a preceding daily phase is still insufficient.

This report is concerned with a comparison of the results of treatment of two groups of patients treated up to one year with regimens including in the intermittent phase low or high dosages of rifampicin, as a part of studies of chemotherapy on various rifampicin and ethambutol two phase regimens of chronic poly-resistant pulmonary tuberculosis.

Regimens of Chemotherapy

In the initial first phase for 3 months all patients were treated with ethambutol (EMB-E) 25 mg/kg body weight plus rifampicin (RMP-R) 600 mg administered daily in one single dose on an empty stomach. During the second phase, randomly allocated to supervised intermittent regimens with ethambutol 50 mg/kg body weight plus rifampicin 600 mg, the same as in the initial daily phase, once or twice weekly (Regimen A), or the patients continued their intermittent treatment with ethambutol 50 mg/kg body weight plus rifampicin 1200 mg, once or twice weekly (Regimen B). The individual dose sizes were thus the same for the once or twice weekly application in all regimens. After 4 months of treatment in hospital the patients continued their intermittent chemotherapy under supervised out-patient conditions up to 12 months.

Patients admitted to the study fulfilled the following criteria: They were previous chemotherapy failures, sputum positive continuously or periodically for at least 2 years, excreting bacilli resistant to isoniazid and streptomycin, as well as to other drugs, or resistant to isionazid alone, if the use of other drugs was contra-indicated due to toxicity. They had not been previously treated with rifampicin and ethambutol and were assumed to be co-operative. A total of 164 patients were eligible for assessment - 82 patients in the group with Regimen A (low RMP) and 82 patients with Regimen B (high RMP).

The regimens to which the patients were allocated consisted of:

Regimen A	No.
ER/E_1R_1 once weekly 600 mg R	42
ER/E_2R_2 twice weekly 600 mg R	40
Total	82 patients

Regimen B	
ER/E_1R_1 - 1200 mg R	41
ER/E_2R_2 - 1200 mg R	41
Total	82 patients

Pre-treatment distribution of age, sex, body weight, extent of diseases and bacteriological content of sputum were similar for all regimens in both groups, without marked difference. The majority of patients were male (83%), mean age over 48 years, mean weight 60 kg (Regimen A) and 61 kg (Regimen B). Over 75% suffered from pulmonary tuberculosis for more than 10 years, nearly 90% of patients have been treated before unsuccessfully with 5 or more drugs.

72% of patients allocated to Group A and 69% of the Group B suffered from far advanced pulmonary tuberculosis, 96% and 88% of cases had cavitation, 91% in both groups were heavy sputum positive on culture. In generaly the patients in this trial had severe chronic cavitary pulmonary tuberculosis, and were in poor clinical condition, many of them with other concomittant diseases.

Bacteriological results are shown in Table 1. All patients were on three pre-treatment culture sputum positive. After 3 months of daily treatment 83% out of 164 patients of both groups were smear and 91% culture negative (89% culture negative in Group A and 94% of patients in Group B respectively). At 6 months 98% of 82 patients with the Regimen A and 97% of 78 patients with the Regimen B were culture negative. The proportion of patients

TABLE 1

COMPARISON OF ONCE AND TWICE WEEKLY INTERMITTENT REGIMENS WITH LOW (600 MG) AND HIGH (1200 MG) DOSAGE OF RIFAMPICIN

	Culture Negative - Percentage					
	RMP 600 mg EMB 50 mg/kg			RMP 1200 mg EMB 50 mg/kg		
Month	E_1R_1	E_2R_2	Total	E_1R_1	E_2R_2	Total
3	95	83	89	95	95	94
6	98	98	98	97	97	97
9	97	95	96	97	100	99
12	95	98	96	97	93	95
Patients on assessment (range)	38-42	40	78-82	35-41	30-41	65-82

with negative cultures did not change significantly thereafter during the treatment up to 12 months.

Bacteriological status at 12 months based on culture results at 10, 11 and 12 months provided the patients had at least 6 cultures showed 95% of 78 patients completing one year chemotherapy with Regimen A 95% E_1R_1 and 95% E_2R_2 and 95% of 65 patients with Regiman B 97% E_1R_1 and 93% E_2R_2, having a favourable status (all culture negative or only one positive) at 12 months (Table 2). The bacteriological results in both the groups appeared equally highly effective without difference related to the low 600 mg or high 1200 mg dosage of rifampicin or the rhythm of application of the drugs once or twice weekly.

At one year a total of 7 patients (4 Regimen A and 3 Regimen B) remained with unfavourable bacteriological status. Four of them had sensitive bacilli to rifampicin and ethambutol (2 patients of Regimen A and 2 patients of Regimen B), the other 2 patients (Regimen A) were excreting bacilli resistant to rifampicin,one of them also to ethambutol. The sensitivity tests of one patient were not known for technical reasons.

TABLE 2

STATUS AT 12 MONTHS BASED ON 6 CULTURE RESULTS AT 10, 11 AND 12 MONTHS

Treatment Series	Regimen A				Regimen B			
	ER/E_1R_1 600 mg		ER/E_2R_2 600 mg		ER/E_1R_1 1200 mg		ER/E_2R_2 1200 mg	
	No.	%	No.	%	No.	%	No.	%
Patients with all cultures negative or one positive	36	95	38	95	34	97	28	93
Two or more cultures positive	2	5	2	5	1	3	2	7
Patients on assessment at 12 months	38	100	40	100	35	100	30	100

Premature interruption of treatment before 1 year

21 (12%) of 164 patients stopped their treatment prematurely before one year. There were 4 (5%) patients out of 82 treated intermitten with the low rifampicin doses of the Group A and 16 (19%) out of 80 treated in the Group B with 1200 high rifampicin intermittent. The difference is statistically significant. In nearly 10% the reason for premature interruption of treatment was drug toxicity caused mainly by rifampicin 1200 mg doses occurring during the intermittent phase of treatment. Only 5 (3%) patients were non-co-operative and refused to continue treatment, a very small number considering that many of the patients had been labelled as asocial or undisciplined before admission to the study.

Adverse Reactions

Adverse reactions during the daily 3 months phase were noted in 17 (10%) patients. They were of mild and transient character. Mainly transient hepatic disturbances, without jaundice, with elevated transaminases, mostly symptomless. No indications for permanent withdrawal of the drugs was necessary in this phase of treatment.

Particular attention is required to adverse reactions in the intermittent phase, especially when rifampicin was given in the higher 1200 mg doses.

Systemic adverse reactions of various types occurred in 26 (33%) of patients treated with Regimen B (1200 mg rifampicin plus ethambutol 50 mg/kg body weight once or twice weekly) and 5 (6%) of patients with Regimen A (600 mg rifampicin plus ethambutol 50 mg/kg body weight). A marked difference of statistical significance in favour of Regimen A with intermittent lower 600 mg rifampicin dose once or twice weekly.

Ethambutol appeared to be an excellent companion drug, being tolerated well and having a very limited risk of toxicity. Only 1 (0.6%) patient on E_2R_2 Regimen B showed at 4 months some optic disturbances. They disappeared when treatment with ethambutol was stopped. Other mild hepatic gastrointestinal disturbances, being mainly characterised by transient elevations of transaminases not connected with "systemic syndromes" were noted in few patients, mostly with previous history of liver dysfunction.

The total classification

The overall response to the applied regimens of both groups of patients analysed from two points (a) on the basis of bacteriological effectiveness, and (b) chemotherapy failures due to toxicity and premature discontinuation of assigned treatment were as follows. Excluded from this analysis were patients who stopped treatment due to other reasons than bacteriological or toxicity. 94% was the total effectivity with Regimen A (600 mg ER/E_1R_1 and E_2R_2) and 87% of Regimen B (1200 mg ER/E_1R_1 and E_2R_2) (Table 3).

TABLE 3

THE OVERALL RESPONSE (BASED ON RESULTS OF 152 PATIENTS)

	600 ER $\frac{E_1R_1}{E_2R_2}$ No.	%	1200 ER $\frac{E_1R_1}{E_2R}$ No.	%
Total patients assessed	79	100	73	100
Favourable bacteriologically at one year	74	95	62	96
Unfavourable bacteriologically	4	5	3	4
Unfavourable toxicity	1	1	8	9
Total patients with unfavourable response	5	6	11	13
Total effectivity	74	94	62	87

The rifampicin 600 mg low dosage intermittent regimen applied once or twice weekly after preceded 3 month daily regimen in continuation with ethambutol is of the same high bacteriological effectivity as the regimens with higher 1200 mg rifampicin dosage once or twice weekly in the intermittency. But the practical effectiveness of the lower 600 mg rifampicin doses in the intermittency once or twice weekly appeared to be considerably higher with regard to bacteriological effectivity and acceptable very low hazard of toxicity.

The encouraging results obtained with regimen including lower dosage of rifampicin in the intermittent phase seem to open new prospects of further improvement of chemotherapy of pulmonary tuberculosis - very effective as well as safe and less expensive, than regimens including higher 900 or 1200 mg doses of rifampicin in the intermittent phase.

SUMMARY

A total of 164 patients with chronic advanced pulmonary tuberculosis that represented previous treatment failures, as initially treated with rifampicin (600 mg) plus ethambutol (25 mg/kg per body weight) in a single daily dose for 12 weeks in hospital afterwards. The patients were allocated at random to either once or twice weekly with high (1200 mg) or low (600 mg) rifampicin dosage plus ethambutol (50 mg/kg body weight) for 52 weeks as ambulatory patients. After the 3 months daily phase 85% were culture negative. An 12 months 95% were culture negative with 1200 mg rifampicin once or twice weekly and 95% with 600 mg rifampicin once or twice weekly regimens. The bacteriological results were similar in the once weekly administration of 600 mg or 1200 mg of rifampicin, as with the twice weekly low or high dosage regimens. No significant differences were seen in the time sputum conversion rates between the regimens. 11% adverse reactions episodes were observed in the daily phase. In the intermittent phase, 33% of systemic reactions syndromes with high rifampicin 1200 mg dose and only in 6% with the low 600 mg rifampicin dose. Due to toxicity to rifampicin intermittent treatment was stopped in 8% in the high rifampicin group, and in 1% of the low rifampicin group (a significant difference). The rifampicin low dosage regimens gave favourable clinical and bacteriological response of better total effectivity, than in the high dosage rifampicin group in which adverse reactions and losses due to premature stopping of treatment were of higher frequency. It is concluded that the routinely applied daily dose of 600 mg rifampicin should not be increased in the once or twice weekly intermittent application of this drug in combination with ethambutol. This regimen and dosage schedule appeared bacteriologically to be highly effective, of very good acceptance diminishing considerably both the risk of untoward reactions during the intermittent application and the cost of treatment.

INCIDENCE OF DRUG RESISTANCE ON THE MYCOBACTERIAL STRAINS ISOLATED FROM TREATED AND UNTREATED PATIENTS

J.A. GARCIA, M.C. SAENZ, J. PRIETO, F. MARTIN

Microbiology Department, Faculty of Medicine

University of Salamanca. Fonseca, 2 (SPAIN)

SUMMARY

The resistances of 308 strains of mycobacteria were studied by means of the technique of Canetti, Rist and Grosset, against seven antituberculosis drugs. Two hundred and ninety-four of the strains were identified as *M. tuberculosis*, and fourteen as atypical mycobacteria. All strains were of human origin.

The strains of *M. tuberculosis* isolated from untreated patients (110 strains) were sensitive to Rifampicin and Ethambutol, while those isolated from treated patients showed variable resistance to the drugs used. The highest percentages of resistances were those of Isoniazid (42.3%), Streptomycin (29.8%) and p-Aminosalicylic acid (22%).

The atypical mycobacteria strains showed a higher resistance disregarding their origin from treated or untreated patients.

INTRODUCTION

Even though endemic tuberculosis has considerably diminished in our country, the prevalence and incidence index are still too high to think of the disease as a subject not worth studying.

The causes are essentially iatrogenic, since in the clinic most patients are still being treated with the three tuberculostatics recommended at the Rome Conference. This has compelled the Spanish sanitary authorities to impose a treatment exclusively based on bacteriological standards, to which end reference laboratories specializing in this field have been created throughout the country. These allow for an accurate isolation and identification and make possible the performance of in vitro sensitivity tests; and have thereby avoided, as far as possible, the occurrence of resistances through the application of the most specific treatment in each case.

Our work deals with the study of resistance in a group of mycobacteria strains isolated from treated and untreated patients. The high percentages of resistance found, particularly in the group of strains isolated from treated patients, leads us to consider the necessity of performing sensitivity tests once the strains have been isolated.

MATERIAL AND METHODS

We have studied the activity of seven antituberculosis drugs against a total of 304 strains of mycobacteria isolated from pathological products of human origin.

The depuration technique used, for most of the products studied, was the Sodium Lauryl Sulfate technique (Tacquet, A., Tison, F., 1961).

For the sensitivity tests, the proportions method was used (Canetti et al. 1963).

Bacterial suspension at 1 mg/ml. in distilled water, together with 10^{-3} and 10^{-4} dilutions from it, were used for each strain.

The medium used for the study of sensitivities was Lowenstein-Jensen, in which the drugs were incorporated, prior to coagulation.

Table I indicates the drugs used, their concentrations, and the criteria by which the resistances were established.

For each strain, a set of tubes of Lowenstein-Jensen containing suitable graded concentrations of the drugs mentioned, was smeared with 0.2 ml. of the 1: 1000 dilutions; two tubes of Lowenstein-Jensen, drug-free, acting as controls, were equally inoculated

Another similar set was inoculated with 2 ml. of the 1 : 10.000 dilution; two tubes of drug-free Lowenstein-Jensen were also smeared, acting as control tubes.

Once inoculated, the cultures were incubated at 37º C., in a horizontal position.

For most of the strains, the reading was done four weeks after the incubation. For the atypical strains, it was always done prior to the fourth week. For some strains of M. tuberculosis showing dysgonic growth, the results were read seven weeks later.

The identification of the mycobacteria strains was done according to growth characters: rate of growth, aspect of the colonies, and presence or absence of pigmentation before and after their

Table I : Drugs, Concentrations and Criteria of Resistance

Drugs and Concentration (mcgr/ml.)		Criteria of Resistance
Isoniazid	0.1	10%
	0.2	1%
	1	
Streptomycin	2	50 to 100%
	4	1%
	10	
p-Aminosalicylic acid	0.25	10%
	0.5	1%
	1	0.1%
Ethionamide	10	50 to 100%
	20	10%
	30	1%
Rifampicin	10	7%
	20	0.1%
	40	0.01%
Ethambutol	1	30%
	2	0.1%
	3	0.01%
Capreomycin	20	50 to 100%
	30	10%
	40	1%

exposure to light. Various biochemical tests were also used to determine the mycobacteria species.

RESULTS

Out of the 308 strains of mycobacteria which were isolated, 294 were identified as M. tuberculosis; the remaining were identified as atypical, 4 of them being M. kansasii; 3 M. avium; 1 M. intracellulare; 2 M. gordonae and 4 M. fortuitum. One hundred and ten strains out of 294 strains of M. tuberculosis were isolated from untreated patients, and 184 from patients who had been receiving antituberculosis therapy.

Of the 14 strains of atypical mycobacteria, 9 were isolated from treated patients, and 5 from patients who had not been under treatment.

The resistances found in the group of 110 strains of M. tuberculosis from untreated patients, are shown in table 2.

Not one strain resistant to Rifampicin was found, nor to Ethambutol; 4 strains were resistant to Isoniazid, 6 to Streptomycin, and 2 to p-Aminosalicylic acid. Two strains showed resistance both to Isoniazid and p-Aminosalicylic acid.

For the second group of M. tuberculosis strains, that is, those isolated from treated patients, the resistances found are detailed in table 3.

Table 2 : Primary Resistance (Untreated Patients)

Antituberculosis Drugs	No.of Resistant strains	%
Isoniazid	4	3.6
Streptomycin	6	5.4
p-Aminosalicylic acid	2	2.2
Rifampicin	-	-
Ethambutol	-	-
Isoniazid + Streptomycin	2	2.2
Total resistance	10	9

Table 3 : Secondary Resistance (Treated Patients)

Antituberculosis Drugs	No.of Resistant strains	%
Isoniazid	78	42.3
Streptomycin	55	29.8
p-Aminosalicilic acid	42	22
Rifampicin	8	4.3
Ethambutol	15	8.4
Ethionamide	25	13.5
Capreomycin	11	5.9
Isoniazid + Streptomycin	40	21.7
Isoniazid + Ethionamide	10	4.8
Isoniazid + p-Aminosalicilic acid	14	5.4
Streptomycin + p-Aminosalicylic acid + Isoniazid	24	13

The drugs against which greater resistances were observed are the following : Isoniazid (42.3% of the strains), Streptomycin (29.8%) and p-Aminosalicylic acid (22%).

The resistances found in the group of atypical mycobacteria are detailed in table 4.

Table 4 : Resistance of Atypical Strains

Atypical Strains	Antituberculosis Drugs						
	INH	SM	PAS	ETH	RAMP	EMB	CM
M. kansasii (4)[a]	4[b]	2	4	0	0	1	1
M. intracellulare (1)	1	1	1	0	0	1	0
M. avium (3)	3	2	3	2	1	3	2
M. gordonae (2)	2	1	2	1	0	1	0
M. fortuitum (4)	4	4	4	4	4	4	4

a). No. of isolated strains.
b). No. of resistant strains.

All strains of atypical mycobacteria were resistant to Isoniazid and to p-Aminosalicylic acid.

The four strains of M. fortuitum were resistant to all the drugs.

DISCUSSION

Although our sample is not excessively large, we believe, on the basis of the results obtained, that in those cases in which the isolation of the strains, and consequently, the study of sensitivities cannot be made, it would be advisable, whenever the patient has not received antituberculosis drugs, to apply Rifampicin and/or Ethambutol, together with Isoniazid and/or Streptomycin, since the primary resistance to the former two drugs are rare, or at least lower than the rest of the antituberculosis drugs. In our case, we found no primary resistances to these drugs.

In those patients who have received previous treatment with unsuccessful results, it would be of most value to study the resistances of the strain, in order to guarantee an effective therapy.

REFERENCES

CANETTI, G.; RIST, N., and GROSSET, J. - (1963). - "Mesure de la sensibilité du bacille tuberculeux aux drogues antibacillaires par la méthode des proportions. Méthodologie, critères de résistance, résultats interprétation". - Rev. Tub. Pneumol. 27. 217.

TACQUET, A., and TISON, F. - (1961). "Nouvelle téchnique d'isolement des mycobactéries par le lauryl-sulfate de sodium". Ann. Inst. Pasteur 100, 676.

INTRAUTERINE ADMINISTRATION OF STREPTOMYCIN FOR GENITAL-TUBERCULOSIS

G. Franz, M. Kaether and R. Reimann

2000 Hamburg 76, Finkenau 35
Frauenklinik Finkenau Hamburg
Hamburgisches Seehospital, Cuxhaven, West Germany

In cases of endometrial tuberculosis (T.B.) it appears logical to influence the specific inflammatory and chronic process by the additional intrauterine application of drugs. This method of treatment has been given up for the following reasons:

1. Adverse side-effects appeared.
2. The effectiveness of this method was doubtful.
3. Systemic drug-therapy and adequate rehabilitation procedures could finally lead to complete cure of T.B.

Adverse side-effects appeared when drugs were applied as a substance: Foreign-bodies-granulomatosis developed and often caused bleeding-anomalies. Depending on the severity of the bleeding, in some cases abrasions were necessary, in others even extirpation of the uterus. Because of genital T.B., the latter procedure involved the removal of much parametrial tissue.

A histological section of the uterine wall shows foreign-body granulomatosis. Another histological section, photographed in half-polarised light, shows the foreign bodies deep in the uterine wall, which are easily detected because of the double refraction.

When applying drugs in liquid form into the uterine cavity, (in cases of T.B. for example a Streptomycine-solution), no effect could be obtained, because the cavum uteri is not a cavity in the strict sense, but rather to be compared with a capillary space communicating via the cervical canal with the vagina. When solutions are applied, they are discharged from the cavity into the vagina and there is not enough time to achieve an effect at the place of application. We have developed a new method allowing the application of Streptomycine to the endometrium in such a way, that topical influence will result. A loop, similar to those used as an intrauterine device for birth-control, was connected with a polyvinyl-catheter. The loop served for anchoring the catheter in proper position within the uterine cavity. Furthermore, when the application was finished, the catheter could be removed, when the loop was withdrawn. That part of the catheter to be placed into the cavity was pierced all over via the use of a thin canula. With the aid of a BRAUN-perfusion-pump it was possible to irrigate the endometrium slowly and continuously through hours. For 8-12 days 1.0 mg of Streptomycine was administered daily, the duration of irrigation was 2-7 hours. Systemic therapy with tuberculostatic agents (generally with a changing drug-regimen) was continued.

In a slide showing the uterus cut open, the loop-like anchor connected with the catheter can be seen. Another slide shows the distribution of a blue liquid applied via the catheter. In the uterus the liquid spreads quickly all over the cavity and passes quickly through the cervical canal. A roentgengram shows the loop-like anchor and the catheter in proper position. A contrast medium is applied. It is to be observed how the uterine cavity is continuously filled more and more. In the last picture the copious contrast medium has already left the cavity. X-ray shadows are seen in the vaginal vault. It is important to note that all these pictures are taken in extremely short intervals. Between the taking of the first picture and the last there are but a few seconds. Another slide shows a patient with the irrigation apparatus in place. The BRAUN-perfusion-pump is seen, by the aid of which the drug in aqueous solution is applied continuously for a prolonged period of time.

We used this method in 76 cases of genital T.B., that were treated partly at the womens hospital Finkenau and, to a larger extent, at the Hamburgean Seehospital, Nordheim Foundation, Cuxhaven.

59 cases had T.B. of the endometrium. The diagnosis was verified in 10 cases by histopathology and bacteriology, in 36 cases by histopathology and in 13 cases by bacteriology.

In 25 of these 59 cases with T.B. of the endometrium, concomitant T.B. of the adnexa could be diagnosed, in 4 cases concomitant peritoneal T.B. was present, 3 cases had both. 17 patients had T.B. of the adnexa without evidence of T.B. of the endometrium. After the application of Streptomycine all cases were controlled by repeated bacteriological examinations: All controls proved to be T.B. negative. In 21 cases histological control was indicated or possible 4-6 weeks after the end of treatment: All but one were negative for T.B. In this one case - she was one of the first patients so treated - one has to consider whether the loop was in the right position: In the first series we had to position the loop-like anchor with some difficulties using a Fehling-canula. Furthermore, the patient did not tolerate the tuberculostatic agents well, and apparently she had not taken the prescribed medication.

On the other hand, we are afraid, that she herself had removed the applicator.

In 24 of the 59 cases of endometrial T.B., correspondent findings could be obtained by palpation: These findings were normalised in 17 patients up to the time of control after 4 to 6 weeks, in 7 patients significant improvement was observed.

12 out of 17 cases of genital T.B. without evident endometrial T.B. showed corresponding findings by palpation: Normalisation was obtained during the period stated above in 9 cases, improvement was seen in 3 cases.

This method of treatment was found useful also in cases of pyometra of nontubercolous origin. We applied in this way antibiotica as well as fibrinolytic agents.

We would like to mention one case of endometrial carcinoma. Before surgery the patient had to undergo intensive pretreatment. In this case we applied 0.2 mg Trenimon for a period of 10 days daily into the uterine cavity. After the operation we could observe in histological sections an influence of the drug on the cancerous cells.

In conclusion it should be said that the method described offers new aspects for the treatment of tubercular, inflammatory and neoplastic processes by the intrauterine application of drugs. It appears possible to shorten the course of treatment, since also processes outside the uterine wall area, for example the adnexae, are influenced as well. It remains to be hoped that in some cases of genital T.B., fertility may be maintained or resotred.

GENETICS OF LOW-LEVEL ANTIBIOTIC RESISTANCE IN NEISSERIA GONORRHOEAE

P.F. SPARLING, F.A. SARUBBI, Jr., and E. BLACKMAN

University of North Carolina, Chapel Hill, N.C.

SUMMARY

The Genetics of resistance in the gonococcus was studied by mutation and transformation, in laboratory and clinical strains. Low-level penicillin resistance was the result of mutations at penA, ery and penB, which additively resulted in an approximate 100-fold increase in penicillin resistance, to an MIC of 1.0 μg/ml. Mutation at ery resulted in very-low level increases in resistance (two to eight fold) to diverse drugs, detergents and dyes, probably by decreasing cell envelope permeability, Mutations at loci designated envA and envB resulted in increased sensitivity to the same drugs, detergents and dyes, probably by increasing cell envelope permeability. All studied genes were chromosomal, and no evidence was found for drug-inactivating enzymes.

INTRODUCTION

Sensitivity of the gonococcus to penicillin and other antibiotics decreased gradually between 1950 and 1970 in many areas of the world (Sparling 1972). The "Resistance" which developed to most clinically useful drugs was only relative, and does not currently pose serious problems to therapy if adequate doseages are given. Nevertheless, it seemed relevant to understand the genetics and biochemistry of low-level resistance in the gonococcus, in order to help formulate rational guidelines for therapy, and for limiting selection of still more resistant strains.

The methods we have used have been presented in detail elsewhere (Sparling 1966, Maness and Sparling 1973, Sarubbi et al 1974). Most genetic studies were done by introducing transforming DNA from a donor strain (usually relatively antibiotic resistant) into a competent recipient (usually antibiotic sensitive) with selection for one donor resistance marker. Purified transformants were then scored for resistance to the selected drug and others. Two strains were studied intensively: FA48, a multiply-drug resistant mutant selected in several steps in vitro (Maness and Sparling 1973, Sarubbi et al 1974), and FA5, an equally resistant clinical isolate obtained initially from a patient in Los Angeles. Results were nearly identical with these two strains.

PENICILLIN RESISTANCE

Resistance to penicillin was shown to result from mutations at a minimum of three loci (Sparling et al 1975). Each locus resulted in small increases in penicillin resistance, of approximately 8-fold, 2-4 fold, and 4-fold, respectively for <u>pen</u>A, <u>ery</u>, and <u>pen</u>B. When the three loci were introduced sequentially in successive transformation steps into an initially sensitive recipient, the MIC for penicillin increased from 0.007 μg/ml to a final value of 1.0 μg/ml (Table I).

Table I

Additive Effects of Penicillin Resistance Loci in the Gonococcus

Strain		MIC Penicillin (μg/ml)
FA19	(a)	0.007
FA102	(<u>penA2</u>)	0.06
FA171	(<u>ery-2</u>)	0.015
FA136	(<u>penA2</u> <u>ery-2</u>)	0.25
FA212	(<u>ery-2</u> <u>penB2</u>)	0.06
FA140	(<u>penA2</u> <u>ery-2</u> <u>penB2</u>)	1.0

(a) FA19 was recipient for DNA from multiply resistant strain FA48 which has an MIC (penicillin) of 2.0 μg/ml.

The three loci affecting penicillins resistance were unlinked to each other, or to any of 9 studied auxotrophic markers. One of the penicillin loci was linked to the cluster of gonococcal ribosomal genes (Sarubbi et al 1974, Maness et al 1974) as evidenced by 10% to 20% co-transformation between <u>pen</u>B and a locus (<u>spc</u>) for high-level (ribosomal) resistance to spectinomycin.

In many attempts, we were unable to select <u>pen</u>B2 transformants unless the recipient strain already carried <u>ery</u>-2, which suggested that <u>ery</u>-2 was a type of modifier mutation, necessary for the phenotypic expression of <u>pen</u>B2 (Sparling et al, 1975).

Two of the penicillin loci also resulted in resistance to drugs besides the penicillins (Table 2). Transformants selected for ery became somewhat more resistant to a wide variety of antibiotics of different chemical structure and mode of action, and also to several dyes and detergents. Interestingly, ery did not result in significant increases in resistance to ampicillin or the new amidino penicillin FL1060. Introduction of ery also resulted in decreased uptake of crystal violet, decreased rates of autolysis, and decreased sensitivity to lysozyme (Guymon and Sparling 1975). It seems reasonable therefore, that ery causes resistance to penicillin and other drugs by reducing the permeability of the outer envelope. A similar gonococcal locus (designated mtr) for non-specific resistance has also been described by Maier et al (1975).

Loci Resulting in non-specific changes in Drug Resistance in the Gonococcus

Drug	Fold increase (decrease) due to mutation at		
	ery-2	penB2	envA(a)
Penicillin G	2-4	4	(8-16)
Ampicillin	-	2	(2)
Amidinopenicillin	-	2	-
Erythromycin	8-16	-	(64)
Tetracycline	1-2	2-4	(4)
Chloramphenicol	2	1-2	(4)
Rifampin	4	-	(16)
Fusidic Acid	8	-	(32)
Deoxycholate	2	-	(8)
Triton X-100	32	-	(256)
Acridine orange	4	-	(4)
Crystal violet	4	-	(8)

(a) Effects of envA1 were determined by introducing the envA1 locus by transformation into penA2 ery-2 penB2 strain FA140. When the env loci were introduced into penA2 ery^+ $penB^+$ strain FA102, smaller relative decreases in resistance to most drugs were noted.

The biochemistry of penicillin resistance is incompletely understood. No beta-lactamases or other penicillinases were found by micro iodometric methods or bioassays (Sparling et al 1975). Moreover, no evidence has been found for enzymatic inactivation of other drugs by extracts or whole cells of isolates resistant to the respective drugs, including streptomycin, spectinomycin, chloramphenicol, tetracycline, and erythromycin. The limitation of these latter studies is that only a few strains have been tested, and the only method used was a bioassay. (Maness et al 1974, Sparling et al

1975). No major alterations in lipopolysaccharides, phospholipids or fatty acids have been found yet in strains carrying ery-2 or penB2 (Guymon et al, unpublished) or in genetically uncharacterized penicillin-insensitive strains from Denmark (Wolf-Watz et al 1975).

Our demonstration that penicillin resistance in the gonococcus is due to additive effects of several genes is consistent with studies of sensitivities of large populations of clinical isolates, which have shown several discreet peaks separated in penicillin sensitivity by four-fold increments (Olsen, 1973). That some of these genes, most noteably ery also result in cross-resistance to other classes of drugs is consistent with (indeed, explains) the frequent observation that relatively penicillin-resistant isolates are often relatively resistant to many other drugs, including some not used in clinical medicine (Reyn and Bentzon 1969, Maness and Sparling 1973, Maier et al 1974).

LOSS OF RESISTANCE: ENV MUTATIONS

Multiply resistant clinical isolates may also lose resistance to many drugs in a single mutational step (Maness and Sparling 1973). These mutations result in complete phenotypic suppression of low-level resistance determined by ery and penB (Sarubbi et al 1975), probably by increasing permeability of the outer envelope (Guymon and Sparling 1975). By transformation crosses, two similar loci have been identified, designated envA and envB. The effects of envA1 on a resistant strain are shown in Table 2.

Since the env mutations result in greater than normal sensitivity ("hypersensitivity") to certain drugs, including erythromycin, rifampin, fusidic acid and most detergents, their prevalence in clinical isolates can be estimated. Initial study suggests that up to 10% of North Carolina isolates carry env mutations (Sarubbi et al 1975). These may account for failure of some strains to grow on selective media, because envA mutations result in an approximate 4-fold increase in sensitivity to vancomycin, to an MIC near the 3 µg/ml concentration employed in Thayer-Martin medium. The relatively frequent occurrence of env mutations in clinical isolates implies that env mutations result in selective advantage to the host cell, but there is little clue as to its nature. All studied env mutations result in increased sensitivity to antibiotics, detergents, and lysozyme; more rapid autolysis under conditions of divalent cation depletion; and often in relatively poor growth in vitro, perhaps due to increased sensitivity to the fatty acids present in most media.

CHROMOSOMAL LOCI

Most gonococci contain plasmids, which has raised the possibility that some resistance loci might be carried on plasmids similar to those found in many other species. However, several groups have found no differences in the plasmids present in antibiotic resistant and sensitive clinical isolates. In addition, comparison of transformation frequencies for each of the str, tet, chl, penA, penB, ery, and envA loci showed 10^4 more transforming activity with chromosomal DNA from resistant clinical strain FA5 than with carefully purified plasmid DNA from the same strain.

Although gonococci do not apparently contain R-factors, they do easily transfer drug resistance in mixed culture experiments in vitro (Sarubbi and Sparling 1974). This transfer is due to autolysis and liberation of transforming DNA into the culture medium. It is possible that drug resistance transfer between gonococci or other Neisseria occurs in nature although there is no evidence by which to judge the actual occurrence of such events.

Mutants with higher levels of penicillin resistance (MIC 6 ug/ml or more) are relatively easily selected in vitro. It is hoped that use of recommended treatment schedules, which provide high serum levels of penicillin may be less likely to select mutants to increased resistance than was the therapy employed in past decades.

REFERENCES

GUYMON, L. and P.F. SPARLING 1975. Altered crystal violet permeability and lytic behaviour in antibiotic-resistant and sensitive mutants of Neisseria gonorrhoeae. J. Bacteriol. (in press).

MAIER, T.W., H.R. BEILSTEIN, and L. ZUBRZYCKI 1974. Multiple antibiotic resistance in Neisseria gonorrhoeae. Antimicrob. Agents Chemother. 6: 22-28.

MAIER, T.W., L. ZUBRZCKI and M.B. COYLE 1975. Genetic analysis of drug resistance in Neisseria gonorrhoeae: identification and linkage relationships of loci controlling drug resistance. Antimicrob. Agents Chemother. 7: 676-681.

MANESS, M.J., G.C. FOSTER and P.F. SPARLING 1974. Ribosomal resistance to streptomycin and spectinomycin in Neisseria gonorrhoeae J. Bacteriol. 120: 1293-1299.

MANESS, M.J. and P.F. SPARLING 1973. Multiple antibiotic resistance due to a single mutation in Neisseria gonorrhoeae. J. Infect. Dis. 128: 321-330.

OLSEN, G.A. 1973. Consumption of antibiotics in Greenland, 1964-70 IV. Changes in sensitivity of Neisseria gonorrhoeae to antibiotics. Brit. J. Vener. Dis. 49: 33-40.

REYN, A., and M.W. BENTZON, 1969. Relationships between the snesitivities in vitro of Neisseria gonorrhoeae to spiramycin, penicillin, streptomycin, tetracycline and erythromycin. Brit. J. Vener. Dis. 45: 223-227.

SARUBBI, F.A.,Jr., E. BLACKMAN, and P.F. SPARLING 1974. Genetic mapping of linked antibiotic resistance loci in Neisseria gonorrhoeae. J. Bacteriol. 120: 1284-1292.

SARUBBI, F.A.,Jr., and P.F. SPARLING 1974. Transfer of antibiotic resistance in mixed cultures of Neisseria gonorrhoeae. J. Infect. Dis. 130: 660-663.

SARUBBI, F.A.,Jr., P.F. SPARLING and E. BLACKMAN 1975. Loss of low-level antibiotic resistance in Neisseria gonorrhoeae due to mutation at envA or envB. J. Bacteriol. (in press).

SPARLING, P.F. 1966. Genetic transformation of Neisseria gonorrhoeae to streptomycin resistance. J. Bacteriol. 92: 1364-1371.

SPARLING, P.F. 1972. Antibiotic resistance in Neisseria gonorrhoeae. Med. Clin. N.A. 56: 1133-1144.

SPARLING, P.F., F.A. SARUBBI,Jr., and E. BLACKMAN 1975. The inheritance of low-level resistance to penicillin, tetracycline, and chloramphenicol in Neisseria gonorrhoeae. J. Bacteriol. (in press).

WOLF-WATZ, H., T. ELMROS, S. NORMARK, and G.D. BLOOM 1975. Cell envelope of Neisseria gonorrhoeae: outer membrane and peptidoglycan composition of penicillin - sensitive and resistant strains. Infect. Immun. 11: 1332-1341.

A DOUBLE-BLIND PLACEBO-CONTROLLED TRIAL OF MINOCYCLINE IN THE TREATMENT OF NON-SPECIFIC URETHRITIS

M.J. PRENTICE, D. TAYLOR-ROBINSON and G.W. CSONKA

Clinical Research Centre, Harrow and Central Middlesex Hospital, Park Royal

The cause of non-specific urethritis (N.S.U.) is, by definition, unknown. The suspected agents include tetracycline-sensitive organisms such as chlamydiae, ureaplasmas (T mycoplasmas) and corynebacteria, which could be responsible either individually or synergistically.

The evidence that chlamydiae cause some cases is strong but Koch's postulates have not been fulfilled for any organism in man, nor has the relationship of chlamydiae to self-limited disease been established. The role of ureaplasmas is controversial due partly to a similar lack of information. To study the aetiology of N.S.U., the effect of tetracycline on the isolation of these organisms in relation to symptoms might not only clarify their role in the disease but also indicate whether an antibiotic resistant, isolate-negative group of cases exists. If this were so, these are the patients in whom to seek further aetiological factors, whether viral, bacterial, physical or immunological. In an attempt to elucidate these points, a double blind, placebo-controlled trial of minocycline in the treatment of N.S.U. was undertaken in conjunction with the isolation of chlamydiae and mycoplasmas.

MATERIALS AND METHODS

MINOCYCLINE. Minocycline is a long acting tetracycline. Therapeutic blood levels of approx. 2 µg/ml are maintained by 12 hourly oral administration which reduces the problem of inadequate therapy in these patients. A loading dose of 200 mg was followed by 100 mg 12 hourly for 6 days, a total dose of 1.3 gm.

PATIENTS. Gram-stained smears of urethral discharge from consecutive patients suffering from urethritis were examined. If gonococci or yeasts were not seen and more than 15 polymorphonuclear leucocytes were present in one microscopic field (magnification 800-1000x) the patient was admitted to the trial. Patients who had received any antibiotics in the previous week, passed urine within the last 4 hours, or who had been in recent contact with gonorrhoea or trichomonal infections were excluded.

EXPERIMENTAL DESIGN. Tablets of minocycline and lactose placebo were packed identically and administered so that neither the patient, the clinician nor the microbiologist knew the contents. The patients were instructed to abstain from taking alcohol and having sexual contact at least until the next visit a week later. Any patient who admitted to intercourse before that time was rejected from the trial. If a discharge persisted after treatment the patient was re-treated with a similar course of minocycline. The treatment code was not broken until all specimens had been tested.

COLLECTION OF SPECIMENS. At the first visit, urethral specimens were taken for culture of gonococci, chlamydiae and mycoplasmas. Patients were asked to re-attend 7 days later, when they were questioned about symptoms and examined for discharge. If this was present, a Gram-stained smear was used to confirm the persistence of urethritis and a wet-film was examined for trichomonads. In all patients, specimens were taken again for culture of chlamydiae and mycoplasmas at this time. If re-treatment was necessary, a third set of specimens was taken after completion.

ISOLATION OF MICROORGANISMS

a) Gonococci. A swab or bacteriological loop was used to inoculate urethral discharge onto chocolate agar, or more frequently, "GC selective agar medium" (Oxoid). The plates were transported to the laboratory in a candle jar, incubated in 2% CO_2 for 48 hours and examined for the presence of Gram-negative, oxidase-positive diplococci.

b) Mycoplasmas. A meatal swab was expressed into mycoplasma liquid medium which was stored at -70°. These specimens were later titrated in urea-containing medium for the detection of ureaplasmas and in arginine-containing media for M. hominis (1), the identity of which was confirmed by the use of specific antiserum in the disc growth-inhibition test.

c) Chlamydiae. A meatal specimen, taken with an abrasive plastic-tipped swab, was expressed into sucrose-phosphate transport medium which was plunged into liquid nitrogen. The McCoy cell culture method was used (2). In some cases the cell monolayers were treated with 30 µg/ml of 5-iodo-2'-deoxyuridine for 3 days instead of γ-irradiation.

RESULTS

CLINICAL RESPONSE TO TREATMENT. Of 179 patients seen initially, satisfactory paired specimens were obtained from 81 men suffering from N.S.U. Minocycline was given to 47 patients. A week later, 41 (87.2%) were symptom free but 6 (12.8%) still had a discharge. Placebo was given to 34 patients. A week later, 10 (30.3%) were symptom free and 24 (69.7%) had a persistent discharge.

MICROORGANISMS INITIALLY ISOLATED. Of 81 patients, chlamydiae were isolated from 26 (32%), ureaplasmas from 47 (58%) and *M. hominis* from 6 (7.4%). Both chlamydiae and ureaplasmas were isolated from 10 (12.5%), and none of these organisms were cultured from 18 patients.

RESPONSE OF INITIALLY CHLAMYDIA-POSITIVE PATIENTS TO TREATMENT

a) Clinical response. As shown in the Table (A), there is a significant correlation between the disappearance of symptoms and minocycline therapy, in contrast to placebo ($p < 0.002$). From 10 of the 26 chlamydiae-positive patients, ureaplasmas were also isolated, but, as shown in the Table (B), the correlation mentioned above still exists if the patients from whom only chlamydiae were isolated are considered ($p < 0.01$).

b) Microbiological response. From only 1 of 13 initially chlamydia-positive patients given minocycline were chlamydiae isolated after treatment, whereas the organisms were recovered from 9 of 13 placebo-treated patients. This correlation between the isolation of organisms and treatment is significant ($p < 0.005$), and the association is still seen if we consider patients from whom only chlamydiae were isolated ($p = 0.007$).

After treatment, the presence or absence of symptoms correlated with the persistence of or failure to isolate chlamydiae in 21 of 26 initially chlamydiae-positive patients ($p < 0.005$). Similarly, in the group of patients from whom only chlamydiae were isolated the association was still observed ($p < 0.02$).

RESPONSE OF INITIALLY UREAPLASMA-POSITIVE PATIENTS TO TREATMENT

a) Clinical response. As shown in the Table (C), there is a significant correlation between the disappearance of symptoms and minocycline therapy, in contrast to placebo ($p = 0.0002$). From 10 of the 47 ureaplasma-positive patients, chlamydiae were also isolated, but, as shown in the Table (D), the correlation mentioned above still exists if the patients from whom only ureaplasmas were isolated are considered ($p < 0.02$).

RESPONSE OF INITIALLY CHLAMYDIA AND UREAPLASMA CULTURE-POSITIVE PATIENTS TO TREATMENT

Treatment	No. of patients	Symptom free	Persistent discharge
A. TOTAL CHLAMYDIA POSITIVE			
Minocycline	13	11 (84.4%)	2 (15.6%)
Placebo	13	2 (15.6%)	11 (84.4%)
			(p <0.002)
B. ONLY CHLAMYDIA POSITIVE			
Minocycline	8	8 (100%)	0
Placebo	8	2 (25%)	6 (75%)
			(p <0.01)
C. TOTAL UREAPLASMA POSITIVE			
Minocycline	25	20 (80%)	5 (20%)
Placebo	22	5 (22.6%)	17 (77.4%)
			(p = 0.0002)
D. ONLY UREAPLASMA POSITIVE			
Minocycline	17	14 (82.5%)	3 (17.5%)
Placebo	13	5 (38.5%)	8 (61.5%)
			(p <0.02)

b) Microbiological response. Five of 25 initially ureaplasma-positive patients given minocycline yielded ureaplasmas after treatment, whereas the organisms were recovered from 18 of 22 placebo-treated patients. This correlation between the isolation of organisms and treatment is significant ($p < 0.001$), and the association is still seen if we consider patients from whom only ureaplasmas were isolated ($p < 0.02$).

After treatment, the presence or absence of symptoms correlated with the persistence of or failure to isolate ureaplasmas in 37 of 47 initially ureaplasma-positive patients ($p = 0.0002$). However, in the group of patients from whom only ureaplasmas were isolated this association was not statistically significant ($p = 0.1$), a result different from that observed for chlamydiae.

RESPONSE OF INITIALLY ISOLATE-NEGATIVE PATIENTS TO TREATMENT

Of 18 isolate-negative patients, 14 were given minocycline and 4 placebo. Only one patient in each group had symptoms a week later, and all but one were still isolate negative. The exception was the symptomatic placebo-treated patient from whom ureaplasmas were cultured. Unfortunately, the small size of the placebo group prevents statistical analysis of these results.

DISCUSSION

The association between minocycline treatment and the subsequent failure to isolate chlamydiae does not, of course, indicate that these organisms are pathogenic in the urethra. On the other hand, the correlation between the presence of symptoms after treatment and the isolation of chlamydiae in the absence of mycoplasmas, is strongly suggestive that chlamydiae are a cause of urethritis.

The initial chlamydial isolation rate of 32% in this study is lower than that obtained by some other workers. Our use of meatal, instead of endourethral, swabs to collect specimens may have been a less sensitive technique. If we assume that 50% of the patients did, in fact, harbour chlamydiae, we should have found 40/81 to be isolate positive, that is 14 more than we detected. Considering as a group all the patients from whom we failed to isolate chlamydiae, the disappearance of their symptoms is significantly related to minocycline treatment ($p < 0.001$). If 14 patients are removed from this "chlamydia negative" group, according to the distribution of results in the Table (B) (which shows the symptomatic response to treatment of patients from whom only chlamydiae were isolated), statistical analysis of the remainder still indicates that minocycline is clinically more effective than placebo ($p < 0.002$). This is evidence that minocycline-sensitive aetiological agent(s) other than chlamydiae exist. This calculation is based on the assumption that our chlamydial isolation procedure is inefficient. Although there are no reports of an isolation rate exceeding 50%, it is possible that a much greater incidence of infection exists and extension of this reasoning would result in the conclusion that all cases of minocycline-responsive N.S.U. are caused by chlamydiae. Of course, this cannot be proved at the moment and it is no reason to neglect other possible aetiological agents.

There is no statistical correlation between the presence of symptoms and the isolation of ureaplasmas, in the absence of chlamydiae, after treatment. Therefore, the evidence for these organisms being pathogens is certainly not as obvious as that for chlamydiae. Nevertheless, it has been shown that some ureaplasma strains are pathogenic in animals whereas others are not (3). If this situation existed in man, we would expect the organisms to disappear after minocycline treatment, but the clinical response to therapy to be unpredictable because of the unknown ratio of pathogenic to non-pathogenic strains. For the same reason, there would be no obvious association between the isolation of ureaplasmas and the presence of symptoms, especially after placebo treatment. Clearly, a search for markers of pathogenicity, initially in an animal model, is warranted.

It is noteworthy that a good symptomatic response occurs in minocycline treated, isolate-negative, patients. This implies that the aetiological agent or agents are antibiotic sensitive and may be either the organisms already considered or other bacteria. However, the disappearance of symptoms may have been spontaneous and unrelated to minocycline therapy. Unfortunately, the number of patients in our placebo-treated, isolate-negative group was insufficient to resolve this point.

Infection by many microorganisms, irrespective of their minocycline sensitivity, could theoretically result in a self-limited disease, and so be a cause of symptoms in the 30% of all patients who apparently responded clinically to the placebo. Therefore, the possibility that a virus or minocycline-resistant bacterium, either alone or by synergism, causes urethritis in a minority of patients cannot be excluded.

SUMMARY

The results of a double-blind therapeutic trial show minocycline to be more effective than a placebo in the treatment of N.S.U. There is evidence that chlamydiae are a cause of urethritis and indications that ureaplasmas may also be pathogenic. Although there is no supportive evidence, the existence of a minocycline-resistant aetiological agent cannot be excluded.

REFERENCES

1. Taylor-Robinson, D., Williams, M.H. and Haig, D.A. J. gen. Microbiol. 54, 33, 1968.

2. Darougar, S., Kinnison, J.R. and Jones, B.R. Trachoma and related disorders. Ed. R.L. Nichols. Excerpta Medica, Amsterdam and New York, p. 63, 1971.

3. Gourlay, R.N., Howard, C.J. and Brownlie, J. J. Hyg., Camb., 70, 511, 1972.

EPIDEMIOLOGY AND ETIOLOGY OF NONGONOCOCCAL URETHRITIS IN MEN

King K. Holmes, William O. Harrison, Richard Hooper, and E. Russell Alexander

From the University of Washington Schools of Medicine and Public Health, and the U.S. Public Health Service Hospital, Seattle; the Venereal Disease Control Division, Center for Disease Control, Atlanta; and the U.S. Navy E.P.M.U. No. 6, Honolulu.

This research was supported by Contract No. HSM 21-73-535 with the Center for Disease Control, Health Services and Mental Health Administration, Department of Health, Education, and Welfare; U.S.P.H.S. N.I.A.I.D. Training Grants AI-146 and AI-00191; and U.S.P.H.S. Research Grants EY-00219 from the National Eye Institute and AI-12192 and AI-06311 from the N.I.A.I.D.

Presented in part before the Twelfth Interscience Conference on Antimicrobial Agents and Chemotherapy, Atlantic City, New Jersey, September 28, 1972.

Correspondence to: Dr. Holmes, U.S. Public Health Service Hospital, 1131 Fourteenth Avenue South, Seattle, Washington 98114

The epidemiology of nongonococcal urethritis (NGU) refers to the study of NGU as it occurs in populations of men, while etiology encompasses study of microbial as well as nonmicrobial causation. The meager existing state of knowledge about NGU dictates that epidemiologic studies of NGU be linked closely with studies of causation. Current interest is stimulated by the increasing incidence of NGU apparent in many countries. This interest is further heightened by the wide range of opinions concerning NGU which are firmly held by practicing physicians. Opinions differ on such basic issues as whether the syndrome is or is not usually sexually acquired, whether it is infectious or noninfectious, and what microbial pathogens might cause it. These differences are due to the lack of controlled research employing concomitant epidemiologic and etiologic study methods until very recently. This paper presents a preliminary analysis of a cohort study of the epidemiology of NGU, conducted by the U.S. Public Health Service, the U.S. Navy, and the University of Washington; and a review of case-control studies of the etiology of NGU, conducted in London and Seattle.

COHORT STUDY

This study was conducted among the crew aboard an aircraft carrier. As the ship was en route from the West Coast of the United states to Southeast Asia, the men aboard the ship were asked to volunteer to undergo an initial interview, blood test, and urethral cultures for *N. gonorrhoeae* and *Chlamydia trachomatis*. 1,896 men agreed to participate. During the next seven months, the ship operated in Southeast Asia and made frequent port calls in the Philippines, Japan, Hong Kong, and Singapore. During the seven month period, the total incidence of urethritis exceeded one case per man per year.

Before and after the first three port calls, an attempt was made to determine whether NGU was sexually transmitted and if so, was NGU caused by an infectious agent? The latter question may seem unnecessary, since it has been proven that antibiotics such as tetracycline suppress NGU, at least temporarily. However, it has been argued that the suppressive effect of tetracycline may represent a nonspecific effect, rather than a specific antibacterial effect. We reasoned, therefore, that if *prophylactic* administration of tetracycline was effective in *preventing* NGU, this would provide convincing evidence that NGU was caused by an infectious agent.

NGU was uncommon prior to the first port call, but an outbreak of NGU cases occurred following each port call. In the cohort group, these outbreaks of NGU, like the outbreaks of gonorrhea, were almost entirely limited to men who had intercourse, and NGU was rarely found among men who later underwent routine screening examination and who denied having intercourse.

The results of the prophylaxis study showed that 200 mg of minocycline given following exposure prevented at least 85% of cases of NGU acquired during the first two port calls, and thus indicated that most NGU was caused by an infectious agent (Harrison WO. Presented at the 101st meeting of the American Public Health Association, New Orleans, October 20-23, 1974). I will now turn to a review of etiologic studies of NGU which have involved a case-control design, rather than a cohort design.

CASE-CONTROL STUDIES OF ETIOLOGY

It must be acknowledged at the onset that no rigorous case-control studies of the etiology of NGU have actually been reported. This would require matching of NGU cases and controls without urethritis with respect to age, race, sexual experience, and venereal disease history, at a minimum. However, recent studies involving comparison of NGU patients with other nonsymptomatic patients selected from the same clinic population (i.e., V.D. Clinic patients) have permitted some conclusions regarding the probable association of Chlamydia trachomatis with NGU. The most noteworthy studies of this type are those of Oriel, Reeve, and their co-workers,[1] and Richmond and her colleagues,[2] in London. Both studies showed that the prevalence of C. trachomatis in the urethra of men with NGU was nearly 40%, and this was significantly higher than among male V.D. Clinic patients with no urethritis. Dunlop, Jones, Darougar, and their associates have pioneered in studies of the relationship of C. trachomatis to NGU, and have also shown that about 45% of V.D. Clinic patients with NGU have urethral chlamydial infection.[3] Schachter, et al, have made similar observations in the United States.[4]

It might be helpful to very briefly review the current status of methods for isolation and classification of C. trachomatis. The development by Gordon and Quan[5] of the method for isolation of C. trachomatis by centrifuging the clinical specimen onto irradiated McCoy cell cultures greatly facilitated clinical and epidemiologic studies of genital chlamydial infection. Use of irradiated cells is no longer considered necessary, and we employ McCoy cells which have been treated with IUDR, as described by Wentworth and Alexander.[6]

The most reliable method of typing C. trachomatis is the immunofluorescent (IF) method developed by San-Pin Wang.[7,8] This IF technique is also the basis for an indirect IF method for quantitating serum antibody to chlamydia.[9] In most patients, it is possible to identify the immunotype-specificity of antibody, that is, to determine which immunotype stimulated the antibody to be formed.

A second agent which has been linked with NGU by some researchers is Ureaplasma urealyticum, or T-mycoplasma. Although evidence is contradictory, most researchers have found that the prevalence of T-mycoplasmas in the urethra of men with NGU is the same as that observed in male V.D. Clinic patients who have no urethritis - and is generally higher than 50% in both groups. The development of the differential agar medium by Shepard,[10] which permits ready recognition and differentiation of Mycoplasma hominis and T-mycoplasmas on primary isolation, has facilitated studies of these mycoplasmas in relation to NGU.

Table 1. Prevalence of urethral infection with Chlmaydia trachomatis, Mycoplasma hominis, Ureaplasma urealyticum (T-mycoplasma), Herpesvirus hominis, and cytomegalovirus in men with nongonococcal urethritis (NGU), gonorrhea (GC), or no urethritis (NU).

	NGU	GC	NU
C. trachomatis	48/113 (42%)	13/69 (19%)	4/58 (7%)
M. hominis	16/112 (14%)	8/49 (16%)	26/62 (42%)
U. urealyticum	70/112 (63%)	23/49 (47%)	36/62 (58%)
H. hominis	2/115 (2%)	3/53 (6%)	2/62 (3%)
Cytomegalovirus	0/60 ---	0/28 ---	0/20 ---

I would like to turn now to case-control studies conducted in Seattle, in which we have employed urethral cultures and serology to assess the role of C. trachomatis in NGU; and have also compared the prevalence of T-mycoplasma and other agents in men with chlamydia-positive and chlamydia-negative NGU. The results of all cultures from these patients are shown in Table 1.

A higher rate of recovery of chlamydia from patients with gonorrhea has been noted by Richmond, et al,[2] who suggested that chlamydia might exist as a latent urethral infection in large numbers of individuals, and then become detectable only when inflammation caused by some other primary pathogen or by trauma "stirs up" a latent chlamydial infection. This interpretation represents the principal argument against the inductive inference that because C. trachomatis is known to cause conjunctivitis in humans, and because NGU is associated with urethral chlamydia infection, chlamydia therefore causes NGU.

I should point out that chlamydia were found significantly more often among patients with NGU than among those with gonorrhea in our study; Dr. Reeve will subsequently discuss the significance of chlamydia infection in patients with gonorrhea, so I will not pursue this question any further.

However, there is additional evidence that the association of chlamydia with NGU is causal rather than secondary, at least in some patients. First, a fourfold or greater rise in immunofluorescent antibody titre to chlamydia was noted in 11 of 36 paired sera from NGU patients who had positive cultures and from only two of 50 pairs from NGU patients who had negative cultures for C. trachomatis ($p<0.005$).

The development of IF antibody to chlamydia, among patients who were initially seronegative, termed seroconversion, occurred in seven of 13 patients who had positive cultures for chlamydia and only one of 25 who had negative cultures. This suggests that chlamydia infection was acquired concomitantly with the occurrence of NGU in these patients. The immunoglobulin class of antibody detected in the IF test was determined in two of these seroconversion cases. In both patients, the initial antibody was predominantly IgM, while antibody detected later on was IgG, which is consistent with a primary immune response. Reeve and Philip and their colleagues[11,12] have reported that IgM IF antibody to chlamydia is more common among chlamydia-positive NGU cases than among chlamydia-negative cases.

It is of further interest that the prevalence of antibody to *C. trachomatis* among culture-negative patients in all three V.D. Clinic groups was related to previous history of NGU. Antibody was detected in 47% of those with no past history of NGU, 57% of those with one previous episode of NGU, and 91% of those with two or more previous episodes of NGU ($p<0.05$).[13] It has also been noted that antibody to chlamydia in patients with negative urethral cultures is related to previous sexual experience.[13] This suggests that previous chlamydial infection in this population of young adults in Seattle was sexually transmitted. We have obtained further evidence that the differentiation between chlamydia-positive and chlamydia-negative NGU is meaningful by comparing the response of these two forms of urethritis to antibiotic therapy. Since Dr. Oriel and Dr. Taylor-Robinson will be discussing the therapy of NGU, I will defer to them on this discussion.

Finally, if one concludes, as we do, that chlamydia are probably responsible for a certain proportion of urethritis cases, what causes the chlamydia-negative cases?

Some data suggests that a certain proportion of cases with chlamydia infection who present early in the course of their disease may be missed by culture. Chlamydia may become easier to detect by culture after symptoms have been present for longer than one week. In our study, chlamydia were recovered from 31% of NGU patients whose symptoms of urethritis had been present from one to seven days, and from 56% of patients who had symptoms of over one week's duration. Similarly, Richmond, et al,[2] recovered chlamydia from 61% of NGU patients who had had symptoms longer than seven days.

However, we do not believe that the majority of NGU patients with negative cultures for chlamydia actually have undetected chlamydia infection. There are at least two reasons for this. First, as mentioned previously, seroconversion occurred in seven of 13 patients who had positive cultures for chlamydia and only one of 25 who had negative cultures for chlamydia. Secondly, when the female sex partners of men with NGU were examined, chlamydia were recovered from the endocervix of the sex partner of 15 of 22 men who had chlamydia-positive NGU and only 2 of 24 NGU patients who were chlamydia-negative. Oriel, et al,[1] had very similar data. In our study, immunotypes recovered from two sex partners were identical in 85% of cases.[13] Again, if chlamydia-positive and chlamydia-negative NGU cases responded differently to therapy, this would provide further evidence that the chlamydia-negative cases were distinctive.

If most chlamydia-negative cases are not due to undetected chlamydia infection, what are they due to? We believe that *T. vaginalis*, *Herpesvirus hominis*, and cytomegalovirus have been excluded as major causes of chlamydia-negative NGU, although *T. vaginalis* and *H. hominis* undoubtedly do cause occasional cases. Further studies being conducted by Dr. William Bowie in Seattle, appear to show that *H. vaginalis*, anaerobic bacteria, and T-mycoplasma all are very common in the urethras of patients with NGU and in asymptomatic controls with no urethritis, but neither the *prevalence* nor the *quantity* of *H. vaginalis* or of *anaerobes* appears to be higher among men with chlamydia-negative NGU than among asymptomatic controls. Similarly, the *prevalence* of T-mycoplasma infection is *not* significantly higher among men with chlamydia-negative NGU than among those with chlamydia-positive NGU or among asymptomatic controls. However, we are not prepared to discount the possible role of T-mycoplasma in causing NGU. Shepard has previously suggested that the *quantity* of T-mycoplasma in the urethra may be higher in men with NGU than in asymptomatic men. At this meeting, Dr. Rangoonwala and his colleagues from Munich also reported quantitative differences in the number of T-mycoplasma recoverable from men with and without NGU. Neither Shepard nor the group from Munich apparently studied men who were matched for sexual experience or history of NGU. Nonetheless, these observations are of interest, and quantitative studies of *Ureaplasma urealyticum* infection among men with chlamydia-positive and chlamydia-negative NGU and men without NGU who have been matched for sexual experience and for previous V.D. history are required.

In conclusion, the past three years have been very interesting ones for research involving the epidemiology and etiology of NGU, and it seems likely that the same level of interest will persist for some time in the future.

REFERENCES

1. Oriel JD, Reeve P, Powis P, et al: Chlamydial infection. Isolation of Chlamydia from patients with non-specific genital infection. Brit J Vener Dis 48:429-436, 1972
2. Richmond SJ, Hilton AL, Clarke SKR: Chlamydial infection. Role of Chlamydiae subgroup A in non-gonococcal and post-gonococcal urethritis. Brit J Vener Dis 48:437-444, 1972
3. Dunlop EMC, Vaughan-Jackson JD, Darougar S, et al: Chlamydial infection. Incidence in "non-specific" urethritis. Brit J Vener Dis 48:425-428, 1972
4. Schacter J, Hanna L, Hill EC, et al: Are chlamydial infections the most prevalent venereal disease? JAMA 231:1252-1255, 1975
5. Gordon FB, Quan AL: Isolation of the trachoma agent in cell culture. Proc Soc Exp Biol 118:354-359, 1965
6. Wentworth BB, Alexander ER: Isolation of *Chlamydia trachomatis* by use of 5-IODO-2-Deoxyuridine-treated cells. Appl Microbiol 27:912-916, 1974
7. Wang SP, Kuo CC, Grayston JT: A simplified method for immunological typing of trachoma-inclusion conjunctivitis-lymphogranuloma venereum organisms. Infect Immun 7:356-360, 1973
8. Wang SP, Grayston JT, Gale JC: Three new immunologic types of trachoma-inclusion conjunctivitis organisms. J Immunol 110:873-879, 1973
9. Wang SP, Grayston JT: Human serology with TRIC-LGV (*Chlamydia trachomatis*) infection with microimmunofluorescence. J Infect Dis 130:388-397, 1974
10. Shepard MC, Lunceford CD: Differential agar medium for identification of "T" mycoplasmas in primary cultures. Bacteriol Proc 70:83, 1970
11. Reeve P, Gerloff Rk, Casper E, et al: Serologic studies on the role of chlamydia in the aetiology of nonspecific urethritis. Brit J Vener Dis 50:136-139, 1974
12. Philip RN, Casper EA, Gordon FB, et al: Fluorescent antibody responses to chlamydial infection in patients with lymphogranuloma venereum and urethritis. J Immunol 112:2126-2134, 1974
13. Holmes KK, Handsfield HH, Wang SP, et al: Etiology of nongonococcal urethritis. N Engl J Med 292:1199-1205, 1975
14. Hofstetter A, Blank H, Rangoonwala R: Tetracyclines for treatment of mycoplasma-prostate-urethritis. Presented at the 9th International Congress of Chemotherapy, London, July 13, 1975

SURFACE STRUCTURES AND ANTIBIOTIC TARGETS IN THE GONOCOCCUS

M. R. J. Salton, K. S. Kim, R. Davis and K. Y. Cho

New York University School of Medicine

550 First Avenue, New York, NY 10016 U. S. A.

Summary: All four colony types of N. gonorrhoeae possess pit-like structures in the outer membrane of their envelopes. A stable, piliated strain GC1 of intermediate colony morphology also possesses this structural feature. Isolated envelopes of gonococcal strain GC1 and T1 have an active D-alanine carboxypeptidase. This membrane-bound enzyme in GC1 has an alkaline pH optimum, a K_m of 0.25 mM and is sensitive to inhibition by penicillin G, ampicillin, cloxacillin and methicillin. An active phospholipase A is present in GC1, T1 and T4 envelopes, the activity is stimulated by methanol (30%) and the enzyme converts phosphatidylethanolamine to lysophosphatidylethanolamine. It is suggested that such an enzyme could modulate barrier properties of the outer membrane.

Surface wall or envelope structures of Neisseria gonorrhoeae were first isolated by Salton (1951) using the techniques applicable to other Gram-negative species. The structural and biochemical properties of this organism had been largely neglected until comparatively recently but with the increased incidence of gonorrhea in recent years a fuller understanding of all aspects of this pathogen has become imperative. Investigations in our laboratory have been primarily directed towards the characterization of the surface properties of the envelopes of the gonococcus and the identification of key, cell-surface membrane enzyme markers and penicillin-sensitive enzyme target(s). The organisms we have used in our studies include Kellogg's types (Kellogg et al.,

1963, 1968) T1, T2, T3 and T4 selected from a T1 clinical isolate kindly provided by Dr. Yvonne C. Faur of the Public Health Laboratory Services, City of New York, Department of Health, together with a stable, piliated strain (our strain GC1) which has a colonial morphology intermediate between that of types T1 and T4. All cultures have been checked for colony morphology on N. Y. C. Medium described by Faur et al. (1973), the presence of the outer membrane (OM) pit-like structures reported by Swanson et al. (1971) have been observed by electron microscopy in all strains and pili detected in types T1, T2 and our strain GC1 but not in T3 and T4 as reported by other investigators (Swanson et al., 1971; Jephcott et al., 1971). Moreover, the presence of plasmids in the gonococcus first indicated by Maness and Sparling (1972) and Engelkirk and Schoenhard (1973) has been confirmed in our strains by direct isolation and measurement of the plasmid contour lengths by electron microscopy (Palchaudhuri et al., 1975). Some of the properties of the isolates used, together with their sensitivity to penicillin are summarized in Table 1.

Although the presence of pili is restricted to the type T1, T2 cultures and our GC1 strain, the pitted structures are found in all strains of the gonococcus we have examined. The characteristic appearance of these structures seen in negatively stained preparations examined in the electron microscope is illustrated in Figs. 1 and 2. These structures are rather unique in Gram-negative envelopes and apart from the meningococcus are not generally seen in other *Neisseria* species nor in other Gram-negative species (Kim and Salton, unpublished observations). The origins and functions of these "pits" are unknown at the present time. They do not appear to be correlated with the presence or absence of pili. These pit-like structures are reminiscent of the "holes" observed in the envelopes of Gram-negative organisms treated with antiboty and complement (Bladen et al., 1966). One possible mechanism for the formation of these structures which we are investigating involves the role of outer membrane phospholipase A activity. Evidence for the activity of such an enzyme during the normal growth of the gonococcus was reported by Walstad et al. (1974) when they reported the inhibitory effects of the products (fatty acid and lysophosphatidylethanolamine). Some of the features of envelope phospholipase A of the gonococcus will be presented in this paper. This enzyme now appears to be one of the major outer membrane markers of the Gram-negative envelope (Scandella and Kornberg, 1971; Bell et al., 1971; White et al., 1971).

Table 1. Properties of Some Neisseria gonorrhoeae Strains Used for Studies of D-alanine Carboxypeptidase and Phospholipase A.

Strain and colony type			MIC penicillin G μg/ml
T1	Piliated	Pitted OM	0.6
T2	Piliated	"	0.6
T3	Non-piliated	"	0.6
T4	Non-piliated	"	0.6
GC1*	Piliated	"	0.3

* Intermediate colonial appearance.

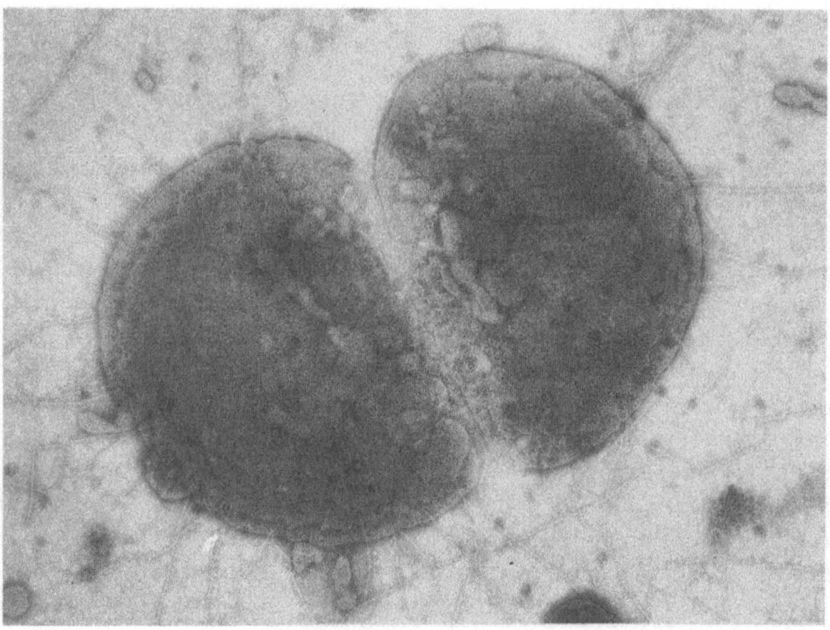

Figure 1. Negatively stained crude envelope fraction of N. gonorrhoeae strain GC1 showing pili and outer membrane pits.

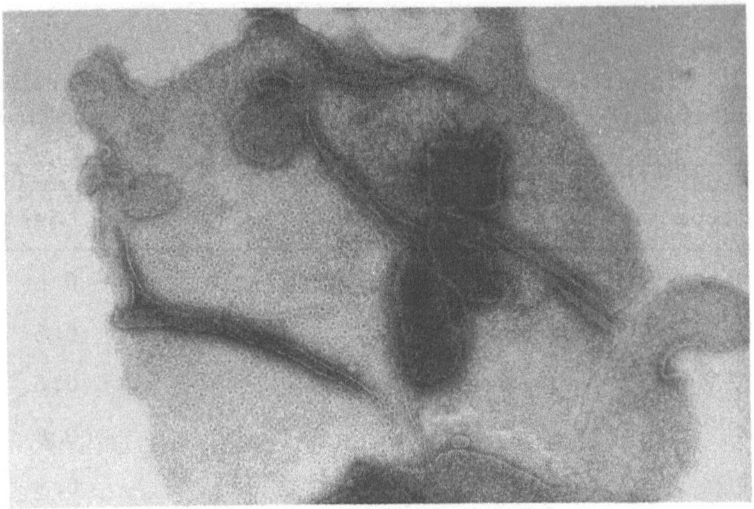

Figure 2. Negatively stained envelope fragment of N. gonorrhoeae strain GC1 showing pitted structures.

Penicillin Target in the Gonococcus

The development of low-level and multiple antibiotic resistance in N. gonorrhoeae (Maness and Sparling, 1973; Maier et al., 1974) has focused much interest in attempts to elucidate the mechanisms involved. Because of the development of multiple drug resistance it has been suggested that envelope permeability is involved (Maness and Sparling, 1973). Although recent work by Wolf-Watz et al. (1975) failed to detect any significant differences in envelope components between a sensitive and resistant (non-isogenic) strain of N. gonorrhoeae, it is evident that more sensitive means of determining altered envelope barrier properties are needed before this mechanism can be ruled out. Our investigations have therefore focused on the penicillin-sensitive enzyme targets as potential probes in assessing their accessibility in sensitive and low-level resistant strains of N. gonorrhoeae. To this end we have detected the presence of an active D-alanine carboxypeptidase in gonococcal envelopes isolated from our strain GC1 and also from the T1 isolate. Most of the work on the properties of the membrane-bound D-alanine carboxypeptidase has been performed with the GC1 strain.

The substrate used throughout our investigations is UDP-N-acetylmuramyl-L-alanyl-D-iso-glutamyl-meso-diaminopimelyl-D-alanyl-D-alanine isolated from Bacillus cereus T as described by Lugtenberg et al. (1971) and purified according to the method of Anderson et al. (1966). Envelope preparations catalyze a steady release of the terminal D-alanine from the substrate. When tested in buffers over the range pH 5-10, the D-alanine carboxypeptidase activity exhibited a broad optimum in Tris and veronal buffers in the alkaline range pH 8-9.8. In Tris-HCl buffer (pH 8.56) maximal activity was observed with molarities of 0.2-0.4 M. The activity was relatively insensitive to ionic strength adjusted by the addition of NaCl to veronal buffer (pH 8.95) over a wide range of 50-300 mM NaCl. The presence of 20-40 mM Mg^{2+} increased the level of activity to 135% that of the control level (i.e. no added Mg^{2+}). The Michaelis constant K_m of the gonococcal D-alanine carboxypeptidase determined by the Lineweaver-Burk plot was 0.25 mM, a value very similar to that reported for Bacillus subtilis (0.26-0.33 mM) by Umbreit and Strominger (1973). Some of the properties of the GC1 gonococcal D-alanine carboxypeptidase are summarized in Table 2.

The sensitivity of the envelope D-alanine carboxypeptidase to several penicillins was determined and the 50% inhibitory levels are presented in Table 3. The correlation between the MIC for the GC1 strain and the inhibition levels for the enzyme is quite good. Thus the MIC for penicillin G (0.52 unit/ml) agrees well with the level of antibiotic needed for maximal inhibition of activity (85% inhibition with 10^{-6} M penicillin G, equivalent to 0.527 unit/ml). So far we have been unable to demonstrate any transpeptidase activity in these preparations using UDP-muramyl pentapeptide as donor and glycine as acceptor. Purification of the D-alanine carboxypeptidase and/or transpeptidase from the gonococcal membranes would provide essential penicillin-sensitive enzymes as probes for investigating their accessibility and/or different characteristics in sensitive and partially resistant strains of N. gonorrhoeae. Studies on the release and purification of the D-alanine carboxypeptidase are being pursued in our laboratory.

Envelope Phospholipase A

In view of the remarkable similarity of the pit-like structures of the gonococcal envelope to those generated in Gram-negative bacteria by the antibody-complement bactericidal system we

Table 2. Properties of the Envelope D-alanine Carboxypeptidase of *N. gonorrhoeae* Strain GC1

pH optimum	8.0-9.8
Tris molarity optimum	0.2-0.4 M
Mg^{2+} optimum	20-60 mM
Michaelis constant K_m	0.25 mM

Table 3. 50% Inhibition Levels of D-alanine carboxypeptidase by Penicillins

Antibiotic	50% Inhibition
Penicillin G	10^{-8} M
Ampicillin	10^{-8} M
Cloxacillin	10^{-5} M
Methicillin	5×10^{-7} M

have wondered whether these pits may result from unregulated phospholipase activity, producing localized 'lesions' in the outer membrane. To gain further insight into the possible role of phospholipase A in modulating the barrier properties of the gonococcal envelope we began a study of the properties of this enzyme in *N. gonorrhoeae*. Phospholipase A activity in isolated envelopes has been assayed by using ^{32}P-labelled phosphatidylethanolamine (^{32}PE) and as shown in fig. 3, the envelopes will catalyze the conversion of ^{32}PE isolated from either *N. gonorrhoeae* or from *E. coli* K12. The course of conversion PE to lysophosphatidylethanolamine (LPE) can be followed simply by chromatography and autoradiography to separate ^{32}PE from L^{32}PE and by counting the radioactivity in substrate and product as shown in fig. 4. Phospholipase A activity appears to be greater in the envelope preparations from the gonococcus than corresponding envelope fractions from *E. coli* K12 as illustrated in fig. 5 (1, ^{32}PE, no envelopes; 2 and 3, *E. coli* envelopes; 4, 5 type T1 gonococcal envelopes; 6, type T4 envelopes; reaction mixtures 2, 4 and 6 were assayed in the presence of 0.03% SDS in 0.05 M Tris pH 7.6 and mixtures 3 and 5 were supplemented with methanol at 30% v/v final concentration). There was a progressive increase in activity when envelopes of T1 were assayed in 0.05 M Tris buffers containing 30% v/v methanol, 2 mM Ca^{2+} over the pH range 7.0 to 9.0. Work on the release and characterization of this outer membrane enzyme marker is in progress to determine its potential role in the function of this surface barrier of the gonococcal cell.

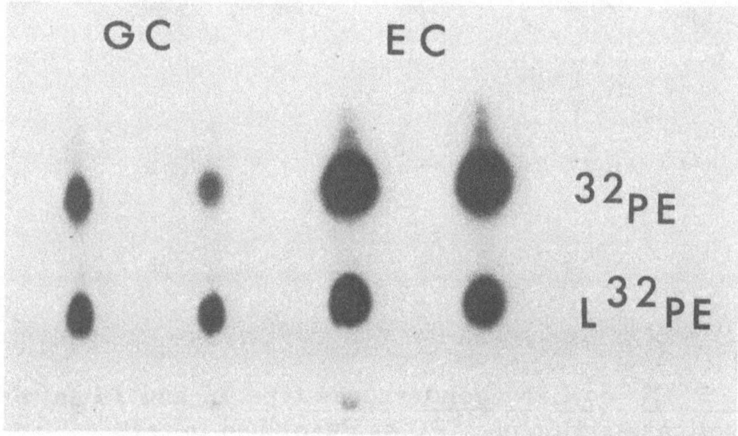

Figure 3. Autoradiogram of gonococcal envelope phospholipase action on N. gonorrhoeae ^{32}PE (GC) and E. coli ^{32}PE (EC).

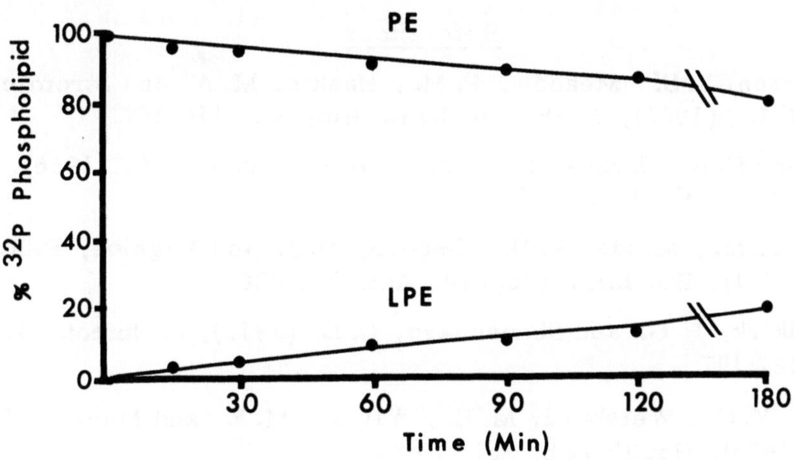

Figure 4. Course of gonococcal envelope phospholipase A action on ^{32}PE.

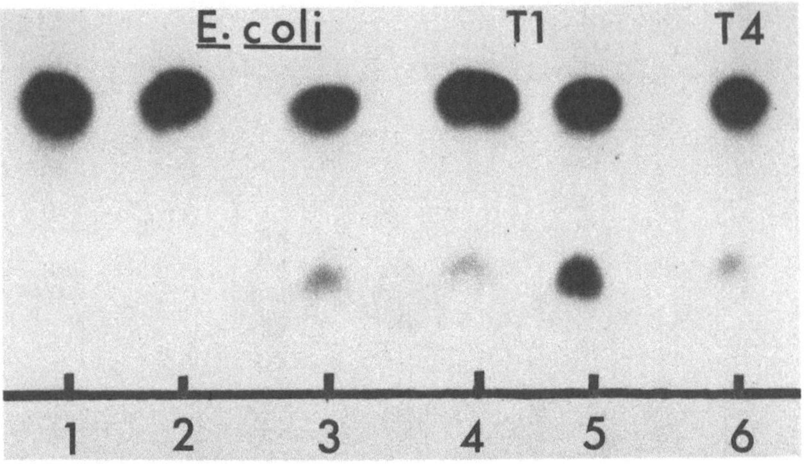

Figure 5. E. coli, N. gonorrhoeae type T1 and T4 envelope phospholipase action on ^{32}PE as described in text.

Investigations were supported by a grant (U 2235) from the Health Research Council of the City of New York.

References

Anderson, J. S., Meadow, P. M., Haskin, M. A. and Strominger, J. L. (1966), Arch. Biochem. Biophys. 116:487.

Bladen, H. A., Evans, R. T. and Mergenhagen, S. E. (1966), J. Bacteriol. 91:2377.

Bell, R. M., Mavis, R. D., Osborn, M. J. and Vagelos, P. R. (1971), Biochim. Biophys. Acta 249:628.

Engelkirk, P. G. and Schoenhard, D. E. (1973), J. Infect. Dis. 127:197.

Faur, Y. C., Weisburd, M. H., Wilson, M. E. and May, P. S. (1973), Health Lab. Sci. 10:44.

Jephcott, A. E., Reyn, A. and Birch-Andersen, A. (1971), Acta Pathol. Microbiol. Scand. Sect. B. 79:437.

Kellogg, D. S., Jr., Peacock, W. L., Jr., Deacon, W. E., Brown, L. and Pirkle, C. I. (1963), J. Bacteriol. 85:1274.

Kellogg, D. S., Jr., Cohen, I. R., Norins, L. C., Schroeter, A. L. and Reising, G. (1968) J. Bacteriol. 96:596.

Lugtenberg, E. J. J., van Schijndel-van Dam, A. and van Bellegem, T. H. M. (1971), J. Bacteriol. 108:20.

Maier, T. W., Beilstein, H. R. and Zubrycki, L. (1974), Antimicrob. Agents Chemother. 6:22.

Maness, M. J. and Sparling, P. F. (1972), Clin. Res. 20:52.

Maness, M. J. and Sparling, P. F. (1973), J. Infect. Dis. 128:321.

Salton, M. R. J. (1951), Some properties of the bacterial cell envelope, Ph. D. Dissertation, University of Cambridge.

Scandella, C. J. and Kornberg, A. (1971), Biochemistry 10:4447.

Swanson, J., Kraus, S. J. and Gotschlich, E. C. (1971), J. Exp. Med. 134:886.

Umbreit, J. N. and Strominger, J. L. (1973), J. Biol. Chem. 248:6759.

Walstad, D. L., Reitz, R. C. and Sparling, P. F. (1974), Infect. Immun. 10:481.

White, D. A., Albright, F. R., Lennarz, W. J. and Schnaitman, C. A. (1971) Biochim. Biophys. Acta 249:636.

Wolf-Watz, H., Elmros, T., Normark, S. and Bloom, G. D. (1975), Inf. Immun. 11:1332.

EVALUATION OF THE AMES NEISSERIA GONORRHOEAE CULTURE SYSTEM

G.W. Csonka and S.H. Qureshi

Central Middlesex Hospital, London N.W.10. U.K.

A Neisseria gonorrhoeae detection system has been developed by the Ames Co. aiming at a simple culture method for the isolation of gonococci from bacterially contaminated sites such as the rectum. Our aim in this study was to compare the Ames culture system with the routine Thayer-Martin cultures in men with presumed gonorrhoea.

METHODS

The Ames culture system consits of a slide cassette with two culture areas not based on agar which contains antibiotics and antifungal agents and is sealed in a dehydrated form in a foil pouch. To activate it, the cassette is removed from the pouch, hydrated and both culture areas are inoculated with material from the same site. The cassette is then closed, returned to the pouch with a CO_2-releasing tablet and incubated at 37° for 24-48 hours. It is important to place the preparation lid down to prevent drying out in the incubator. The whole procedure takes on average 3-4 minutes.

After 24 hours incubation, the cytochrome oxidase test is performed by placing a test strip impregnated with tetramethyl-paraphenylenediamine on to one culture area. If positive, blue/purple spots develop indicating the colonies. If negative, incubation is continued for a further 24 hours and then the second culture area is tested for oxidase reaction. Smears from the blue areas can also be taken for Gram staining. As the oxidase reagent is toxic to N.gonorrhoeae, subcultures from areas affected by the oxidase reaction are not possible.

Specimens were taken in parallel from each of 95 men with presumed gonorrhoea and 25 men with non-gonococcal urethritis for culture on Thayer-Martin plates and the Ames system.

RESULTS

The results in men with presumed gonorrhoea are given in Table I, indicating that the Ames system is reliable in the diagnosis of gonorrhoea in this group of patients giving a satisfactory 95.7% positive results after 48 hours incubation. It is noteworthy that the bulk of positive reactions could already be read after 24 hours incubation, which constitutes a considerable saving of time over conventional cultures. Comparison of the two culture systems used is shown in Table II. Thus the Ames culture system had the edge over the Thayer-Martin cultures. When the positive results of both are combined, only one patient (1.1%) would have escaped correct diagnosis by cultures. 89 specimens came from the urethra and 6 from the rectum in rectal gonorrhoea; these 6 were positive by both types of culture. Four cases of urethral gonorrhoea were asymptomatic carriers with their sexual contacts having proven gonorrhoea and urethral scraping showing Gram negative intracellular diplococci, of these four, the Ames cultures were positive in all and the Thayer-Martin plates in two.

The group with non-gonococcal urethritis were negative by both culture systems.

It was noted, however, that occasionally a slight uniform blueing would develop after application of the cytochrome strip which was non-specific and could be produced on inoculated and non-inoculated culture areas and at first caused some confusion.

TABLE I

COMPARISON OF AMES CULTURE SYSTEM WITH THAYER-MARTIN ROUTINE CULTURE IN MALE GONORRHOEA

Total No. of patients	Positive: Ames System 24 h	Positive: Ames System 48 h	Positive: Thayer-Martin
95*	87 (91.5%)	91 (95.7%)	84 (88.4%)

* 6 rectal gonorrhoea, the rest urethral gonorrhoea.

TABLE II

A = AMES CULTURE SYSTEM

TM = THAYER-MARTIN PLATES

	A +	TM +	A +	TM -	A -	TM +	A -	TM -
NUMBERS	81		10		3		1	

DISCUSSION

The Ames culture system is not expected to be reliable for oropharyngeal cultures as it cannot differentiate gonococci from meningococci. It would clearly be an advantage if the system were modified so as to allow easy subculturing for fermentation and sensitivity tests.

We found the Ames culture system to be simple, quick and easily taught to bacteriologically untrained nurses. Its specificity is as good as the combination of selection of sites, presence of Gram negative diplococci and a positive oxidase test. The certain proof of specificity by fermentation and/or immunofluorescence tests is not yet possible using this system.

The next step will be to explore its value in women where the need for a rapid, simple and reliable culture for the detection of gonorrhoea is especially pressing. The results in the small number of rectal gonorrhoea suggests that the system is suitable for heavily contaminated sites. Its use as a transport medium will also be investigated.

In conclusion, it is believed that if these results are confirmed and found to be successful in women, the culture system should prove valuable in clinics throughout the world which have no access to competent laboratories and in communities where the general practitioner commonly manages these infections. It might also be of use in laboratories as a fairly rapid and simple screening procedure for gonococci.

TREATMENT OF GONORRHOEA WITH "GONOCOCKTAIL", A SINGLE DOSE OF AMPICILLIN PLUS PROBENICID

A. Lassus, O-V Renkonen, R. Suhonen

Department of Dermato-Genereology

University of Helsinki, Finland

Ampicillin in one or two doses or in combination with probenicid is an established effective mode of treatment of acute, uncomplicated anogenital gonorrhoea (Eriksson, 1971; Bro-Jørgensen and Jensen, 1971). The present study is an evaluation of a new type of administration, the so-called genococktail, which is a mixture of 3.5g of ampicillin and 1g probenicid, as a treatment of acute, uncomplicated gonorrhoea in males and females.

MATERIAL AND METHODS

257 patients, 184 males and 73 females, with acute anogenital gonorrhoea were treated. The diagnosis was in all cases based on microscopical examination of methylene-blue stained smears from urethra and cervix and culture of gonococci from the urethra and in female cases also from the rectal mucosa. The culture was carried out on a Thayer-Martin medium containing trimethoprim. Gonococcal isolates were identified by colonial morphology, oxidase reaction, and sugar fermentation tests. The isolates were tested for their sensitivity to ampicillin using the plate dilution method described by Reyn et al (1958).

After a microscopical diagnosis of gonorrhoea the patients were served a drink containing 3.5g ampicillin and 1g probenicid and asked to return for re-examination one week later. The same examinations as before treatment were carried out during the re-examination.

RESULTS

One of the patients returned on the day after treatment presenting a rash, which obviously was due to ampicillin. He had no earlier experience of allergic reactions to penicillins. Two patients complained that they had suffered from nausea on the day of drug administration.

An evaluation of the sensitivity of the isolated gonococcal strains to ampicillin showed that about 67% of the strains were inhibited by 0.05 mcg/ml of ampicillin, but six strains (2.3%) were resistant to 0.5 mcg/ml.

196 patients (132 males and 64 females) returned for re-examination. This means that 76% of the treated patients were re-examined. Three male patients were found to have a positive gonococcal culture when re-examined. The mean inhibitory concentration (MIC) value to ampicillin was 0.05 mcg/ml in two cases and 0.1 mcg/ml in one case. Two of these three patients denied the possibility of a re-infection. Four of the six patients with highly resistant strains, i.e. with a MIC value of 1.0 mcg/ml or more, were re-examined and they were all cured.

COMMENTS

The gonococktail seems to be well tolerated since there was a minimum of gastric reactions after treatment. The treatment is definitely effective as only three of the 196 re-examined patients had a positive culture for gonococci one week after treatment. If these three male patients actually had re-infections or true treatment failures is difficult to define. One of them admitted the possibility of re-infection.

Gonococktail seemed to be more effective in female cases, which is in agreement with the findings of Putkonen et al (1968), that a highly efficient treatment regimen seems to produce more treatment failures in males, because of their higher promiscuity and higher rate of re-infections. If a less effective treatment is used, this difference is less evident because of true treatment failures in both groups.

SUMMARY

184 males and 73 females with acute, uncomplicated anogenital gonorrhoea, were treated with gonococktail, a mixture of 3.5g ampicillin and 1.0g probenicid. 67% of the gonococcal strains isolated had a MIC value $\leqq$ 0?05 mcg/ml of ampicillin, while six strains (2.3%) had a MIC value $\geqq$ 1.0 mcg/ml. 196 patients were re-examined one week after the treatment and three of them had a positive culture when re-examined, which did not agree with the low MIC values of the strains in these cases.

TREATMENT OF UNCOMPLICATED GONORRHOEA WITH A SINGLE DOSE OF AMOXYCILLIN

A. Lassus, O-V. Renkonen, T. Rostila
Department of Dermato-Venereology and Department of Serology and Bacteriology
University of Helsinki
Snellmanink. 14, Helsinki 17, Finland

Amoxycillin is a semi-synthetic penicillin with a broad spectrum of activity similar to that of ampicillin. Amoxycillin given orally is better absorbed than ampicillin and gives serum levels approximately twice as high as those obtained with the same dose of ampicillin (Rolinson). As ampicillin, alone in one or two doses or combined with probenicid, has proved highly effective in the treatment of uncomplicated gonorrhoea in males and females (Eriksson) it is quite natural that also amoxycillin has been evaluated for the treatment of gonorrhoea. Several studies (Alergant 1973, Braff 1974, Deal et al. 1974, Gurwith et al. 1974, Karney et al 1974, Roberts 1974, Willcox 1974 and Wolk 1974) have shown that a dose of 3 g of amoxycillin alone, or a smaller dose combined with probenicid, is very effective in the treatment of uncomplicated gonorrhoea.

In the present study a single dose of amoxycillin was used to treat uncomplicated gonorrhoea in both male and female patients and the results were compared with the sensitivity of the isolated strains to amoxycillin.

Material

Ninety-four males and fifty-nine females with acute uncomplicated gonorrhoea were treated with 3 g amoxycillin as a single oral dose. Thirteen of the females had also rectal gonorrhoea. Patients suspected to have pharyngeal gonorrhoea were not included in the series.

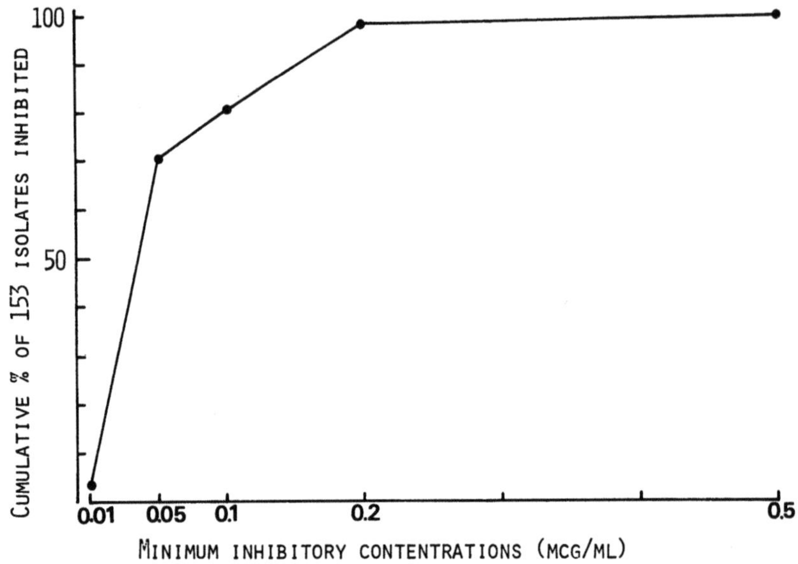

Fig.1. Cumulative Percentage of 153 Isolates of N.Gonorrhoeae Inhibited by Increasing Concentrations of Amoxicillin.

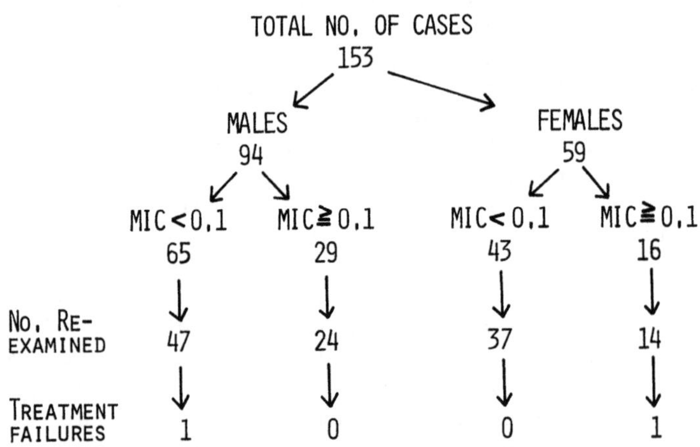

Fig.2. Results of the Treatment of 153 Patients with Anogenital Gonococcal Infection with Amoxicillin as a Single Dose.

Methods

Neisseria gonorrhoea was in all cases identified by microscopical examination of a methylene-blue stained smear from the urethra and cervix. Cultures were carried out in all cases, in males from the urethra and in females from the urethra, cervix and rectum. The species were cultured on a Thayer-Martin medium and identified by oxidase and fermentation procedures. All isolated strains were tested for their sensitivity to amoxycillin using the plate dilution method described by Reyn et al. (1958).

After the microscopical diagnosis of gonorrhoea the patients swallowed eight capsules of 375 mg amoxycillin each in the presence of a nurse. They were asked to return after seven days when a new microscopical examination and culture were performed.

Results

As illustrated in Figure 1, about 70 per cent of the gonococcal strains were inhibited by 0.05 mcg/ml of amoxycillin while 1.3 per cent required 0.5mcg/ml.

Seventy-one of the 94 males and 51 of the 59 females returned for re-examination one week after the treatment (Figure 2). One man and one woman were still found to have gonococci. The sensitivities of the gonococcal strains to amoxycillin were 0.05 an 0.1 mcg/ml respectively. Both patients admitted a possible re-infection.

None of the re-examined patients had vomitted or had any gastric problems after the administration of the drug, and no allergic reactions were seen.

Comment

The sensitivity pattern of the present gonococcal strains to amoxycillin compares with that of gonococci to penicillin in Finland, since about 30 per cent of the strains require at least 0.2 U/ml for inhibition (Lassus et al.). The present treatment results seem to be somewhat better than those obtained with the standard treatment of 2.4 mega units ofporcaine penicillin plus 1 g of probenicid, which on an average gives a treatment failure of about 5 per cent. About one-fifth of the patients of the present series failed to return for re-examination. Only two of those who returned still had an infection, which in both cases probably was a re-infection. However, one is always concerned about the patients not re-examined, who constitute a possible pitfall in most studies on the treatment of gonorrhoea.

In conclusion amoxycillin in a single dose of 3 g seems to be a highly efficient and well tolerated mode of treatment for acute, uncomplicated gonorrhoea both in males and females.

Summary

Hundred and fifty-three patients, 94 males and 59 females, with acute, uncomplicated gonorrhoea were treated with a single oral dose of amoxycillin. About 70 per cent of the isolated gonococcal strains were sensitive to 0.05 mcg/ml of amoxycillin. Two of the 122 re-examined patients still harboured gonococci when re-examined one week after treatment and both admitted a possible re-infection. It was concluded that 3 g amoxycillin as a single oral dose seems to be a highly efficient and well tolerated mode of treatment for acute,-uncomplicated gonorrhoea both males and females.

References

Alergant, C.D.: Treatment of gonorrhoea with amoxycillin. Brit. J. vener. Dis. 49:274, 1973.

Braff, E.H.:Amoxycillin in the treatment of gonorrhoea. J. Infect. Dis. 129: Suppl. June 1974, p. 254.

Deal, W.B., Polly, S.M. & Zellner, S.R.: Therapy of uncomplicated gonococcal urethritis in the male with a single dose of amoxycillin. J. Infect. Dis. 129: Suppl. June 1974, p. 256.

Eriksson, G.: Oral ampicillin in uncomplicated gonorrhoea. IV. Comparison of pharmacological and clinical results. Acta Derm. Venereol. (Stockh.) 51:467, 1971.

Gurwith, M.J., McGinnis, S., Ronald, A.R. & Henry,R.: Treatment of uncomplicated gonorrhoea in woman with a single oral dose of amoxycillin.J. Infect. Dis. 129: Suppl. June 1974, p.258.

Karney, W.W., Turck, M. & Holmes, K.K.: Single-Dose oral therapy for uncomplicated gonorrhoea: Comparison of amoxycillin and ampicillin given with and without probenicid. J. Infect. Dis. 129: Suppl. June 1974, p. 250.

Lassus, A., Renkonen, O.-V, Johansson, E.A. & Foerstroem, L: Sensitivity of gonococcal strains to penicillin G, ampicillin and doxycycline in a Finnish metropolitan material in 1971. Acta Derm. Venereol. (Stockh.) 53:233, 1973.

Reyn, A., Korner, B. & Bentzon, M.W. : Effects of penicillin, streptomycin, and tetracycline on N. gonorrhoea isolated in 1944 and in 1957. Brit. J. vener. Dis. 34:227, 1958.

Roberts, F.L.: Treatment of uncomplicated gonorrhoea with amoxycillin. J. Infect. Dis. 129: Suppl. June 1974, p. 262.

Rolinson, G.N.: Laboratory evaluation of amoxycillin. Chemotherapy 18: Suppl. 1-10, 1973.

Willcox, R.R.: Effective treatment of gonorrhoea in London with two oral doses of amoxycillin. Brit. J. vener. Dis. 50:120, 1974.

Wolk, E.: Amoxycillin in the treatment of uncomplicated Dis. 129: Suppl. June 1974, p. 264.

TETRACYCLINE IN TREATMENT OF MYCOPLASMA-INDUCED PROSTATO-URETHRITIS

A. Hofstetter, H. Blenk, and R. Rangoonwala

Department of Urology

University of Munich

During the years of 1973/1974 we could not identify any bacteria either in prostatic or seminal fluid in 2/3 of the total number of our patients with inflammatory affections of the male adnexa. On the other hand, we found in approximately 49 % of those abacterial inflammations only mycoplasmens in colony forming units at a rate of more than 10^6/ml examined material.

Although the pathogenetic importance of genital mycoplasma-strains until to-day is not ascertained, we are convinced due to our more than 6 years clinical experiences, based on controlled biopsie and immunological investigations, with an aimed evaluation of therapeutic results, that there is at least a facultative pathogenicity of genital mycoplasma-strains.

Our therapeutic experiences of the last years are essentially based on the use of Doxycycline and Minocycline. In this paper, we would like to discuss the results of the following investigations:

1.) the MIC of the different Tetracyclines against various Mycoplasmen-strains isolated from clinical material,

2.) the therapeutic results with Hostacyclin(R) a Tetracyclin-HCl-preparation by the indication mycoplasma-induced prostato-urethritis

and 3.) tetracycline-titres in serum and prostatic-fluid.

MATERIAL AND METHODS

1.) The minimal inhibition concentrations of the different tetracyclines against various mycoplasmen-strains isolated from clinical material were estimated by aid of dilution test series and agar-diffusion-test.

The test platelets were uniformly impregnated with 30 mcg respectively.

Since the value of twice the logarithm MIC (1) is in correlation with the diameters of the inhibition zones of the agar-diffusion-test, it was possible to draw conclusions regarding the MIC-values. The mycoplasma-strains were assumed to be sensible against tetracyclines, if their growth was inhibited by 2 mcg/ml or less, moderately sensible between 2 and 8 mcg/ml $>$ 8 mcg/ml to be resistant.

2.) From September 1973 till December 1974 we treated 82 patients, aged 22 to 41, having mycoplasma-induced prostato-urethritis, with 2 x 500 mg Hostacyclin (R)/die over 10 days. 8 days after therapy was ceased, corresponding microscopical, bacteriological and partly immunological tests of the prostatic-fluid were performed. If the results led to the conclusion that the mycoplasma-infection still persisted, Hostacyclin (R) in the same dosage was given for 10 more days; 8 days after termination of therapy the corresponding controls were repeated. Before treatment was started, adequate resistance-tests on antibiotic-free culture media were carried out by means of diffusion-test.

3.) Moreover by 10 patients with chronic adnexitis (prostato-urethritis) the tetracycline titres were estimated in serum and prostatic fluid.

RESULTS

1.) From 82 cases of mycoplasma-induced prostato-urethritis, we could isolate 39 time mycoplasma hominis and 43 times ureaplasmas. Corresponding to our definition only 1 strain of ureaplasma was resistant, whilst 3 strains moderately sensible to Tetracycline. Amongst the strains of mycoplasma hominis 38 were sensible and only one moderately sensible.

2.) From the 39 patients with prostato-urethritis 6 caused by M. hominis and treated with 2 x 500 mg Hostacyclin/die over 10 days and the first control after an interval of 8 days without therapy, we could identify in 3 patients M. hominis more than 10^4/ml in colony forming units in prostatic-fluid.

Both the number of leucocytes in prostatic-fluid and immuno-electrophoresis of the ejaculate led to the conclusion of an inflammatory process. After a repeated treatment of 10 days the inflammatory condition persisted in two patients.

In 43 cases with infection caused by ureaplasma, 4 were seen without clinical improvement - after 10 days therapy with Hostacyclin and after a therapy over 20 days by 2 patients

3.) The tetracyclines-titer in serum and prostatic-fluid. 6 h after application of the different Tetracyclin-derivates drugs are shown. The difference in the concentrations levels were not statistically significant.

DISCUSSION

Corresponding to our earlier investigations (4) and that of Schmid, Price and Krech (5), we could demonstrate in vitro-tests that the examinated mycoplasmens were significantly sensitive against tetracycline. This very fact and the furthermore the pharmacokinetic properties of tetracyclines which are described by Hessel and Stamey (3) concerning their concentrations in prostatic-fluid, explains the efficacy of tetracyclines by genital-urinary infections caused by mycoplasmens.

In spite of a certain differences in pharmacokinetic behaviour between the so-called basic-tetracyclines and the long-acting tetracyclines, according to our dosage scheme, we could not find any significant differences in the clinical results between 2 x 500 mg Hostacyclin (R)/die and in our earlier studies with 2 x 100 mg Doxycyclin or 2 x 200 mg Minocycline.

Although the urinconcentrations after tetracyclin HCl is considerably higher than after Doxycycline or Minocycline, the fact that the levels of concentration in prostatic-fluid are about the same dimension, we would like to emphasize that the Tetracyclines concentrations in the prostatic-fluid plays an important role by mycoplasma-induced prostato-urethritis.

SUMMARY

The administration of tetracycline-hydrochloride (Hostacycline (R)) in a oral daily dosage of 2 x 500 mg by 82 patients with mycoplasma-induced prostato-urethritis, proved to be of a noteworthy therapeutical efficacy. These clinical results corresponds to that of in vitro-tests and the titre-estimations in serum and prostatic-fluid. Among the therapy-resistant cases we found one strain which was primary and the other developed during the treatment. The reasons for the remaining might be due to unfavourable conditions of absorption, insufficient takings of the drug or neglecting the treatment of the female partner.

ASSESSMENT OF MYCOPLASMAS AND INFERTILITY AND THE EFFECT OF DOXYCYCLINE

G.L. RIDGWAY, V. LITTLE, E. RADWANSKA, AND G.I.M. SWYER

UNIVERSITY COLLEGE HOSPITAL
GOWER STREET, LONDON, W.C.1

INTRODUCTION:

The role of T-mycoplasmas as pathogens of the urinary and genital systems is still largely undetermined. SHEPARD (1954) first isolated T-mycoplasmas from patients with non-gonococcal urethritis, and since then some surveys have suggested a causal relationship SHEPARD (1960), CSONKA ET AL.(1966), whilst other surveys have not supported this view. TAYLOR-ROBINSON ET AL (1969). With regard to women, marked variation in carriage rate have been noted; with a possible relationship to sexual activity. ARCHER (1968) studied 100 pregnant women, 94 women attending an Infertility Clinic, 98 women in a Geriatric Unit, and 106 nuns in an enclosed order, and found carriage rates of 58,51, 29 and 8 per cent respectively. Similarly, MÅRDH & WESTRÖM (1968) found that the carriage of T-mycoplasmas was significantly higher in pregnancy. (68.4% against 45.8% and 55.4% in non-pregnant females and females with signs of genital infection respectively). The possibility of an association between low birth weight and T-mycoplasma infection during pregnancy was considered and investigated by KLEIN ET AL(1969)and investigated and confirmed by BRAUN ET AL(1971.) KUNDSIN & DRISCOLL(1970)postulated an aetiological role for T-mycoplasma in human reproductive failure and premature birth. A pathogenic role for genital mycoplasmas was demonstrated by SOLOMAN ET Al(1973)in a review of 11 cases of gynaecological sepsis, 3 due to T-strains, and the remainder *M.hominis.*

A further facet of T-mycoplasmas was revealed by GNARPE AND FRIBERG (1972)(1972a) (1973) concerning human infertility. They isolated T-mycoplasmas from 45 of 52 infertile couples, but only from 9 of 40 pregnant females, a result in contrast to the findings of ARCHER. They further demonstrated that 29% of the infertile females became pregnant within a few months of eradication of the T-strains by treatment with doxycycline.

These results were widely publicised (THE TIMES 1973), NATURE (1973), JAMA (1973). As a result, pressure from infertile patients asking for treatment with doxycycline led DE LOUVOIS ET AL(1974)to investigate the relationship between mycoplasma carriage and unexplained infertility, with results which were not consistent with those of GNARPE & FRIBERG. We found ourselves in a similar position at about the same time. We therefore undertook a trial to establish the incidence of T-mycoplasma and M.hominis carriage in our practice and further to establish the effect, or lack of effect of treatment with doxycycline on infertility in T-mycoplasma positive patients.

METHOD

The culture technique was based on that of **TAYLOR-ROBINSON ET AL** (1969a), involving primary isolation in liquid medium containing urea for T-strains, and arginine for M.hominis, with a chemical indicator. Isolates were confirmed on solid media. M.fermentans was also looked for, but not found. To avoid any bias, the source of specimen was unknown to the microbiologist.

Specimens were taken onto standard cotton wool swabs, and placed in a transport medium, and delivered to the laboratory within one hour. They were either immediately put up in culture, or on a few occasions deep frozen at -70°C until they could be cultured.

PATIENTS

A total of 303 patients were investigated, all attending the infertility clinic. Cervical swabs were taken from the women, and where possible from their husband's seminal fluid. The distribution is as shown on the table, patients included in the unknown cause group having been fully screened for a possible cause of infertility.

TABLE 1 - Distribution of Patients.

	Unknown	Adequate cause	Pregnant
Couples	66	59	8
Wife only	1	11	20
Husband only	0	5	0
Total number of patients	133	134	36

RESULTS

The distribution of T-mycoplasmas in the infertile couples is shown in Table II. This gives an overall isolation rate of 39% in the non-pregnant groups. Both cervix and seminal fluid were positive in 31 out of 49 T-mycoplasma positive couples.

TABLE II - Distribution of T-mycoplasmas

	Unknown	Adequate cause
Wife positive. Husband positive	15	16
Wife positive. Husband negative	9	4
Wife negative. Husband positive	3	2
Number of couples with positive culture	27	22

TABLE III. In 17 couples, M.hominis was also isolated, always in association with T-strains (Table III). In only 4 cases were husband and wife positive for M.hominis

TABLE III - Distribution of M.hominis in couples carrying T-Mycoplasmas

	Unknown	Adequate cause
Wife positive: Husband positive	2	2
Wife positive: Husband negative	4	4
Wife negative: Husband positive	4	1
Wife negative: Husband negative	17	15
% T-Mycoplasmas positive couples with positive M.hominis culture	37	31.8

The carriage rates of T-mycoplasma and M. hominis were not significantly different in the two groups (TABLE IV and V). The carriage rate in the pregnant group was 35%.

TABLE IV - Incidence of T-Mycoplasmas in cervix or semen of couples

	Unknown	Adequate cause
T-Mycoplasmas cultured	27	22
T-Mycoplasmas absent	39	37
% positive cultures	39.4	37.2

TABLE V - Incidence of M.hominis in cervix or semen of couples

	Unknown	Adequate cause
M.hominis cultured	10	7
M.hominis absent	56	52
% positive cultures	17.9	11.9

21 couples in the unknown group, and 13 couples in the adequate cause group received doxycycline. On the first day 200mg, then 100mg, daily for 9 days. In 2 couples a further course was necessary to eliminate T-strains. Further, concurrent therapy for relevant causes of infertility was given in the adequate cause group. TABLE VI. 8 women who were T-mycoplasma positive conceived before doxycycline could be given, 4 in each group. One patient conceived who was negative for T-mycoplasma, but the husband's semen was positive, he had not received doxycycline. Thus, elimination of T-mycoplasmas did not result in a higher rate of pregnancy than in those untreated, nor was the rate higher in couples negative for T-mycoplasma.

Further, in the pregnant group, (TABLE VII) where no doxycycline was used at all, the presence of absence of T-mycoplasma to date had no effect on the outcome. The lowest birth weight was 2.2Kg in a woman who did not harbour T-mycoplasmas.

DISCUSSION

If the existence of T-mycoplasmas were of aetiological significance, the organism would be expected to be present in a higher proportion of the infertile group having no adequate cause of infertility, than in those with a recognisable cause. We have been unable to support this hypothesis.

TABLE VI - Cumulative conceptions in relation to Doxycycline.

	1 year follow up	
	Doxycycline	No Doxycycline
Unknown (Conceived	1	5
Unknown (Did not conceive	2	0
Treated cause (Conceived	3	4
Treated cause (Did not conceive	1	0

TABLE VII - Outcome to date of pregnant group.

	T-mycoplasmas cultured	T-mycoplasmas absent
Total number of women	13	25
Number subsequently aborted	2	3
Normal delivery	3	10
Forceps delivery or Caesarian Section	2	6

TABLE VIII - Percentage isolations of T-mycoplasmas in the groups studied.

Group	T-mycoplasmas %
Infertile (adequate cause)	37.2
Infertile (no cause found)	39.4
Pregnant	35

TABLE VIII - these results are at a variance, both with the high carriage rates in pregnancy (68.4%) of MARDH & WESTRÖM, and the high carriage rate of infertile without cause (90%) of GNARPE & FRIBERG. Further, in contrast to these latter workers, we did not find that the use of doxycycline to eliminate T-mycoplasmas resulted in increase in conception. Of our unknown group, only 1 of 14 women followed up for 6 months after elimination of T-mycoplasmas conceived, whilst 5 women in this group conceived before we were able to give a course of doxycycline for T-mycoplasma infection. 5 out of 7 women pregnant, with T-mycoplasma infection have to date had term deliveries, suggesting no adverse effect of the mycoplasmas on the pregnancy.

We cannot explain the wide variation of results between workers. Isolation techniques have advanced significantly over the years. Geographical variation is a possible further factor.

Thus, we conclude that in our experience the presence or absence of T-mycoplasma in the genital tract has no effect on the ability to conceive, or the outcome of the pregnancy. Further, we found that elimination of genital mycoplasma carriage with doxycycline did not in itself result in an increase in conception rate.

ACKNOWLEDGMENTS

We thank Dr. E.J. Stokes for support and encouragement, Dr. D. Taylor-Robinson for advice on culture technique, and Mr. A. East for technical assistance. The secretarial help of Mrs. A. Harrington is gratefully acknowledged.

REFERENCES

Archer J.F., (1968) Brit.J.Ven.Dis. 44 232.
Braun P., Lee Y.H., Klein J.O., Marcy S.M., Klein T.A., Chales D., Levy P., Kass E.H. (1971). New Eng.J.Med. 284 167.
Csonka G.W., William R.E.S., Corse J., (1966). Lancet 1 1292.
Gnarpe H., Friberg J., (1972) Amer.J.Obst.Gynae 114 727.
Gnarpe H., Friberg J., (1972a). IBID p.963.
Gnarpe H., Friberg J. (1973) Nature 242 120.
Harrison R.F., deLouvois J., Blades M., Hurley R., Stanley V.C., (1974) Lancet 1 1073.
Jama (1972) Leading article 226 3 263-267
Klein J.O., Buckland D., Finland M (1969) New Eng. J. Med. 280 1025.
Kundsin R.B., Driscoll M.D., (1970) Surg.Gynae & Obst. 131 89.
deLouvois J., Blades M., Harrison R.F., Hurley R., Stanley V.C. (1974) Lancet 1 1073.
Mårdh P., Weström L (1970) Acta.Path.Microbiol.Scand. Section B 78 367-374.
Nature (1973) Leading article 242 83.
Shepard M.C., (1954) Amer.J.Syph. 38 113.
Shepard M.C., (1960) Ann.N.Y. Acad. Sci. 79 397.
Solomon F., Caspi E., Bukousky I., Simpolonsky D., (1973) Amer.J.Obst. & Gynae 114 785.
Taylor-Robinson D., Addey J.P., Hare M.J., Dunlop E.M.C. (1969) Brit.J.Ven.Dis. 43 265.
Taylor-Robinson D., Addey J.P., Goodwin C.S., (1969a) Nature 272 275.
The Times (1973) September 15th.

ORAL, VAGINAL AND COMBINED OROVAGINAL THERAPY OF MYCOPLASMOSIS UROGENITALIS

E.R. Weiβenbacher

Women's Clinic of the Munich University

Munich

SUMMARY

Within two years, 150 female patients suffering from chronically recurrent fluor were treated, in whom mycoplasmas could be demonstrated as a possible cause for the fluor. The patients were treated as follows: 50 patients vaginally (5 days 200 mg of chlorotetracycline-hydrochloride); 50 patients orally (10 days 4 x 250 mg of tetracycline-HCl, daily); and 50 patients orally plus vaginally. Control examinations - 8 days and 4 weeks, respectively, after cessation of therapy - had the following results: 7 recidivations after vaginal therapy, one recidivation after oral treatment and no recidivation following the combined therapy.

INTRODUCTION

Different examination results support the assumption of an optional pathogenicity of the mycoplasmas in the male (7, 14, 15, 18) and in the female urogenital tract (1, 2, 5, 6, 10, 11, 12, 19, 20). No clinical picture, however is known that might be typical for an infection by mycoplasmas. Certainly, there are time and again patients with chronically recurrent fluor in whom no other cause for the fluor can be found than mycoplasmas. The women presented degree of vaginal purity II and III (13). In more than 1,500 women suffering from chronically recurrent fluor, we have not be able to fina a patient so far showing an infestation with mycoplasmas while simultaneously presenting a proper Döderlein flora (degree of purity I).

For the restitution of a normal vaginal milieu (degree of purity I), an elimination of the mycoplasmas appears to be unavoidable. Tetracyclines have been found to be trustworthy for the treatment of infections by mycoplasmas in the pulmonary region (3, 4). It is obvious, therefore, to use them also in cases of mycoplasmosis urogenitalis; but the problem arises: In which manner should the tetracyclines be administered so as to make sure success of therapy quickly and permanently? Is mere vaginal or oral application sufficient, or has the therapy to be a combined one?

In our clinic, a treatment of the populating processes with mycoplasmas was carried out in the following cases:

1, patient complaining of fluor where mycoplasmas were recognized as the only possible cause;
2, female patients whose partners were also being treated by a urologist because of mycoplasma infestation of the prostate;
3, female patients who frequently changed their coitus partners and were infested with mycoplasmas.

Altogether, 150 women were treated by us in whom ureas and non-urease-splitting strains of mycoplasmas in the exterior genital tract had been demonstrated. These patients were examined in our special consulting hours for microbiology over a period of two years, and they complained of chornically recurrent fluor. Mycoplasmas were the only possible cause.

MATERIALS AND METHODS

50 patients received tetracycline vaginally, i.e., 100 mg of chlorotetracycline-hydrochloride, each time - in the morning and in the evening - one vaginal suppository, for a period of 5 days. 50 patients were administered orally, tetracycline-HCl, 4 times a day, each time 250 mg, for ten days. 50 patients received tetracycline vaginally as well as tetracycline-HCl orally. Pregnant women were not admitted to this examination. Control tests were carried out 8 days and four weeks, respectively, after the last tablet application, because the frequency of recidivation - owing to danger of re-infection - is increasing according to the growing control intervals. During this period, sexual abstinence was prescribed which could not be demanded for longer than four weeks.

Demonstration of mycoplasmas was made by smears from the cervical canal, the surface of the portio, the laterovaginal walls, as well as from the urethra. Inoculation of the plates used by us (6, 7, 15, 20) was carried out by sterile cotton carriers; subsequently, an aerobic cultivation was done (37°C, addition of nitrogen and CO_2 for at least 24, and at the utmost for 96 hours). We found urea and non-urea-splitting mycoplasmas which had to be classified serologically to the strain M. hominis, type I, and to the urealytics ("t-strains").

RESULTS

In 5 of the 50 women who had received tetracyclines vaginally, we could demonstrate, 8 days after the end of treatment, mycoplasmas in the exterior urogenital tract. Two of the women presented a positive mycoplasma result during the four week control. The control result in those women who had been administered tetracyclines was positive only in one case each. As to the patients with combined vaginal and oral therapy, no recidivations could be stated during the period of observation. Side effects of the treatment were candida albicans infections of the vagina in 9 out of 150 women, however these infections could be removed quickly by longterm nystatin application. Women who had a recidivation received a combined treatment.

We got the following statements from those 150 patients who were treated by us and who did not show any mycoplasmas in the exterior genital tract on cultural control: Questioned whether they think that fluor had improved essentially or deteriorated or remained the same, 82 women stated that their fluor had improved to an essential degree, or even totally ceased (51 patients); 18 women were not able to make statements; 35 women reported that their fluor had not improved essentially; 15 women, 9 of whom presented candidiasis of the exterior urogenital tract, mentioned a deterioration with regard to the time before the treatment of their mycoplasmosis; 62 out of 82 patients showing a subjective amelioration presented, after the end of treatment and additional application of lactic acid, a degree of purity I, 13 women a degree of purity II, and two patients a degree of purity III. No classification concerning the degree of purity could be made in 5 women.

DISCUSSION

Tetracyclines appear to be the remedy of choice in cases of mycoplasma infections (8, 9, 16, 17, 11), a fact known from mycoplasma pneumonia and the in vitro tests. This is, however, valid only for non-pregnant women. A therapeutic test with erythromycin is adviseable for gravidae and children. Furthermore, it is known that in cases of mycoplasma infestation there are resistant factors, as well as in other micro-organisms, against antibiotics e.g. tetracycline. Resistance against tetracyline has been determined for the strains cultivated in our laboratories; during these experiments, single resistant factors against tetracyclines could be observed. It cannot be clarified why recidivations appeared in 7 of 50 women after vaginal tetracycline therapy. Mere vaginal treatment evidently does not suffice, to avoid recidivations. The oral way of application grants a successful therapy with the greatest possible certainty. Strict indication (concomitant candidiasis) and weighing the risks (sensibilization, resistance formation) must be taken into consideration here just as well as in any other antibiotic therapy. Cultural control examinations appear to be unavoidable in the interest of a longterm non-recidivation. A treatment of the respective partner should only be carried out in cases of clearly demonstrated infestation with mycoplasmas (secretion smear of the prostate) . A final substitution of lactic acid is recommendable, for it is possible to attain, thereby, the desirable degree of purity I of the vagina more rapidly.

Every three months we carry out control tests on patients who have suffered from fluor for a number of years.

Intensive research will still be necessary in order to clarify which factors keep up or cause a mycoplasmosis urogenitalis. The vaginal region is protected from pathogenic or optionally pathogenic germs more effectively by a well-developed Döderlein flora than by any antibiotic.

As to our results, 82 women demonstrated in a subjective manner an amelioration of their fluor, and 62 of these simultaneously a restitution, objectively, of the normal vaginal milieu (degree of purity I) .

CONCLUSION

At present, the oral or combined orovaginal therapy using tetracyclines appears to be the treatment of choice in cases of mycoplasmosis urogenitalis of women.

ACKNOWLEDGEMENTS

We are grateful to Mrs. V. Mursik, M.D., and Mr. H. Metz, M.D. for their co-operation. We would also like to thank Mr. Sethi, M.D., Institute of Microbiology and Immunology, University of Bonn.

REFERENCES

1. Bassermann, F.J. (1966). Vorkommen und Bedeutung von Mycoplasmataceen (PPLO) in menschlichen Atemtrakt. Prox. Pneumol. 20, 317.
2. Bredt, W. (1975). Mykoplasmainfektionen des Menschen. Med. Klinik, 70, Nr.1.
3. Chanock, R.M., Hayflick, L., Barile, M.F. (1962). Proc. Nat. Acad. Sci., 48, 41.
4. Eaton, M.D. (1965). Pleuropneumonia-like organisms and related forms. Ann. Rev. Microbiol., 19, 379.
5. Faerber, Witzleb, Sproessig, (1969). Mykoplasmen und Erkrankungen des Urogenitaltraktes. Dtsch. Ges.-Wes., 24, 2054.
6. Hofstetter, A., Schmiedt, E. (1970). Mycoplasmenvorkommen bei entzundlichen Erkrankungen des Urogenitaltraktes. Urologe, 9, 200.
7. Hofstetter, A.(1972). Mykoplasmen als Ursache entzundlicher Erkrankungen des Urogenitaltraktes. Habilitationsschrift, Universität, München.
8. Hubmann, R. (1968). Klinische und experimentelle Untersuchungen zur Chemotherapie der unspezifischen Infektionen im Bereich des Urogenitalsystems. Fortschr. Med., 86, 679.
9. Klieneberger-Nobel, E. (1969). Die Mykoplasmen, Grumbach, A., W. Kikuth: Die Infektionskrankheiten des Menschen und ihre Erreger. G. Thieme, Stuttgart.
10. Kundsin, R.B. (1970). Genital mycoplasmosis in man. New Eng. J. Med., 282, 928.
11. Mardh, P.A., Westroem, L. (1970). T-Mycoplasmas in the genitourinary tract of the female. Acta pathol. Microbiol.Scand., 78, 367.
12. Nocard, E., Roux, E. (1898). Le microbe de la peripneumonie. Ann. Inst. Pasteur, 12, 240.
13. Richter, K. (1971). Erkrankungen der Vagina. In: Schwalm, H., Döderlein, G., Wulf, K.H. Klinik der Frauenheilkunde und Geburtshilfe, Bd. 8, S.573. Urban and Schwarzenberg, Müchen-Berlin-Wien.
14. Shepard, M.C. (1970). Nongonococcal urethritis associated with human strains of T-mycoplasmas. J. Amer. Med. Ass. 211, 1335.
15. Shepard, M.C., Alexander, C.E., Lunceford, C.D., Campell, P.E., Washington, D.C. (1964). Possible role of t-strain Mycoplasma in nongonococcal urethritis - a sixth veneral disease. J. Amer. Med. Ass. 188, 729.
16. Smith, P.F. (1971). The Biology of Mycoplasmas. Academic Press, New York.

17. Smith, Freidewald, W.T., Chanock, R.M. (1967). Shedding of mycoplasma pneumoniae after tetracycline and erythromycin therapy. New Eng. J. Med. 272, 1172.

18. Taylor-Robinson, D., Addey, J.P., Hare, M.J., Dunlop, E. (1969). Mycoplasma and non-specific genital infection. Previous studies and laboratory aspects. Brit. J. Vener. Dis., 45, 265.

19. Weissenbacher, E.R., Frank, S., Penning, W., Heyn, R., Weissmann, J. (1973). Untersuchungen zum Mykoplasmenbefall des weiblichen Urogenitaltraktes. Geburtsh.u.Frauenheilk. 33, 786.

20. Weissenbacher, E.R. (1973). Mykoplasmen im weiblichen urogenitaltrakt. Infection I, 241.

21. Westroem, L., Mardh, P. (1971). The effect of antibiotic therapy on mycoplasmas in the female genital tract, in vitro and in vivo studies on the sensitivity of mycoplasma hominis and t-strain mycoplasmas to tetracycline and other antibiotics. Acta obstet. gyn. 50, 25.

A CLINICAL TRIAL OF TINIDAZOLE IN URO-GENITAL TRICHOMONIASIS

Marc Levrier

College of Gynaecology of Bordeaux and of the South-West

SUMMARY

Trichomonas vaginalis parasitizes the male and female uro-genital tract.

The classical clinical signs are not always present, and specific lesions of the vaginal wall and of the cervix must be sought for by colposcopy, and the organisms must be looked for in the adnexal glands, since it is from these sites that relapses occur.

Nitro-imidazole compounds have proved effective over the past twenty years, with metronidazole at their head, which, however, requires long-term treatment.

A new imidazole derivative, tinidazole, has been shown to be effective at lower doses.

Our own clinical experience has confirmed this effect in human therapeutics.

We have treated 52 women suffering from trichomonal vaginitis, using tinidazole in a single oral dose of 2 g. The partner was also given concurrent treatment, at the same dose, in 32 cases.

The result was good in all cases from the first week, and was confirmed 4 to 6 weeks later, with the exception of three cases, in whom a second single course treatment was necessary.

A certain number of organisms associated with trichomonas vaginalis were sensitive to tinidazole. Associated candidiasis, present in 9 cases, was cured in 4.

Clinical tolerance was satisfactory. There were, however, a few side-effects, mainly affecting the alimentary tract.

In any infective gynaecology practices, vaginitis due to trichomonas vaginalis is still very common, with an incidence of about 10% and, according to different authors, follows or precedes mycotic vaginitis. Non-preferential association with pathogenic organisms is usual, and the tendency for the normal flora to disappear should be emphasized.

Trichomonas vaginalis parasitizes the male and female uro-genital tract.

The incidence of infection is higher in practices confined to prostitutes, indicating the venereal origin of the infection (the seventh venereal disease). The organism has, however, been shown in swimming-pool water, so that this may also present a route of infection.

The obvious clinical signs, with copious frothy, foul-smelling leucorrhoea and painful and itching vaginitis, are not always seen. It is necessary to be able to observe the condition of the vaginal mucosa by colposcopy, with its numerous small areas where the surface epithelium is abraded, and plaques of oedema. Cytology shows lymphocytic and serious infiltration and cellular dysplasia, and may even show nuclear anomalies. Schyler's Lugol test usually shows infection of the cervix, with the yellowish-white spots described by Joseph MAGENDIE, but there may in addition, in advanced stages, be leucoplasia with cellular metatypes, which are regarded as pre-malignant changes. The parasite has been found on the inflamed endometrium and in pyosalpinx. Trichomonas may shelter in the adnexal glands of SKENE and BARTHOLIN, and these locations are the origin of relapses.

Apart from the fact that copious itching leucorrhoea results in the pathological state of dyspareunia, the lesions in the cervical epithelium and the uterine mucosa due to trichomonas vaginalis may compel the gynaecologist to carry out more searching investigations.

Invasion of the urinary tract is common, and occurs via the urethra, the meatus of which is one of the favourite haunts of the parasite.

In the male, infection is more discrete, and there are many healthy carriers. The parasite may lodge in the balano-praeputial fold without producing clinical signs, but may on occasion provoke urethritis and less often a prostatitis.

TREATMENT

In the treatment of uro-genital trichomoniasis, attention should be paid to the severity of the manifestations of the acute stage, the occult, latent character of the chronic stage, and of the risk of re-infestation from a non-treated partner.

The nitro-imidazoles have proved their trichomonicidal activity over twenty years, with metronidazole (FLAGYL) at their head, but this substance has to be given for long periods, both orally and topically.

A new nitro-imidazole derivative, nimorazol (or NAXOGYN) is more effective with a shorter period of oral administration.

More recently, a new imidazole derivative, tinidazole, the chemical structure of which is similar to that of metronidazole, has been investigated in vitro against trichomonas foetus and trichomonas vaginalis, and in infected animals, and has been shown to be effective at a dose eight times lower. At a concentration of 5 mcg/ml, tinidazole immobilized all the trophozoites of fifty strains of trichomonas vaginalis isolated, cultured and tested in vitro at the Institute of Parasitology of the Faculty of Medicine, Strasbourg.

Numerous clinical studies since this time have confirmed this potent action in human therapy.

We used tinidazole by mouth alone, at a single dose of 2 g (4 tablets each containing 500 mg given as a single dose after a meal) to treat 52 women suffering from trichomonal vaginitis, who had come for consultation with a complaint of leucorrhoea, which was often the principal symptom, sometimes associated with vulvo-vaginitis. The patients' ages varied between 18 and 68 years. 24 patients had already undergone a number of different treatments, all of which had been ineffective or which had produced only a short period of improvement. The partner was treated at the same dose in 32 of the cases.

A course of FASIGYN-MINUTE was not prescribed for pregnant women, since teratological investigations have not yet been completed.

No associated treatment was prescribed.

BACTERIOLOGY AND PARASITOLOGY EXAMINATIONS

Bacteriology and parasitology investigations were carried out as follows :

- before treatment,
- on the 7th day of treatment,
- between the 28th and 42nd days of treatment.

In each case, the following examinations were carried out on vaginal and cervical secretions, with particular reference to the posterior fornix :

- direct examination in physiological saline, with determination of the vaginal pH (which is invariably alkaline in cases of trichomoniasis).
- on a swab :
  - . Gram staining to identify the bacterial flora.
  - . May-Grun-Giemsa staining to show cellular density, particularly the histiocytes and the percentage of eosinophil polymorphs, and to show trichomonas, although these appear somewhat deformed.
  - . Culture of Deschiens modification of Dobbel-Laidlaw medium (disappointing result).
  - . Culture on Sabouraud's medium .

. Culture on dishes of lactose agar and blood.
. Culture in a tube of broth.
. Analysis of the precipitate following centrifugation of the urine, which in many cases reveals the parasite.

EFFECTIVENESS AND TOLERANCE

EFFECTIVENESS

Whether the infestation was an old one, chronic over many years, had relapsed some months previously, was due to a re-infestation or was recent, the result was in all cases favourable from the first week, and was confirmed 4 to 6 weeks afterwards, with the exception of three cases.

These three cases required a second single-dose treatment, since direct examination showed the presence of trichomonas on the seventh day, in spite of a marked reduction in leucorrhoea.

Bacteriological examination before treatment was negative in 7 cases.

Various pathogens were found before treatment in the other 45 cases.

It was noted that a certain number of these organisms were sensitive to FASIGYN, either at the first week's examination or at the second examination. In particular :

- pathogenic staphylococci disappeared in 5 cases.
- enterococcus disappeared in 11 cases.
- pyogenic streptococcus disappeared in 7 cases.
- diphtheroids disappeared in 1 case.
- escherichia coli with colibacilli and coliforms disappeared in 16 cases.

Trichomonas was associated with candida albicans (+++) in 9 cases : treatment with FASIGYN led to the disappearance of both organisms in 4 cases.

TOLERANCE

Overall, clinical tolerance was good. 21 patients complained of mild side-effects, mainly digestive in nature, but in no case did these continue after the day of administration. They included : nausea : 5 cases ; vomiting : 1 case ; dry mouth : 4 cases ; indigestion : 1 case ; bitter taste in mouth : 3 cases ; coating of the tongue : 1 case ; gastric pain : 1 case ; abdominal discomfort : 2 cases + 3 cases combined with other symptoms ; black stools : 1 case ; polyuria on the first day : 1 case associated with other symptoms ; liverishness on the day after administration : 1 case associated with other symptoms ; headache : 1 case ; drowsiness : 1 case.

Signs of mycotic infection were seen at the first examination in three cases. These were not seen again in 2 cases at the examination at 6 weeks. It may be assumed that the seven cases of mycotic infection which were recognised only at the second examination, i.e. 4 to 6 weeks after treatment with FASIGYN, were the result of a fresh infection.

CONCLUSION

FASIGYN, administered orally in a single dose of 2 g (consisting of 4 tablets each of 500 mg) to women suffering from vaginal trichomoniasis, was shown by clinical and parasitological examination to be a rapid and effective trichomonicidal agent.

A second single-dose treatment was necessary in 3 out of 52 cases.

Yeasts which were found at the first examination in three cases were not present in 2 cases after six weeks.

The concomitant effect of FASIGYN on various pathogens, which in many cases were present in combination, should be noted.

In the case of candida albicans, there was a favourable effect in 4 cases, where this organism was found together with trichomonas before treatment, and no effect in 5 cases.

Clinical tolerance overall was good, apart from a few mild digestive complaints, none of which were present 12 hours after the administration of the product.

No serious side-effects were seen.

No contra-indication was found.

Our patients appeared to be particularly appreciative of the dosage and the ease of absorption of FASIGYN and of its rapid effect on leucorrhoea.

The gynaecologist now has available a trichomonicidal agent, the effectiveness of which particularly impressed us, and the administration of which, by the systemic route, allows for the ubiquitous presence of the parasite in different segments of the uro-genital tract.

REFERENCES

BANDTLOW, K. and FRICK, J. : The treatment of trichomoniasis in men. Proceedings of the 7th International Congress of Chemotherapy, Prague 1972.

COSAR, C. and JULOU, L. : The effect of (hydroxy-2-ethyl) I methyl 2 nitro imidazole (8.823 R.P.) in experimental infections with trichomonas.

COSAR, C. ; GANTER, P. and JULOU, L.: Experimental study of metronidazole : its trichomonicidal and amoebicidal activity. Toxicity and general pharmacological properties.

DIAMOND, L.S. : The establishment of various Trichomonads of animals and man in exenic cultures. J. Parasit. 43, 488-89, 1957.

DIWALD, J. : Treatment of trichomoniasis in women with Tinidazole. (Trichomonasis Behand-lung das Frau mit Tinidazol) - Wiener Medie - Wichr. 1971, n° 24, pages 492-494.

JIROVEC, O. and PETRU, M. : Trichomonas vaginalis and Trichomoniasis. Advances in parasitology, 6, 117-188. Ben Dawes ed. Academic Press London and New-York, 1968.

LAM-SALINAS, P., M.D. : Tinidazole (CP 12,574) in the treatment of vaginal trichomoniasis. Spain Medical Report, August-September 1971.

LATRILLE, J. ; VEAUX, R. ; RIGOU, R. ; DULONG DE ROSNAY, C. ; BOINEAU, J. and PHOLOPPE, P. : Infective vaginitis. Bordeaux Medical n° 10 - October 1969, pages 1981-2002.

MANDOUL, R. ; DARGELOS, R. and MILLAN, J. : The destruction of intestinal protozoa in mice by a nitro derivative of imidazole. Bulletin de la Société de Pathologie Exotique, 54, n° 1, Jan. Fev. 1961, pp. 12-16.

MILTGEN, F. ; KREMER, M. ; DELLENBACH, P. and CRUGNOLA, B. : The isolation and investigation of the "in vitro" sensitivity of trichomonas vaginalis to CP-12,574. Extrait du Journal de Med. de Strasbourg, n° 11, Nov. 1971.

RUSTIA, M. and SHUBIK, P. : Induction of lung tumours and malignant lymphomas in mice by Metronidazole. The Eppley Institute for Research in Cancer. University of Nebraska College of Medicine, Omaha, Nebraska 68105.

THABAUT, A. ; DUROSOIR, J.L. ; DELACROIX, P. and ANGLADE, J.P. : The bacterial flora of the vagina as shown in 995 specimens. Mémoire, Médecine et Armées, 1974, 2, 6, pages 513-521.

WINSTON, R.M.L. : The relation between size and pathogenicity of Trichomonas vaginalis. J. Obst. Gyn. Brit. Comm. 1974, 81, 399-404.

TRICHOMONAS VAGINITIS, AND ITS TREATMENT WITH TINIDAZOLE

P.E.R.RHEMREV AND F.KOSASIH

Dept.for Gynaecology and Obstetrics

St. Elisabeth Gasthuis, Haarlem

ABSTRACT

Fifty-one patients with trichomonal vaginitis diagnosed by microscopicevaluation of the vaginal fluor were treated with Fasigyn (tinidazole)either in a cure of seven days 150mg. b.i.d., or in a single dose of2000mg. Both groups showed a cure-rate of 100% one week after initiation of the treatment. In the 7 day-group the cure-rate was still 100% 4 weeks after treatment as was the case in the single dose group on the 10th dayof the menstrual cycle following treatment. Eight weeks after treatment the cure-rates were 92% and 73%.
In the single dose group 3 patients showed nausea. As most patients from both groups had either recidivating or chronic vaginitis which had already been treated before these results are certainly warranting the use of Fasigyn as a first choice agent in the treatment of Trichomonas vaginalis infections.

The number of patients refered to the gynaecologist for vaginal discharge due to a Trichomonas vaginalis infection has increased steadily over the last years. Various drugs have been used in the treatment of this ailment (3).
The recognition of the sexual transmittance of the disease has proved a major step forward, because it showed the necessity of co-treatment of the infecting sexual partner. The devellopment of orally active trichomonacidal agents has made this treatment regimen possible.

One of the latest devellopments in this group of agents is tinidazole (Fasigyn), a nitro- imidazole dervative that showed better activity in vitro and in vivo over metronidazole (5,7,8,9).

We want to report on two studies we did with this new drug. The first study concerns the treatment of patients and their sexual partners with tinidazole 150 mg. two times daily for seven days. After termination of this study farmacokinetic investigations had shown that tinidazole might be as effective in a single dose of 2000 mg.(8,9). We decided to test the drug in this dose regimen as well.

METHOD

A. first study

Twenty-five female outpatients in whom the diagnosis Trichomonal vaginitis was confirmed by microscopic examination of the vaginal discharge were selected. Excluded were pregnent women, patients with an active organic illness of the C.N.S.,patients with a history of blood dyscrasia and lactating mothers. The treatment results were checked right after the termination of treatment, and after four and eight weeks. Both the patients and their sexual partners were treated with tinidazole 150 mg.b.i.d. in 7 days.

B. second study

Twenty-six female outpatients fullfilling the same criteria as those mentioned under A were selected and treated with tinidazole 2000 mg. in one single dose. The male sexual partners received the same treatment.

RESULTS

A. The 25 selected female outpatients had a mean age of 32 (18-50yrs). In 18 cases (72%) it concerned patients with a recurrent infection, in 5 (20%) the patients presented with a chronic persistent infection while in 2 cases the infection was of recent date.
Table 1. gives the results eight weeks after treatment for the above mentioned groups. The treatment was succesfull in 92 % of all cases.
Table 2. gives a comparison between the results directly after treatment and four weeks after treatment. The two patients who had a positive smear four weeks after treatment received a second course of tinidazole,this time the results were favourable.

Twenty-three of the patients received earlier treatment for the same ailment which was proven ineffective in 11 cases, and which failed in the other 12 because of either recidive or re-infection. Side- effects were not seen in any of the treated patients, nor reproted from the sexual partners.

B. The mean age of the treated patients was 33 yrs(21-55). In 22 patients (85%) a recurrent infection was diagnosed and in the rest (4 patients) a chronic persistent trichomonal vaginitis.
Table 3. gives the results 10 weeks after treatment. The cure rate at this point is 73%.
Table 4. compares the cure- rates one week after treament on the 10th day of the next mentrual cycle and at 10 weeks after treatment. It shows that on the 10th day of the menstrual cycle following treatment the cure-rate is still 100%. Five of the seven patients that had a positive smear by the 10th week were on oral contraceptives of all patients 17 were on oral contraceptives.
Side effects were seen in 3 patients: in concerned 2 cases of mild and 1 case of moderate nausea.
Laboratory test of Hct, Hb, leuco's, thromboc.,SGOT, SGPT, Alk.fosf,serum creatinin, urea, billirubin,sodium, potassium ans calcium showed no drug related abnormalities.

DISCUSSION

We treated 51 female outpatients for trichomonal vaginitis with tinidazole either in a regimen of 150 mg. b.i d. for 7 days (25 cases) or 2000 mg. in a single dose (26 cases). With both treatment regimens all patients had a clean vaginal smear directly after treatment. In the multiple dose group the patients were still cured four weeks after treatment, which was also the case in the single dose group on the 10th day of the menstrual cycle following treatment. Either recidivation or re-infection occured in both groups by 8th week after treatment.
In the multiple dose treated group this occured in 2 cases in the single dose group in 7 . We can not be sure of the significance of these figures, because we do not know whether this concerns re-infection or whether these are cases of true recidivation by non-eradicated germs. In our opinion however the first hypothesis is more probable then the second because non- eradicated germs from the mucosal glands would have become apparent by the 10th day of the cycle following treatment.

Table 1

RESULTS

TRICHOMONIASIS

Results at 8 weeks	of recent date	chronic presistent	recurrent	total
cured	2	5	16	23
not cured	0	0	2	2
TOTAL	2	5	18	25

Table 2

RESULTS

TRICHOMONIASIS	directly after treatment	4 weeks after treatment
Cured	25	23
Not cured	0	2

RESULTS

Table3

	TRICHOMONIASIS		
results at 10 weeks	chronic persistent	recurent	total
CURED	3	16	19
not cured	1	6	7
Total	4	22	26

Table 4

TRICHOMONIASIS	1 week after treatment	day 10 next menstrual cycle	8-10 weeks after treatment
Cured	26	26	19
not cured	0	0	7

CONCLUSION

Tinidazole (Fasigyn) proved to be an effective treatment for trichomonal vaginitis. The possibility to administer this drug as a single 2000mg. dose ensures a perfect patient adherance to the therapy, while the male partner is also more apt to take this one dose then a seven day cure.

ACKNOWLEDGEMENTS

We want to thank Mr. W.L.Hengeveld of the medical dept. Pfizer B.V. Rotterdam who made the drug available to us and assisted us in editing the manuscript.

REFERENCES

1. Trichomonas-Vaginitis. Nadere behandelingsmogelijkheden.
J.Daels et al.
Tijdschrift voor Geneeskunde 15-26e jaargang-1.8.70.

2. Trichomoniasis - Behandelung der Frau mit Tinidazole.
J.Diwald.
Wiener Medizinische Wochenschrift.121 (1971) no.24 (492)

3. History of the treatment of trichomoniasis.
Robert Forgan.
Brit.J.vener. Dis. (1972) 48,522.

4. Zur Behandlung der Trichomoniasis beim Mann.
J.Frick et al.
Therapie Woche 21,6,472 (1971).

5. Tinidazole, a New Antiprotozoal Agent: Effect on Trichomonas and other Protozoa.
H.L.Howes, Jr.,et al.
Antimicrobial Agents and Chemotherapy- 1969,p.261.

6. Perorale Behanlung der Trichomonadenkolpitis mit Fasigyn.
R.Liechti.
Schweiz.Z.Gynäk.Geburtsh. 2,229 - 235 (1971).

7. Tinidazole, a Potent New Antiprozoal Agent.
M.W.Miller et al.
Antimicrobial Agents and Chemotherapy - 1969, 257.

8. Tinidazole and Metronidazole Pharmacokinetics in Man and Mouse.
J.A.Taylor et al.
Anticrobial Agents and Chemotherapy - 1969, 267.

9. The Pharmacokinetics of Metronidazole and Tinidazole in Man.
P.G.Welling et al.
Arzneimittel - Forschung (Drug research) 22,2128 - 2132 (1972).

THE PROBLEM OF TRICHOMONIASIS VAGINALIS IN CHILDREN

Dr. E. Soyka

Gynaecological Clinic of the University of Zurich and

Paediatric Hospital, Zurich Switzerland

Introduction

Vaginal infections are among the commonest gynaecological conditions in children. In this study we shall deal with vaginal trichomoniasis in children and its treatment.

Material and Methods

Our patients were little girls attending the Paediatric Gynaecology Consulting Service. In each child referred on account of suspected vaginal infection, we aspirated the vaginal contents with a suction catheter (which was originally made for suction of the newborn trachea). In this way we obtained sufficient material to carry out culture, cytological examination and investigation of an unstained preparation. In children in whom trichomonads were found in the unstained preparation we calculated the body surface area and we determined the white blood count.

Tinidazole (R) in a single dose was used for treatment*, the dose itself being calculated on the basis of the surface area of the body. An unstained preparation of the vaginal contents was examined, and the white blood count determined, one week after treatment and again four weeks later.

* Trade name in Switzerland: FASIGYN 500 (R) Pfizer AG

Results and Discussion

Table 1

Vaginal discharge in patients seen at the Paediatric Gynaecology Consultation Service, November 1973 - April 1975 inclusive.

All new patients	247	100 %
Vaginal infection	127	51.4 %
Trichomonal infection	20	8.1 %

Over a period of 18 months we investigated 247 new patients. 127 of these children were suffering from vaginal infection, and in 20 of these 127 children we were able to demonstrate trichomonads in the vaginal secretion, an incidence of 8.1 %.

The existence of vaginal trichomoniasis in some of the age-periods surprised us, since it is contrary to general experience.

The authors of most monographs on paediatric gynaecology agree that vaginal infections in children occur according to a definite pattern. The age-periods of small girls are divided into three:

1. Hormonal neonatal period, which lasts for about two weeks after birth, and during which the child is still oestrogenised by maternal hormones.

2. A resting period for the child's genitalia, during which hormones are practically absent.

3. The period of sexual ripening, during which the girl again becomes highly oestrogenised by her endogenous endocrine activity.

These hormonal events may be expected to influence the presence in the immature vagina of the various organisms causing discharge, so that specific or non-specific infection is restricted to one of the three age-periods of childhood (Heinz-Hoyme, Huffmann, Peter-Vesely)

In order to persist and multiply in the vagina, trichomonads require glycogen, the presence of which in the vagina is dependent on oestrogens. The absence of trichomonal infections at the resting period has been explained as being due to this lack of oestrogen. Are these statements still true?

Table 2

Age of patients

0 - 4 years: 1	7 - 8 years: 3	11 - 12 years: -
4 - 5 years: 1	8 - 9 years: 2	12 - 13 years: 2
5 - 6 years: 3	9 - 10 years: 4	13 - 14 years: -
6 - 7 years: 1	10 - 11 years: 2	14 - 15 years: 1

Almost half of our 20 patients were in the resting age-period: none suffered from diabetes mellitus or pubertas praecox; none of them was treated with hormones.

It is usually assumed epidemiologically that infection with trichomonas vaginalis can only occur through sexual intercourse. Other possible routes of infection however, must occur in children.

Perhaps this is associated with changes in the way children are brought up, with a wider social life (gymnastics, swimming in public baths, etc.). The infection may be so massive that the traces of oestrogen in the child's vagina during the resting age-period may suffice for some, more resistant trichomonads, to survive and multiply. Local immunological properties, and changes in these, may also play a part in that the protective action of the local non-specific immune mechanism against infection in the genital tract may be reduced by environmental factors. (Govers).

The diagnosis of vaginal trichomoniasis in children is now easier, so that the diagnosis is made more frequently.

The white blood cell count was determined in order to demonstrate the safety of the drug. There was no case of leucopenia, as was frequently seen as a transient phenomenon in the first studies of metronidazole (Meyer-Herxheimer).

With the introduction of metronidazole by mouth and per vaginam, and later tinidazole by mouth, the previously problematical specific treatment had now become a simple and successful matter.

In children, however, there remains the problem of swallowing tablets over a period of several days, and local vaginal treatment. Large vaginal tablets or ovules cannot be used with the fine, narrow hymen of the small girl, particularly during the resting age-period.

Table 3

Trichomonads in vaginal secretions before and after treatment with tinidazole.

Group	Before treatment	1st follow-up	2nd follow-up	3rd follow-up	4th follow-up	No.
1	positive	negative	negative	--	--	11
2	positive	positive	negative	negative	--	4
3	positive	negative	positive	negative	negative	5

Treatment using a single dose of tinidazole by mouth has solved this problem, and the results of treatment are noteworthy. Treatment was completely successful in the first group.

When trichomonads were still present, at the first follow-up examination one week after treatment or the findings at the first follow-up examination were negative, but were again positive at the second follow-up examination, we treated again with tinidazole. The next two follow-ups were negative in all these children.

The choice of dose gives several points for discussion. In adults a single dose of 2000 mg. tinidazole is regarded as adequate for the treatment of vaginal trichomoniasis, and our own experience agrees with this (Soyka).

Table 4

Comparison of vaginal trichomoniasis in adults and children

	Adults*	Children
Number	70	20
Failures	4	4
Re-infections	4	5

* Personal series, to be published separately (Soyka, E.)

A comparison of the results of treatment in adults, with the results of treatment of children with the single dose of tinidazole calculated on the basis of the body surface area, showed that failure or relapse was commoner in children than in adults.

Table 5

Surface area of body and dose of tinidazole in 20 children

Surface area of body in sq. cm.	Dose of drug administered in mg.	2nd dose in mg.
0.67	900	1200
0.68	900	1000
0.75	1000	--
0.78	1000	1000
0.80	900	1000
0.81	1100	1500
0.81	1000	--
0.89	1000	--
0.90	1000	--
0.93	1500	--
1.05	2000	2000
1.10	1200	1500
1.10	2000	--
1.10	1500	2000
1.12	1800	2000
1.21	1800	--
1.26	1500	--
1.33	2000	--
1.50	2000	--
1.72	2000	--

In the course of the study, therefore, we used a dose higher than that given by the body surface area in some cases, particularly in children in whom the trichomonads in the vagina were not controlled by the first dose of tinidazole. The question, why a relatively larger dose of tinidazole is necessary in some children in comparison with adults is difficult to answer. It may simply be an error due to the small numbers involved. In the case of children, however, one cannot reckon on an increased likelihood of infection but on a reduction in defense mechanisms. Oestrogen lack may play a part since most failures in adults are in women in the later menopausal period.

On the basis of the reports by Varhegyi and Lahon, we had no fears concerning toxic manifestations.

Table 6

Side-effects

	Number of patients
Nil	17
Vomiting	2
Nausea	1

Side-effects were minor, and appeared only in a very small number of children. This fact also encouraged us to consider increasing the dose.

Repeated follow-up examination of children given a fresh course of treatment showed no further trichomonads present, so that we were able to discharge all 20 children as cured.

The treatment of vaginal trichomoniasis in children with a single oral dose of tinidazole thus provides a simple and satisfactory solution of a problem which has previously been a very difficult one.

Summary

Vaginal trichomoniasis as the cause of vaginal discharge was diagnosed in 20 children aged between 3 and 15 years. We wished in our study to test earlier views as to the presence of trichomonas vaginalis during childhood. Childhood is divided into three age-periods, based on whether the child is oestrogenised or not. Trichomonas vaginalis should only occur during the oestrogen periods.

This rule did not apply in our series of 20 patients. The possible reasons for this variation are discussed. We treated vaginal trichomoniasis in children with a single oral dose of tinidazole. The dose itself was calculated on the basis of the body surface area, and between 900 and 2000 mg. were given. As a guide to the dose to be given, we used the dose of 2000 mg. tinidazole, which is administered to adults of average body surface area 1.73 square meters. We increased the dose in some of our patients, or repeated the treatment. The reasons for this are discussed. This was possible since side-effects were rare and minor in nature, and the toxicity of the compound very low. All 20 children were discharged as cured. We regard the treatment of vaginal trichomoniasis in children with a single oral dose of tinidazole as the method of choice.

REFERENCES

1. Andrews P., Schnell J.D. : Gebh. Frhk. 33, 9, 915, 1973

2. Govers J., Girard J.P. : Gynec. Invest. 3, 18, 1972

3. Guay L.A., Kotcher E. : Amer. Journ. Obst. Gyn. 82, 530, 1961

4. Harnack, G.A. von : Kinderheilkunde - Springer, Berlin, Heidelberg, 1971

5. Heinz Marlene, Hoyme S. : Gynäkologie des Kinder- und Jugendalters, Ferdinand Enke, 1974

6. Huffmann Y.W. : Gynäkologie des Kindes, Urban & Schwarzenberg, 1975

7. Jirovec O., Peter R. : Prophylaxe 1, 102, 1954

8. Jirovec O., Vesely K. : Gyn. pratique 4, 1967

9. Kolman J. : Trichomoniasis, Diagnose und Therapie. W. Mandrich, Wien - München - Bern - 1974

10. Komorowska A., Kurnatowska A., Liniecka J. : Ginek. Polska, 32, 229, 1961

11. Korte W. : Gesellsch. für Gynäk. u. Gebh., Berlin 1966, ref. Zbl. Gynäk. 3, 105, 1967

12. Lahon H.F.J. : Adv. in Antimicrob., Antineoplast. chemotherapy 397, 1972

13. Meyer C., Herxheimer A. : Side-effects of Drugs, 6, 328, 1968

14. Meyer C., Herxheimer A. : Side-effects of Drugs, 7, 414, 1972

15. Muller P. : Rev. franc. Gynéc. 63, 7/8, 361, 1968

16. Peter R., Jirovec O. : Praxis 39, 357, 1950

17. Peter R., Vesely K. : Kindergynäkologie, Georg Thieme 1966

18. Rey-Stocker J. : Gynécologie 168 : 413, 1969

19. Soyka E. : im Druck - Therapeutische Umschau

20. Varhegyi M.Th. : Therapie Woche 23, 9, 723, 1973

ORAL TREATMENT OF VAGINAL TRICHOMONIASIS WITH ORNIDAZOLE, A DERIVATIVE OF METRONIDAZOLE

Boris Rubio-Lotvin

American British Cowdray Hospital

Mexico City

SUMMARY

Results of the use of α chloromethyl-2-methyl-5-nitro-imidazole-ethanol in different schedules of oral administration for the treatment of trichomoniasis in couples affected by the parasitic infestation are informed. In a first group of 20 couples were treated with metronidazole. Clinical and parasitological controls were carried out up to the second menstruation after treatment. Very satisfactory results with no relapses were obtained In this group only oral medication was used.

In a second group of 60 couples, 2 g. of the compound were given in 2 doses in a single day treatment adding one vaginal tablet of 500 mg., twice, every 12 hours. Results were excellent as all clinical manifestation in both partners disappeared in 24 to 72 hours. Parasitoscopic studies were negative in 57 couples, with 3 relapses. A second treatment gave immediate satisfactory results in all these cases.

A third group of 30 couples which was given one single oral dose of 2 g. and 1 vaginal application showed excellent results in 3 of these after one month's treatment and 27 couples after 2 months' treatment.

Trichomonad findings were negative in 28 cases and 2 relapses were observed 2 months after treatment. A second treatment gave immediate excellent results.

In the relapsed cases of the two groups, it was impossible to determine whether other partners were involved.

INTRODUCTION

Vaginal trichomoniasis is a frequent and very disturbing parasitic infestation. Many drugs and schedules of treatment have been tried with variable results. Among these, the most common have been metronidazole, nifuratel, nitrimidazine, natamycin, amphotericin B and a mixture of polyethylene glicols, but except for metronidazole comparative trials have failed to confirm their usefulness in this vaginal infestation. (de Carneri, 1969; Evans and Catterall, 1970 and 1971; Paredes and Hawkins, 1973) For well over 12 years, metronidazole has been the treatment of choice. (Evans and Catterall, 1970 and 1971; Davidson, F., 1973).

Recently some derivatives of this compound: tinidazole (Bedoya, 1974; Rustrian and Luyando, 1975; Swarz, 1974) and ornidazole have been reported to be effective in vaginal trichomoniasis. Ornidazole, the α chloromethyl-2-methyl-5-nitro-1-imidazole-ethanol, active as an antiprotozoal agent in animal experiments has shown to be very effective against Entamoeba Histolytica and Trichomonas Vaginalis and Trichomonas Foetus in mice and hamsters. In comparative studies, it proved to be effective in women as well. (Lean and Vengadasalam, 1973; Rubio-Lotvin, et al, 1973). This study was designed in order to assess the efficacy of ornidazole against vaginal trichomoniasis in women.

MATERIAL AND METHODS

Patients who attended the clinic with the usual clinical picture associated with vaginal trichomoniasis and who had a positive trichomonad identification found with the aid of cytology and examination of a wet film were included in the study.

Their partners' urethral secretion was examined on admission, and then together with the patients, after both the first and the second menstruations.

The total group consisted of 110 couples, divided into three different groups: the first one, of 20 couples, was a randomized double blind study to compare results with metronidazole.

The schedule of administration was 250 mg. twice daily for five days. No local treatment was used. A complete battery of laboratory tests was done before and after treatment. These included: red and white blood count, SGOT, SBPT, alkaline phosphatase, creatinine, glucose and complete urine analysis. In this group, 14 women were using hormonal contraception and their mean age was 30 years.

The second group consisted of 60 couples, receiving 1g. twice in one single day, plus one 500 mg. vaginal tablet morning and evening of the same day. In this group 55 patients were on hormonal contraceptives and their mean age was 29.1 years.

The third group, of 30 couples, received one single dose of 2 g. orally, plus one 500 mg. vaginal tablet. Their mean age was 33 years, and 21 of these were on hormonal contraceptives.

In all cases, treatment was given immediately after menstruation and any secondary effects, or clinical changes as well as trichomonad examination were recorded.

RESULTS

Clinical response of the first group is shown in Table 1. It was considered excellent in 7 couples in each of the sub-groups of ten, who were treated with metronidazole or ornidazole, and good in 3 couples in each group. One couple showed up only once after treatment when results were found to be excellent. The other 19 couples did complete their 2 months' follow-up and results remained as indicated.

Wet film examination for trichomonad presence was negative in all cases up to two months after treatment. Results

TABLE 1

Group 1. Double Blind Study. 20 Couples

	CONTROL			
	AFTER TREATMENT		2 MO. FOLLOW UP	
CLINICAL RESPONSE	Ornidazole	Metronidazole 1 Couple	Ornidazole 10 Couples	Metronidazole 9 Couples
Excellent	-	1	7	6
Good	-	-	3	3
Poor	-	-	-	-
TRICHOMONAD IDENTIFICATION				
Negative	-	1	10	9
Positive	-	-	-	-
Relapse	-	-	-	-

Ornidazole - 1 g a day (2 doses of 500 mg each) x 5 days.

TABLE 2

Group 2. Open Study. 60 Couples

CLINICAL RESPONSE	AFTER TREATMENT	2 MO. FOLLOW UP
Excellent	59	1
Good	-	-
Poor	-	-
TRICHOMONAD IDENTIFICATION		
Negative	57	1
Postivie	3	-
Relapse	3*	-

Ornidazole - one day treatment: 2 g (2 doses of 1 g each) plus 2 vaginal tablets of 500 mg each.
*Treatment was repeated and immediate excellent results were obtained.

were considered excellent when original vaginal discharge and discomfort disappeared within 5 days and good when it took up to 10 days. By the second week most patients had complete recovery of their vaginitis.

In the second group, clinical response was excellent in 59 couples within three days of treatment as is shown in Table 2. Only one couple returned for a 2 month follow-up examination and was found to be free of the infestation. Trichomonad identification was negative in 57 couples, 3 of which had positive finding of the parasite. A second treatment gave immediate excellent results. The couple seen 2 months later had negative wet film and cytology.

In 9 cases discreet gastric irritation was mentioned and an antacid was prescribed with satisfactory relief.

Results obtained in the third group were clinically excellent (see Table 3) within 3 days of treatment and remained as such after the first month of follow-up in 3 couples and after 2 months of treatment in the other 27.

Cytology and wet film were negative for trichomonads in all cases save 2 which were positive at the two month follow up. Treatment was repeated in these 2 cases with immediate excellent results.

TABLE 3

Group 3. Open Study. 30 Couples

CLINICAL RESPONSE	CONTROL 1 Mo. Follow Up	2 Mo. Follow Up
Excellent	3	27
Good	-	-
Poor	-	-
TRICHOMONAD IDENTIFICATION		
Negative	3	25
Positive	-	2
Relapse	-	2*

Ornidazole - one single dose 2 g orally plus one 500 mg vaginal tablet.
*Treatment repeated with immediate excellent results.

DISCUSSION

Metronidazole has been for a number of years the best treatment for vaginal and urethral trichomoniasis. Other compounds have shown good in vitro activity but when provided to patients do not seem to be as effective, as in the case of nitrimidazine and other trichomonacidal agents.

Recently a derivative of metronidazole, the α chloromethyl-2-methyl-5-nitro-1-imidazole-ethanol, known as ornidazole, was made available to us for clinical research, after having shown its antiprotozoal properties.

In our first group it was possible to prove that this compound is as effective as metronidazole and it confirmed its trichomonacidal activity when given in divided doses in a single day or in one single dose orally. The use of one or two vaginal applications seemed to be very helpful to give immediate clinical improvement.

A total oral dose of 2 g. proved effective and quite well tolerated. In a total of 100 couples, treated with ornidazole only 9 partners showed some gastric irritation of minimal importance and all patients with the exception of 5 relapses remained free of infestation for 1 or 2 months after treatment. Renewed treatment in these 5 relapsed cases provided immediate excellent results. It was impossible to determine whether other partners were involved in the relapsed cases in the second and third groups.

ACKNOWLEDGMENT.- The author thanks F.Hoffmann-La Roche, and Cie,S.A.for supplies of Ornidazole and support.

BORIS RUBIO LOTVIN, M.D.
SIERRA AMATEPEC 120
MEXICO 10, D.F.
MEXICO

REFERENCES

Bedoya, J. M. (1974): Current Medical Research and Opinion, 2, 165.

de Carneri, I. (1969): Arzneimittel-Forschung, 19, 382.

de Carneri, I. (1971): Proceedings of the Second International Congress of Parasitology, Washington, September 6 to 12, 1970. Part 4, Item. 887. The Journal of Parasitology, 57, No. 4, Section II, Part I, page 9.

Davidson, F. (1973): The Journal of Obstetrics and Gynaecology of the British Commonwealth, 80, 368.

Evans, B.A. and Catterall, R.D. (1970): British Medical Journal, 2, 335.

Evans, B.A. and Catterall, R.D. (1971): British Medical Journal, 4, 146.

Lean, T.H. and Vengadasalam, D. (1973): British Journal of Venereal Diseases, 49, 69.

Paredes, F.R. and Hawkins, D.F. (1973): The Journal of Obstetrics and Gynaecology of the British Commonwealth, 80, 86.

Rubio-Lotvin, B., Ruiz, M. J.A., de Larios, M.N. and Bolio, A.R. (1973): Ginecologia y Obstetricia de Mexico, 34, 397.

Rustrian, A.A. and Luyando, D.H. (1975): Münchener Medizinische Wochenschrift (Mexican Edition) 117, 112.

Swarz, H. (1974): Current Medical Research and Opinion, 2, 181.

SPA-S-222, A NEW ORAL DERIVATIVE FOR SHORT-TERM TREATMENT OF VAGINAL TRICHOMONIASIS

R.Pellegrini - S.Fanciulli

SPA, Division of medical research,(Milano) and Oncology Centre of Provincial Hospital(Viareggio)

SUMMARY

The results obtained in patients with vaginal trichomoniasis, submitted to a short-term treatment by oral route with SPA-S-222, a new soluble derivative of mepartricin, are reported.
These results have demonstrated the effectiveness and the tolerance of the drug.

- - - -

Following the isolation of partricin, a polyene produced from a strain of S.aureofaciens, its methyl ester, mepartricin, was prepared and developed (Bruzzese et al. 1972 - Bruzzese et al.1974). Extensive microbiological (Danesino and Pellegrini 1974 - Mizuba et al.1974 - Perju et al. 1975 - Pucci and Ripa 1973 - Ritzerfeld 1972 - Ruozi et al. 1974 - Simonetti and Strippoli 1971), pharmacological (Riva and Bianchi 1973) and toxicological (Riva and Bianchi 1973) investigations showed the high activity of mepartricin against Candida and T.vaginalis and its good tolerance. These findings were confirmed by several clinical trials, summarized in a recent review (Pellegrini 1974) describing many hundreds of patients with candida and/or trichomonas vaginitis treated with mepartricin by vaginal route only; like other polyenes, in fact, mepartricin is not absorbed and therefore is inactive by oral route.

Further researches have let to the development of SPA-S-222, a product completely water-soluble, containing mepartricin and a surfactant, sodium laurylsolfate, in a weight ratio of about 1 : 2.
After the microbiological and toxicological studies, SPA-S-222, in the form of gastro-resistant tablets of 50.000 Units each, has been assayed in some preliminary clinical trials on patients with cervico-vaginitis due to T.vaginalis. The investigations are still in progress; however, the data so far available and regarding more than 70 cases, are in good agreement with the results, to be reported here, obtained at the Viareggio Hospital in the only pilot trial, completed last March, already over.
This study included 10 patients (average age 36.8 ±2.3); the diagnosis was always ascertained by several microscopic and cultural examinations (May-Grünwald-Giemsa and Papanicolau staining, Kupferberg broth, Lash serum medium). The colposcopic examination performed after the Schiller test, and the degree of cytologic purity, were employed to assess the severity and extension of the inflammatory condition and to follow the relevant changes caused by the treatment. 2 tablets of SPA-S-222 were given every 12 hours for 3 consecutive days, excluding any other local or systemic therapy and advising the patients to avoid intercourse.
In order to assess both the immediate and the long-term efficacy of the treatment, all the abovementioned examinations were repeated on the 2nd and 3rd day of therapy, and then 1 and 30 days after its end.
These examinations demonstrated the very good effects displayed by SPA-S-222. In fact, in all the patients trichomonads were not detectable any more on the 2nd day and at the last follow-up, 1 month later, were still absent; at the same time, the cytologic examinations showed a degree I purity. The signs of inflammation were markedly reduced already on the 3rd day and, at the final follow-up, all the patients had a completely normal pattern.
In our opinion, these results allow to regard SPA-S-222, whose tolerance has always been good, as a drug of promising importance for the oral treatment of vaginal tri-

chomoniasis; this opinion is based on the number of examinations whose consistent changes have demonstrated the effectiveness of the product in all the cases of this small group and on the fact that, as mentioned before, the outcome of these cases is very similar to the first results, available at the present, obtained by other investigators.

REFERENCES

Bruzzese, T., Binda, I., Di Nardo, A., Ghielmetti, G., and Riva,M. (1972), Experientia, 28, 1515.

Bruzzese, T., Binda, I., Ghielmetti, G., and Notarianni, A.F. (1974), Farmaco Edizione Scientifica, 29, 331.

Danesino, V.,and Pellegrini, R. (1974), Pan Minerva Medica, 16, 181.

Mizuba, S., Muir, R.D., Johnson, F., Lee, K., and Ziecina, S. (1974), Development Industrial Microbiology, 15, 338.

Pellegrini, R. (1974), Pan Minerva Medica, 16, 123.

Perju,A., Boteanu, S., and Radulescu, G. (1975), Minerva Ginecologica (in press).

Pucci, G. and Ripa, S. (1973), Farmaco Edizione Pratica, 27, 235.

Ritzerfeld, W. (1972), Farmaco Edizione Scientifica, 27, 235.

Riva M. and Bianchi,C. (1973), Unpublished data.

Ruozi, P., Zara, C. and Pellegrini, R. (1974), Terapia Antibiotica Chemioterapia, 24, 14.

Simonetti, N., and Strippoli,V. (1971), Antibiotica, 9,5.

SHORT-TERM THERAPY OF UROGENITAL TRICHOMONIASIS WITH A NEW NITROIMIDAZOLE DERIVATIVE (ORNIDAZOLE/TIBERAL ROCHE)

S. Granitzka

Universitäts Frauenklinik
6 Frankfurt-am-Main
Theodor Stern Kai 7
West Germany

In our geographical latitudes trichomonas vaginalis infection of urogenital tract is the most frequent parasitosis. Trichomonas vaginalis today is principally taken for a pathogenous parasite (6). The infectivity of this parasite is also present in symptomeless latent trichomoniasis, so that therapy should be instituted in every case.

After the discovery of the trichomonacidal effect of metronidazole a decisive change took place in the treatment of trichomoniasis which so far had been insufficient (6). For the first time a substance active in trichomonas infection had been found that could be administered enterally or vaginally. Besides the good therapeutic effect the new substance was characterised by the absence of severe side-effects (6, 8, 9).

As a dosage guide the intake of two times 250 mg metronidazole per day for 6 days is recommended. During this period in woman additionally a vaginal tablet of 100 mg is inserted.

In every case, treatment of one or more partners is necessary to avoid reinfection.

The mean cure rate is indicated by most authors to be more than 90% (3, 4, 7, 8, 9, 10, 11).

Failures of therapy can be partially explained by

the nonobservance of precautions and by poor absorption or inactivation by pathogenic vaginal flora (1, 3).

A true metronidazole resistance has not, however been detected as yet (6).

During the last years therapy differing from the usual dose scheme has been carried out by several authors (2, 3, 11). In this, the treatment consists in the single administration of 2,0 g metronidazole.

The cure rate of this one-day therapy is found to be 82 - 86% compared to 93 - 96% with prolonged dosage (2, 3, 11).

In the meantime besides METRONIDAZOLE formula on the left side of the slide, new trichomonacidal substances were developed which differ in the lateral chain of the nitrogen-atom 1, like ORNIDAZOLE used by us, see formula on the right hand side of the slide, or TINIDAZOLE.

For the first time, we used ORNIDAZOLE as a one-day therapy in the treatment of trichomoniasis.
After 2-3 hours the blood level after a one-time oral application of 1,0 grams ORNIDAZOLE is 10,4 gamma/ml. The medical half life in plasma is 14,4 hours and this is 6 hours longer as compared to METRONIDAZOLE (5).

Up to now the cure rate in the treatment of trichomoniasis with the intake of 1,0 - 1,5 grams ORNIDAZOLE per day over a span of 5 - 7 days was at 98,3% (5).

We therefore attempted to try a short term therapy with this substance. Up to this point 103 reliable patients which we selected, were treated with ORNIDAZOLE at 2,0 grams during the one-day therapy. Pregnant women were excluded from this treatment.

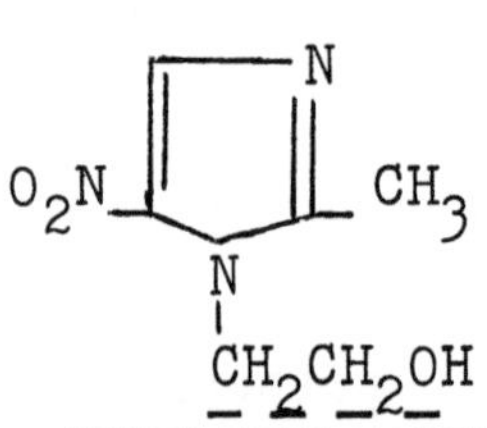

METRONIDAZOLE

1(-hydroxy-ethyl) - 2 methyl -5-nitroimidazole

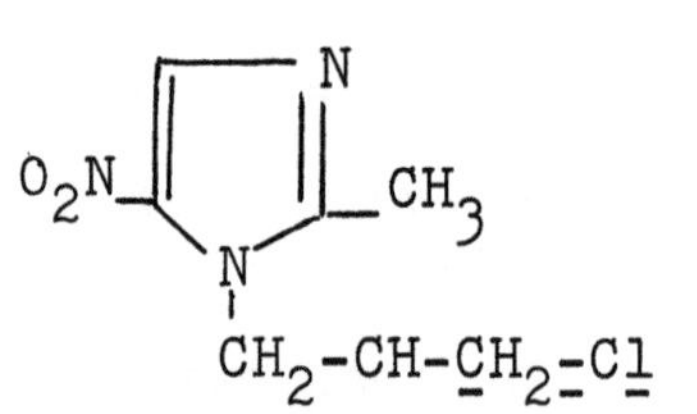

ORNIDAZOLE

(1-chlorhydroxypropyl)

The patients were on the average 38,2 years of age. Oral hormonal contraceptives were taken by 34,9% of the patients.

In the first series patients received 1,0 grams ORNIDAZOLE morning and evening given as two tablets of 500 mg. In addition, in the evening one vaginal tablet of 1,0 g was inserted. In the second series, patients took at noon after lunch 2,0 g ORNIDAZOLE given as four times 500 mg and in the evening one vaginal tablet of 1,0 g.

The treatment of the partner was, in the first series, a dosage of 500 mg per day for five days. In the second series, the partner also received a one-day therapy of a single dose of 2,0 g.

After gynecological investigations which confirmed the presence of trichomoniasis further checks which are summarized in the following slide were done: Macroscopic, parasitological and bacteriological investigations. In addition we performed cultural mycological investigations, which were undertaken before as well as 3 - 5 days after therapy and 4 - 6 weeks after start of therapy. In the second series, we performed during the last check additional cultural investigations on trichomonas.

For the diagnosis of trichomoniasis fresh preparation as well as cytological smear and urine sediment were used. In 103 patients 101 times trichomonas vaginalis was found in the fresh preparation. In two cases who exhibited no trichomonas in the fresh preparation the organisms were found in cytological smears as well as in the urine sediments. 64,0% of the cytological smear were positive for trichomonas.

EXAMINATION OF VAGINAL DISCHARGE
(before treatment 3 - 5 days and 4 - 6 weeks after treatment)

Macroscopic examination	Parasitological examination for trichomonas	Bacterial (culture) examination
Colour, consistency and smell	a) in Na-Cl solution b) in culture c) in cytology preparation d) in urine sediment	Mycological culture test

Urine sediment was positive in 67,9% of the cases. The therapeutic effect was judged by subjective statements of the patients, discharge, pruritus, pain and by objective gynecological examination including parasitological checks.

As you can see in the next slide, subjective freedom of complaints was achieved in 78,6% of the cases. 21,4% of the patients indicated subjective improvement of their complaints. Complete absence of improvement was not observed. More favourable than the clinical results was the parasitological effect. In two patients (1,94%) trichomonas could be found in the checks (slide).

The tolerance of ORNIDAZOLE was indicated good in 102 of the treated women. Only one patient had severe side-effects: vomiting, dizziness, mild impairment of vision.

18 patients (17,5%) complained of mild side-effects (tiredness). Additional laboratory investigations were done before and 3 - 5 days after the therapy.

One day therapy of urogenital trichomoniasis with ornidazole

103 cases

Clinical effect	No. patients	%
cured	81	78,6
improved	22	21,4
failure	0	0,0
Parasitological effect		
negativation	101	98,1
failure	2	1,9

Laboratory tests
(before treatment and 3 - 5 days after treatment)

Haematology	Urinanalysis	Blood chemistry
-Blood sedimentation rate	-Protein	-S.G.O.T.
-Red cell count	-Sugar	-S.G.P.T.
-Reticulocyte count	-Sediment	-Alkaline phosphatase
-White cell count	-Bacteriology	-Serum creatinine
-Neutrophyls, lymphocytes, eosinophyls, basophyls, monocytes	-Bacterial count/ml	
-Thrombocyte count		

33% of the patients showed a slight relative lymphocytosis and a relative reduction of the polymorph neutrophil leucocytes. The total number of the leucocyte counts did not show any significant changes. An inhibition of the hematopoietic system in the bone marrow is not evident from these results. As with metronidazole also with ORNIDAZOLE a check of the white blood-count will be advisable if therapy should be carried out with higher doses and for a longer period of time.

Effects on liver transaminases (GOT, GPT, AP) and on creatinine have not been observed. Also in urinary tests no pathological changes were seen.

Regarding the effect of ORNIDAZOLE on bacteria and fungi: In both organisms no significant activity could be established.

Summary

Derivatives of imidazole have proved effective in the treatment of trichomoniasis. For metronidazole as well as for ORNIDAZOLE which we used, the cure rate lies over 90%.

A one-day treatment principally seems to be possible with all imidazole derivatives having a trichomonacidal effect. With ORNIDAZOLE which we used we found in 103 thoroughly investigated patients two failures of therapy 1,94%. Cure rate was 98,06%.

Side-effects in the high dose one-day treatment with ORNIDAZOLE are mild. Thus, we can see the advantage of such a one-day one-shot therapy in the simple and therefore safe administration in urogenital trichomoniasis.

LITERATURE

1) Benazet, F., L. Guillaume: Lancet 982 (1971) 7731
2) Burslem, R.W.: Prescribers J. 13 (1973) 14
3) Csonka, G.W.: Brit. J. vener. Dis. 47 (1971) 456
4) Fegerl, H., E. Strell: Wien. med. Wschr. 120 (1970) 133
5) Fernex, M., F. Jeunet, R. Richle: 8th Intern. Congr. of Chemotherapy Athens 8th - 14th Sept. 1973
6) Korte, W.: Therapiewoche 23 (1973) 2040
7) Rodin, P., A.J. King, C.S. Nicol, J. Barrow: Brit. J. vener. Dis. 36 (1960) 147
8) Watt, L., R.F. Jennison: Brit.med.J. 1 (1962)276
9) Wiesner, H., K. Fink: Arzneimittel 9 (1966) 361
10) Wisdom, A.R., E.M.C. Dunlop: Brit. J. vener. Dis. 41 (1965) 90
11) Woodcock, K.R.: Brit. J. vener. Dis. 48 (1972) 65

RATIONALE FOR CONTROLLING THE EMERGENCE OF DRUG RESISTANCE

E.J.L. Lowbury

M.R.C. Unit, Birmingham Accident Hospital

Birmingham, U.K.

Nearly thirty years ago, in the halcyon days of the antibiotic era, an eminent virologist told me that, in his opinion, abtibiotics would have fallen into disuse by the end of the century because of the emergence of resistance, and we should then be focussing once again on the healthier pursuits of immunisation. His prophecy was no mere virologist's dig at the current luck of the bacteriologists; for within twenty years we saw the arival (familiar to us all) of an impressive line of antibiotics, to one after the other of which certain bacteria, originally all sensitive, acquired resistance. We saw also the selection of a multi-resistant 'hospital' flora, including resistant variants of staphylococci that were originally sensitive, and Gram-negative 'opportunist' bacilli that were naturally resistant but relatively unimportant until given the chance to emerge through the selective action of antibiotic thereapy - and other methods of treatment that rendered patients more susceptible to such infections. In the general community we saw the emergence of tubercle bacilli resistant to each of the effective chemotherapeutic agents and, more recently, gonococci resistant to penicillin and meningococci resistant to sulphonamides. In tropical countries the emergence in the community of resistant plasmodia created new difficulties in the control of malaria.

The problem however, is more complex than my virologist friend's prediction would suggest. To begin with, there are great differences between different species of bacteria in their tendency to acquire resistance to the same antibiotic; it is well known for example, that while most strains of *Staphylococcus aureus* in hospital - and many in the general community - are today resistant to benzyl penicillin, no penicillin-resistant strains of *Streptococcus pyogenes* have yet been found. There are great differences, too, between different antibiotics in respect of the ease with which the same organisms can acquire resistance to them; to streptomycin, for example, most bacteria readily acquire resistance, while to the related aminoglycoside, kanamycin, resistance emerges much less frequently. And there are other important factors; e.g. some pathogens, such as Clostridium tetani and Actinomyces israeli, rarely encounter antibiotics used in therapy against them, so the sbsence of resistant variants of these bacteria to common antibiotics may simple reflect a lack to opportunity for their selection; a similar reason may underlie the absence hitherto of vancomycin-resistant Staph. aureus - in this case because of the infrequent use of vancomycin.

At least four factors are important in the emergence of antibiotic-resistant infection - the microbe, the antibiotic, the patient and the environment. Mutation, resistance transfer, intrinsic resistance and, in some cases, possibly adaption are the contributing mechanisms of the microbe. Selective encouragement of resistant organisms is the contribution of the antibiotic. The patient adds an important contribution in discriminating against certain resistant variants which are less capable of colonising the human tissues and carrier sites than their sensitive parent strains (e.g. neomycin-resistant staphylococci can be produced with ease on habituation of sensitive strains in vitro, but clinically important neomycin-resistant Staph. aureus did not appear until many years after the introduction of this group of antibiotics). Lastly, the environment the familiar selection of resistant organisms in hospital where antibiotics are used creates the ironic situation that where the antibiotics are most needed the organisms are most likely to be resistant.

In planning our strategy for controlling the emergence of drug resistance we must consider these various factors and use our accumulated knowledge about each antibiotic and about each microbial species in relation to its parasitic, pathogenic and ecological properties. I shall give some examples, particularly from experience which my colleagues and I have had in a burns unit.

EMERGENCE AND CONTROL OF RESISTANCE IN A BURNS UNIT

Patients in burns units are notoriously apt to be infected with multi-resistant bacteria. The reasons are obvious: extensive burns usually become heavily colonised with bacteria acquired by cross infection from other patients, and antibiotics are often used for the treatment of such infections. While Strept. pyogenes, which is highly vulnerable to antibiotics, can usually be well controlled, multi-resistant Staph. aureus and Gram-negative bacilli tend to predominate. During a period since 1950 we have seen the emergence of Staph. aureus resistant to several new antibiotics. In 1954 erythromycin-resistant strains appeared, and their incidence increased in proportion to the amount of the antibiotic in use, at the same time as erythromycin-resistant staphylococci were becoming predominant, there was a reduction in the frequency of isolation of tetracycline-resistant Staph. aureus, apparently due to the replacement of tetracycline by erythromycin as the antibiotic used for routine treatment of infection with Strept. pyogenes (Figure 1). This change in routine treatment for streptococcal infection was prompted by the emergence of tetracycline-resistant Strept. pyogenes, which in 1956 reached the alarming proportion of 60% of isolates, including different serotypes. Stopping the use of tetracycline for treatment of streptococcal infections led to a gradual decline and eventual cessation of tetracycline-resistant streptococcal infections in the Unit, though tetracycline-resistant Strept. pyogenes soon became common in many centres. (2,3,4).

For 9 years we used neomycin without any emergence of resistant Staph. aueus and were inclined to think this would never happen; but in 1963 resistant strains appeared, as they had appeared in some other hospitals both in the U.S.A. and in Britain, and within months they became the predominant staphylococcus in our Burns Unit (5). When we stopped using neomycin and kanamycin in June 1963, these strains declined and disappeared - though later they turned up again.

Other antibiotics against which resistance has emerged in relation to antibiotic usage are methicillin and its homologues; trimethoprim (6); and recently (associated with the successful topical use of silver sulphadiazine in extensive burns) sulphonamides (18). (See Figure 2). Fucidin-resistance emerged in relation to the use of this agent in individual patients, - the same phage type appearing in a burn at first sensitive and then, after treatment of the patient with fucidin, resistant to the antibiotic (7). When fucidin therapy was stopped, the fucidin-resistant strains quickly disappeared (Figure 3). Something similar happened with novobiocin. With that antibiotic an effort was made to check the emergence of resistance by combined use of novobiocin and erythromycin, but though this may have delayed the emergence of novobiocin-resistant strains, it did not prevent their appearance at a later stage (8).

Three factors contribute to the disappearance of resistant strains from a ward: 1) the discharge of patients carrying resistant organisms; 2) the displacement of resistant by sensitive organisms when selection pressure favouring the former is removed; 3) the reversion to sensitivity of some resistant strains; the last is true especially of resistance determined by R factors, though transferable resistance may become stabilised. In the early period of our study, unlinked resistance to a new antibiotic emerging in sensitive strains (or in strains resistant only to penicillin) was selectively encouraged by use of the new antibiotic, and tended to disappear when

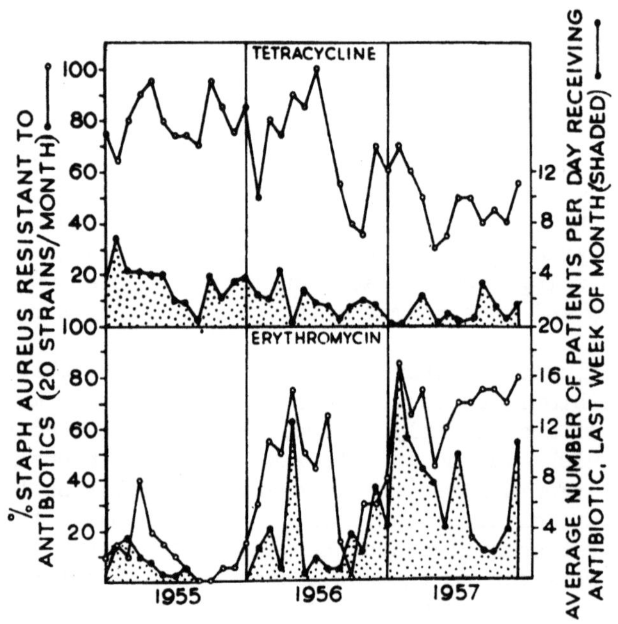

Fig. 1. A monthly record for a period of three years showing the association of antibiotic resistance with use of the antibiotics in a burns unit.

use of the antibiotic was stopped, as I have illustrated. There was evidence, too, that resistance to one antibiotic - e.g. fucidin - was associated with a higher incidence of sensitivity to other antibiotics - e.g. tetracycline and erythromycin (7).

But more recently many hospital strains have been shown to have linked multiple resistance to several antibiotics, so that the use of any of these antibiotics may exert a selection pressure which will maintain the presence of strains resistant to antibiotics that are not being used.

An interesting example of this phenomenon occurred in our Unit several years ago when an R factor (RP_1) which determined linked resistance to tetracycline, kanamycin, carbenicillin, ampicillin and cephaloridine suddenly appeared (9). It was detected first through the emergence of *Ps. aeruginosa* highly resistant to carbencillin. Richmond and his colleagues (10) at Bristol and Fullbrook and his colleagues (11) at Beecham Research Laboratories showed that these strains carried an R factor transferable between *Ps. aeruginosa* and various species of Enterobacteria, and we found that such resistance transfer could occur in burns of mice (12). We tried to eliminate the organism from the Burns Unit by banning the use of carbenicillin, and this led to the elimination of highly carbenicillin-resistant *Ps. aeruginosa*, which was not surprising, because carbenicillin was the only one of the antibiotics in the linked resistance pattern determined by this R factor which was active against *Ps. aeruginosa*, and could therefore exert a selection pressure in favour of strains of *Ps. aeruginosa* carrying the R factor. But when we decided that it was safe to use carbenicillin again, and did so in two patients, there was an almost immediate emergence of carbenicillin-resistant *Ps. aeruginosa* in the burns of these patients - apparently due to transfer of the R factor from Enterobacteria in the same burns; the Enterobacteria, unlike *Ps. aeruginosa*, had remained a reservoir of resistance determined by the R factor, because the use of the tracycline, kanamycin and ampicillin (to which many Enterobacteria are sensitive) exerted a selection pressure in faviour of resistant Klebsiella, Proteus etc. When, in 1972, one virtually banned the use of all five antibiotics in the resistance pattern, Enterobacteria as well as *Ps. aeruginosa* carrying the R factor disappeared from the Unit, and have not returned.

RECOMMENDATIONS

Our experience and that of others has suggested ways in which the emergence of antibiotic resistance can be curbed. The broad strategy is economy in the use of antibiotics, which means not using antibiotics for all infections (including some minor infections which might be helped but which should resolve without chemotherapy). The tactics require consideration of the peculiarities of organisms, antibiotics, patients and the environment. Against the prophets of doom

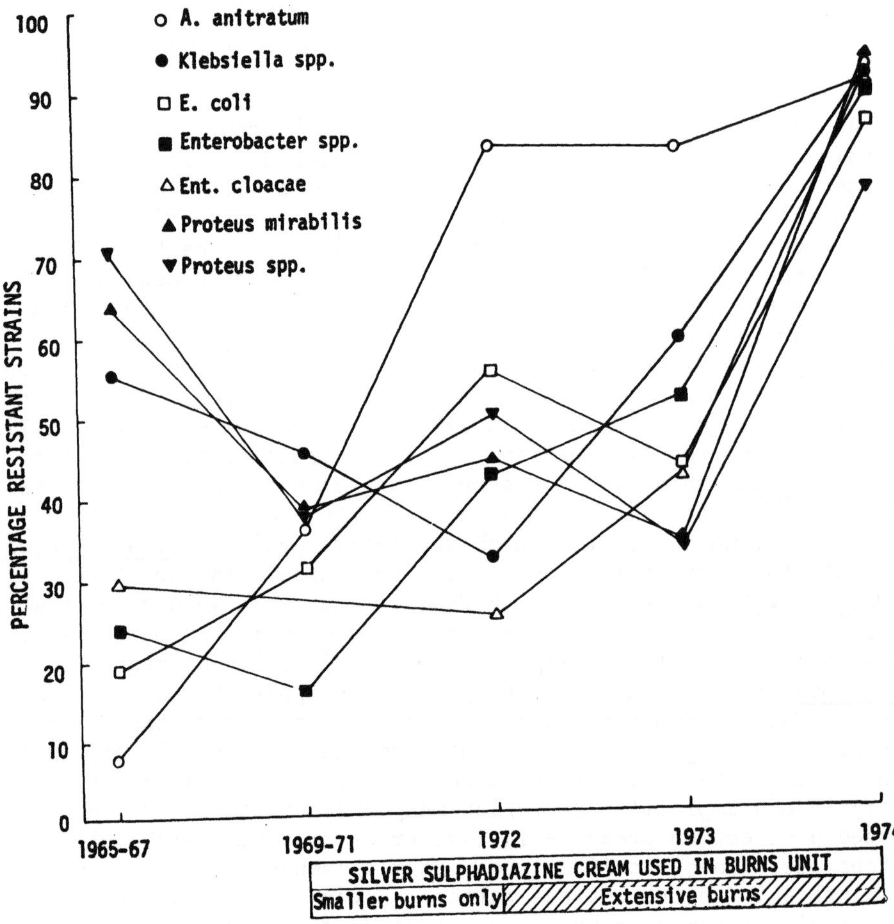

Fig. 2. Increase in Sulphadiazine-Resistant Gram Negative Bacilli

we have good evidence to show than an antibiotic policy based on scientific and clinical considerations can actually reverse the trend towards resistance. I have given an example from a burns unit; two other striking examples are (1) the finding reported by Bulger and Sherris (14) in Seattle, of a reduced incidence of resistance and of infection in a general hospital where a policy of reduced, rational chemotherapy had been adopted, and (2) the findings of Price and Sleigh (15) in a neurosurgery unit where endemic multi-resistant Klebsiella infection was brought to an end by severely limiting the use of antibiotics.

A framework for an antibiotic policy (16) can be presented in the form of a table (see Table 1) showing three categories of availability. 1) relatively unrestricted:i.e. 'safe' antibiotics long in common use, against which there has been little or no increase in resistance in recent times; 2) relatively restricted: i.e. useful antibiotics against which resistance emerges readily, or which carry some hazards of toxicity; and 3) reserved: i.e., valuable antibiotics for severe infections, to which the bacteria causing such infections are still always or virtually always senstivie, to be kept available for use when no other treatment is likely to help; also, valuable antibiotics which have lost their usefulness because of the emergence of resistance or which must not be used until an R factor that they carry has been eliminated from the ward (see example, already discussed above, of R favtor RP_1 determining carbenicillin-resistance of Ps. aeruginosa) The antibiotics that should be placed in these categories will vary with the current incidence of resistance reported (preferably in regular - e.g. quarterly - reports) by the Microbiology Laboratory. E.g. during the time when the R factor RP_1 was endemic in the Burns Unit of the Birmingham Accident Hospital, tetracycline, kanamycin, carbenicillin, ampicillin and cephaloridine were on the reserve list in that hospital (see Table 2). The policy is backed up by tactful advice to clinicians from an expert on the control of infections today.

General principles and recommendations for controlling the emergence of antibiotic-resistant bacteria may be summarised as follows (see also Lowbury and Ayliffe (17)):-

(1) Antiobiotics should be used only where necessary and where likely to be effective; this requires a knowledge of the natural history of the disease and of the sensitivity of the pathogen - or (until and unless that can be known) of its probable sensitivity.
(2) Narrow range antibiotics should be used when broad spectrum antibiotics are not necessary.
(3) Prophylactic use of antibiotics should be restricted to a limited range of specific indictions - i.e. when there is danger in not using them, such as the risk of gas gangrene in operations involving muscle of ischaemic legs; courses of prophylaxis against surgical infection should be very short.

TABLE 1: ANTIBIOTIC POLICIES: CATEGORIES OF AVAILABILITY

Category of Availability	Reason for Allocation
1. relatively UNRESTRICTED	Long in common use Little change in resistance patterns Relatively non toxic Inexpensive.
2. relatively RESTRICTED, (but on general prescription)	Resistance increasing, readily acquired; or because toxic.
3. RESERVED for severe infections, when other antibiotics inadequate (on consultant's signature only)	a) to preserve activity of valuable antibiotic; b) to restore activity when most strains resistant. also because toxic or expensive.

TABLE 2: ANTIBIOTIC POLICIES: CATEGORIES IN RELATION TO RESISTANCE (R) OF GRAM-NEGATIVE BACILLI

Examples from two hospitals, 1971.

Antiobiotic	B.A. Hospital (Burns Unit)			D.R. Hospital (General)		
	% strains R		Category	% strains R		Category
	Proteus sp.	Klebsiella sp.		Proteus sp.	Klebsiella sp.	
Ampicillin	53	76	3	24	98	2
Kanamycin	71	56	3	4	9	2
Streptomycin	11	30	2	36	38	2
Tetracycline	94	72	3	88	46	1
Gentamicin	0.4	5	3	-	-	3
Sulphonamides	38	46	1	17	41	1

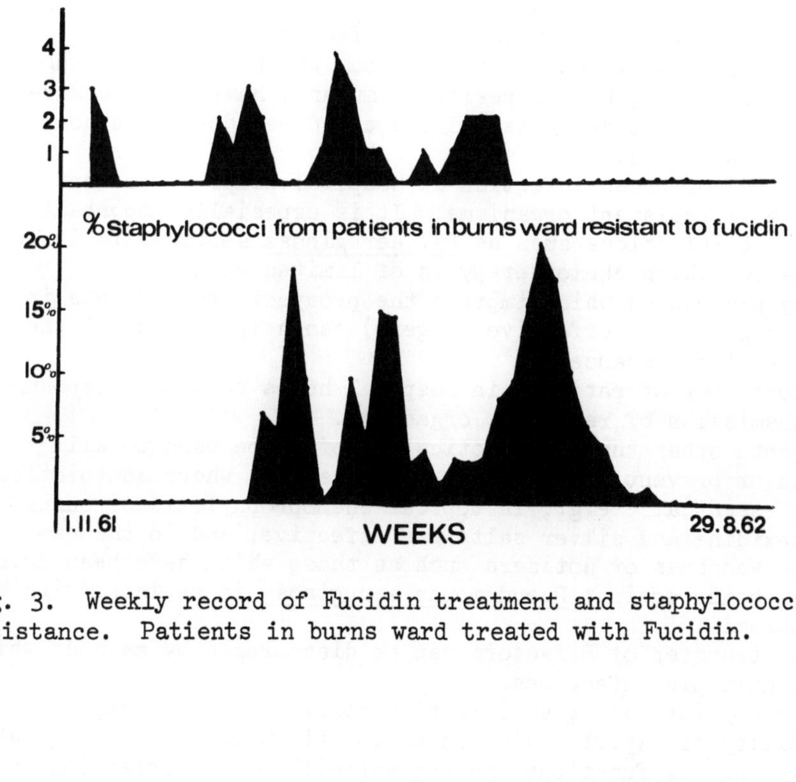

Fig. 3. Weekly record of Fucidin treatment and staphylococcial resistance. Patients in burns ward treated with Fucidin.

(4). Antibiotics used in treatment of infection should be given at full dosage for the minimum period required to achieve elimination or pathogens. Combined use of two antibiotics that exercise synergy may be indicated.
(5) Preference should be given to antibiotics against which resistance rarely or never emerges (e.g., a penicillin or a macrolide rather than tetracycline against Strept. pyogenes.)
(6) In the treatment of tuberculosis, combined therapy with two unrelated compatible antibiotics has proved effective; it depends on the principle that mutants resistant to both antibiotics will rarely emerge. The slow growth rate of tubercle bacilli is an asset in this context. The method has been found less effective in the control of surgical infection, and is irrelevant to the emergence of multi-resistance due to acquisition of an R factor.
(7) The use of antibiotics in rotation, which change of drug after a short period (i.e., before resistant mutants have had a chance to appear), is theoretically useful and could be adopted in hospital antibiotic policies.
(8) Control of cross-infection in hospital helps to prevent the emergence of resistant organisms. It is especially important to try and prevent infections such as Ps. aeruginosa septicaemia in burned patients for which chemotherapy is of limited value).
(9) Any procedures which improve the prospects for success in chemotherapy (e.g., effective surgery) can help to control the emergence of resistance.
(10) Short stay of patients in hospital helps to reduce exposure to and transmission of resistant organisms.
(11) Agents other than antibiotics can often be used to kill bacteria or prevent their growth in situations where antibiotics are not essential - e.g., in topical chemoprophylaxis of burns, where chlorthexidine and silver salts are effective, and in the use of specific vaccines or antisera such as those which have been developed for protection against Pseudomonas aeruginosa in patients with burns and leukaemia.
(12) The transfer of R factors can be discouraged by methods which prevent multiple infections.
(13) The appointment of an infection control team in hospitals and the availability of expert advice on antibiotic therapy is the greatest value; among its functions are the surveillance of infection and of antibiotic resistance patterns.
(14) Education and instruction of doctors on the use of antibiotics in hospital and in general practice should be increased.
(15) The search for new antibiotics must continue; though we must expect 'diminishing returns', promising new agents are still being found, and are needed.

Such a scheme must be flexible, and must be changed in relation to changed sensitivity patterns and new knowledge. The personal factors - supervision, vigilance, good rapport of laboratory and clinical staff - are of prime importance. In attempting to control

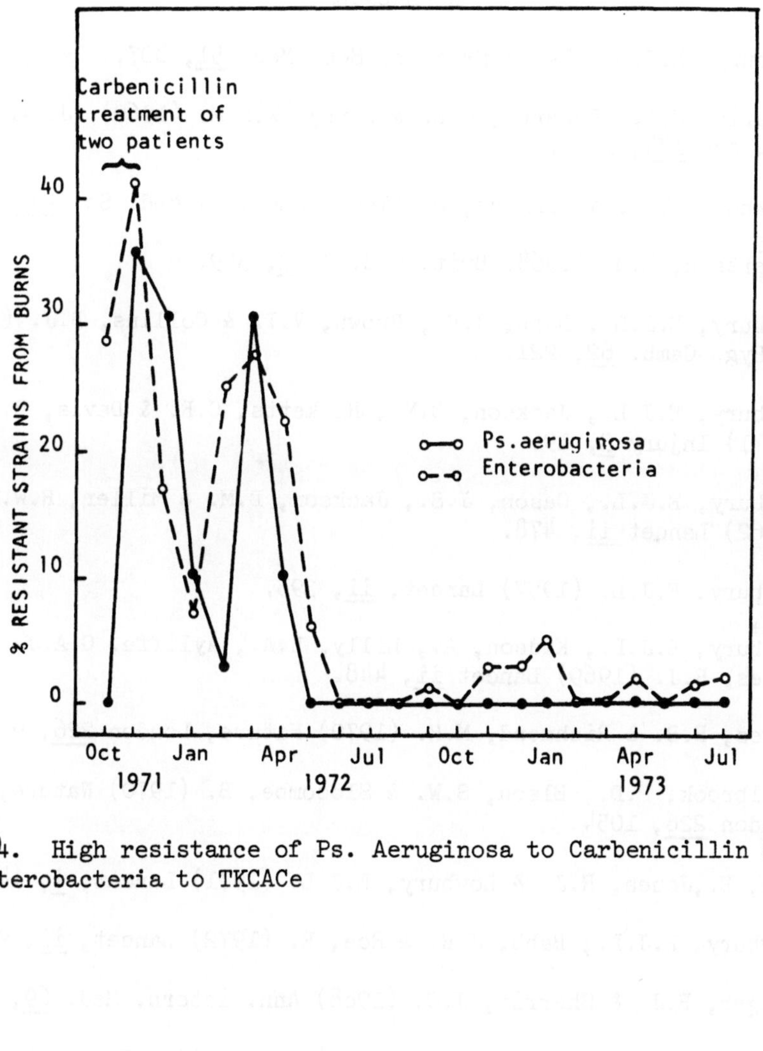

Fig. 4. High resistance of Ps. Aeruginosa to Carbenicillin and of Enterobacteria to TKCACe

the emergence of antibiotic resistant organisms, we must use our wits against evolutionary forces that help the microbial pathogens, and in this battle the microbes, which cannot evade the dictates of their genetic determinants, have a certain advantage over members of hospital staff: at least we know that our efforts can in some measure, succeed, and we have no reason to assume that, by the end of the century, we shall be looking back remorsefully to the antibiotic era as a short and glorious episode in man's continuing war against disease.

REFERENCES

1. Lowbury, E.J.L. (1958) Proc. r. Soc. Med. 51, 807.

2. Kaharic, H.A., Roberts, C.E. & Kirby, W.M.M. (1960). J. Amer. Med. Ass 174, 1779.

3. Eickhoff, T.C. & Finland, M. (1965) Amer. J. Med. Sci 249, 261.

4. Robertson, M.H. (1968) Brit. med. J. 3, 349.

5. Lowbury, E.J.L., Babb, J.R., Brown, V.I. & Collins, B.J. (1964) J. Hyg. Camb. 62, 221.

6. Lowbury, E.J.L., Jackson, D.M., Ricketts, C.R. & Davis, B. (1971) Injury 3, 19.

7. Lowbury, E.J.L., Cason, J.S., Jackson, D.M. & Miller, R.W.S. (1962) Lancet ii, 478.

8. Lowbury, E.J.L. (1957) Lancet, ii, 395.

9. Lowbury, E.J.L., Kidson, A., Lilly, H.A., Ayliffe, G.A.J. & Jones, R.J. (1969) Lancet ii, 448.

10. Sykes, R.B. & Richmond, M.H. (1970) Nature, London 226, 952.

11. Fullbrook, P.D., Elson, S.W. & Slocombe, B. (1970) Nature, London 226, 1054.

12. Roe, E.,Jones, R.J. & Lowbury, E.J.L. (1971) Lancet, i, 149.

13. Lowbury, E.J.L., Babb, J.R. & Roe, E. (1972) Lancet, ii, 941.

14. Bulger, R.J. & Sherris, J.C. (1968) Ann. intern. Med. 69, 1099.

15. Price, D.J.E. & Sleigh, J.D. (1970) Lancet ii, 1213.

16. Lowbury, E.J.L., Ayliffe, G.A.J., Geddes, A.G. & Williams, J.D. (Editors) Control of Hospital Infection: A Practical Handbook (1975) Chapman & Hall, London.

17. Lowbury, E.J.L., & Ayliffe, G.A.J. (1974) Drug Resistance in Antimicrobial Therapy. Charles C. Thomas, Springfield, Illinois.

18. Bridges, K. & Lowbury, E.J.L. (1975) in preparation.

MECHANISM OF THE INHIBITORY EFFECT OF OXACILLIN ON THE BETA-LACTAMASE OF BACILLUS CEREUS

J. Erdei, F. Hernádi, Cs. Jászberényi, T. Gunda, and G. Szabó

Biological Institute, Pharmacological Institute
Medical University of Debrecen
4012 Debrecen, Hungary

In the last decade many studies have been carried out to find synthetic and natural substances which can prevent inactivation of penicillins and cephalosporins by beta-lactamase of pathogenic microorganisms.

The inhibitory effect of semisynthetic penicillins among them the isoxazolyl penicillins: oxacillin and cloxacillin has been demonstrated by Gourevitch et al. /1/ and Smith et al. /2/. Citri and Garber /3/ have found the inhibitory action of the oxacillin to be competetive by its nature.

In our work the inhibitory effect of oxacillin was studied in detail. We investigated whether one or more structural parts of the oxacillin molecule are responsible for the inhibitory action on the hydrolytic enzyme.

MATERIALS AND METHODS

A commercially available B.cereus beta-lactamase Neutrapen /Riker Lab. Loughborough, England/ was used in all experiments. The concentrated enzyme solution was diluted in 0.08 M phosphate buffer. Test tubes and vessels were silicon coated. Enzyme activity was measured with the method of O'Callaghan et al. /4/. Cephaloridine /Ceporin, Glaxo Lab. Ltd. Greenford, England/ was used as substrate. Photometric measurements were carried out with a Unicam SP 1800 spectrophotometer. Ki values were calculated with the method of Lineweaver and Burk, as cited by Webb /5/. Substances tested for inhibitory capacity: Oxacillin /Chinoin Pharmaceutical Works, Hungary/, oxacillinsulfoxyde, oxacillinsulfon, 3,5-dimethylisoxazolylpenicillin, 6-APA, penicillanic acid, different thiazolidine derivatives, 3,5-dimethyloxazol, 3-phenyl-5-methylisoxazole, 3-phenyl-5-methylisoxazole-4-carboxylic acid, and its derivatives, substituted by Cl, Br an I in position 4,3-phenyl-5-methylisoxazole-4-carboxamide, 3-phenyl-5-methylisoxazole-4-carboxamidoacetic acid, and 7-//β-phenyl-5-methylisoxazole-4-carboxamido/-desacetoxycephalosporanic acid, a cephem analogue of oxacillin. Substances listed above were synthesized in the Institute of Organic Chemistry, Kossuth Lajos University, Debrecen.

RESULTS

Among the tested compounds /fig. 1, 2, 3, 4/ those that have inhibitory capacity contain the penam structure as well. The penicillanic acid and the oxacillin analogue of the 7-aminodesacetoxy-cephalosporanic acid had no inhibitory activity. Neither the oxacillinsulfoxide nor the oxacilsulfon were inhibitory even up to 10^{-2} M concentration.

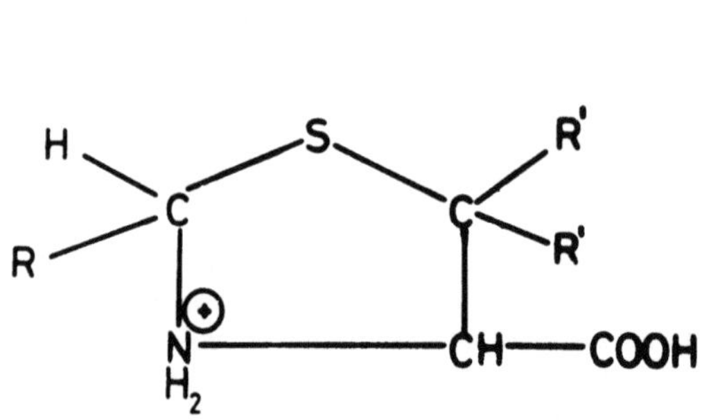

Fig. 1.

R = H R' = H
R = H R' = CH_3

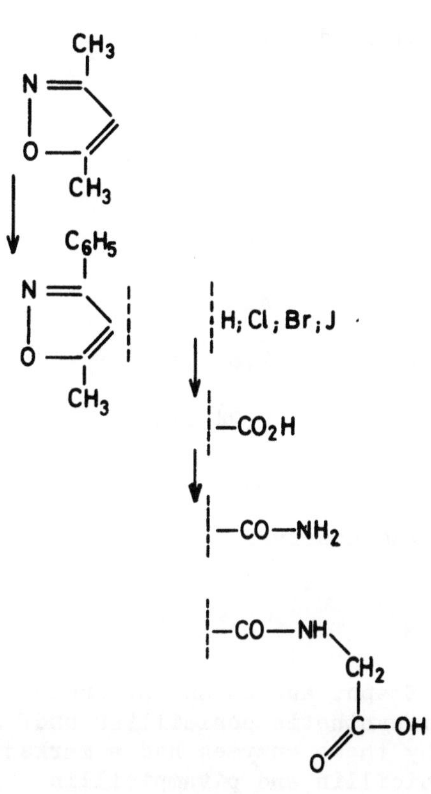

Fig. 2.

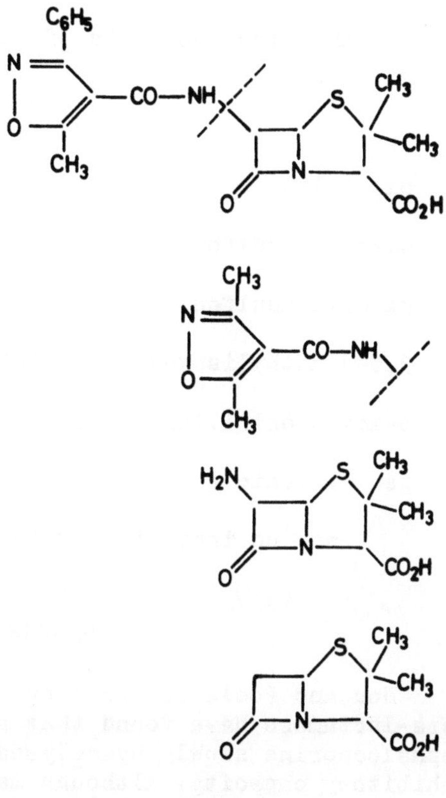

Fig. 3.

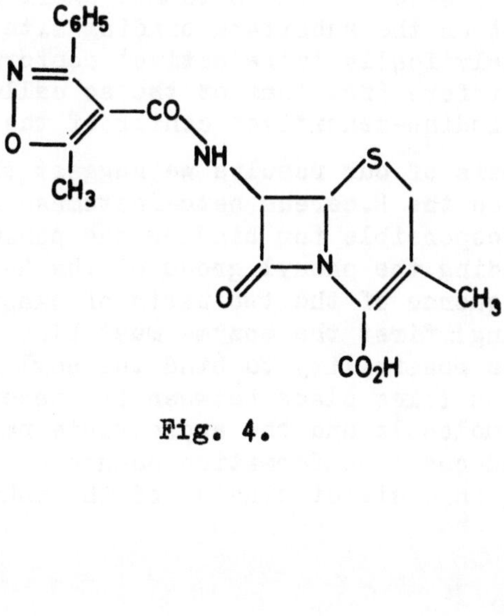

Fig. 4.

Table I

Inhibitor constants of oxacillin derivatives

	Ki / M /
oxacillin	8,8 $.10^{-5}$
oxacillinsulfoxyde	ni
oxacillinsulfon	ni
3,5-dimethylisoxazolylpenicillin	2,0 $.10^{-4}$
6-aminopenicillanic acid	2,24 $.10^{-4}$
penicillanic acid	ni

ni: no inhibitory effect was observed

DISCUSSION

Hou and Poole /6/ working on Staph. aureus and B.cereus beta-lactamase have found that semisynthetic penicillins and cephalosporins slowly hydrolysed by these enzymes had a marked inhibitory capacity. Although methicillin and pivampicillin were resistant to the hydrolytic action of these enzymes they had very low if any inhibitory action. On these basis the theory cited above /6/ seems not to be completely acceptable. Zyk and Citri /7/ showed that penicillins which are good substrates for B.cereus beta-lactamase exert a conformation changing effect on the substrate binding site of the enzyme, inducing a catalytically 'more active' conformation. The effect of oxacillin differs from that of the so called good substrates. It opens the 'iodine-sensitive' center of the enzyme molecule.

On the basis of our results we suggest that there are two binding sites on the B.cereus beta-lactamase for the inhibitor. The first is responsible for binding the penam structure, the second for binding the phenyl group of the N-acyl substituent. The binding sequence of the two parts of oxacillin molecule is the following: first the enzyme must bind the penam nucleus. Then it has the possibility to bind the acyl substituent. When this interaction takes place between the second binding site of the enzyme molecule and the appropriate part of the inhibitor, it induces a conformation change of the enzyme molecule resulting in a strict binding of the inhibitor to the enzyme --changing the conformation of the catalitic //penam-binding// site-- and a decreased catalitic activity. It seems to be realistic because no inhibitory activity was observed with any compound containing the whole acyl part of oxacillin molecule.

Although there are data in the literature reporting marked differences in the aminoacid sequence of beta-lactamases of different origin, this proposed mechanism of the inhibitor action may serve as a basis to design new semisynthetic penicillins exerting inhibitory action on beta-lactamases of pathogenic microorganisms.

REFERENCES

1. Gourevitch, A., Pursiano, T.A., Lein, J.: Nature 195. 496 /1962//
2. Smith, J.T., Hamilton-Miller, J.M.T., Knox, R.: Nature 195. 1300 /1962/
3. Citri, N., Garberg, N.: J. Pharm. Pharmacol. 14. 784 /1962/
4. O'Callaghan, C.H., Muggleton, P.W., Ross, G.W.: Antimicr. Ag. Chemother. 1968. 57 //1969/
5. Webb, J.L.: Enzyme and Metabolic Inhibitors. AP.NY. 1963 Vol. I.
6. Hou, J.P., Poole, J.W.: Chemotherapy 19. 129 //1973//
7. Zyk, N., Citri, N.: BBA. 146, 219 /1967/

MODE OF ACTION OF CHEMOTHERAPEUTIC AGENTS AGAINST BACTERIA GROWING IN A CONTINUOUS FLOW CULTURE WITH SPECIAL REFERENCE TO THE ANTI-BACTERIAL EFFECT OF CEPHALOTHIN, ERYTHROMYCIN AND KANAMYCIN

Hirokazu Otaya,* Atsushi Ozawa,** and Jinsaku Goto **

* Shionogi & Co., Ltd., ** Second National Hospital

* 3-12, Doshomachi Higashi-ku, Osaka, Japan

Summary

The present results show that the antibacterial mode of action of Cephalothin, Erythromycin and Kanamycin to bacteria growing in a continuous flow culture, a dynamic environment which the physiological state is assumed to be constract was significantly different from each other. The results obtained here would provide a useful information on proper dosage schedule of chemotherapeutic agent for *in vivo* study.

In a case of setting a proper dosage schedule of chemotherapy, many characters of drug are considered, especially the value of MIC of drug to causative bacteria is a important factor as a target blood concentration of drug. However, *in vivo*, especially in a case of intermittent administration, a case without a target blood concentration of drug could not maintained, a clinical effect has been expected, this reason may be the comprehensive effect of antibacterial effect of drug and the resistance factors of living organism, that is immunoresistance, phagocytosis etc.

We, therefore, studied relationships between drug concentration and the multiplication of bacteria in a continuous flow culture (CF culture) which is thought to be an *in vivo* experimental model, that is a dynamic eviroment which the physiological state is assumed to be constant and to be free from stated above resistance factors of the living organism.

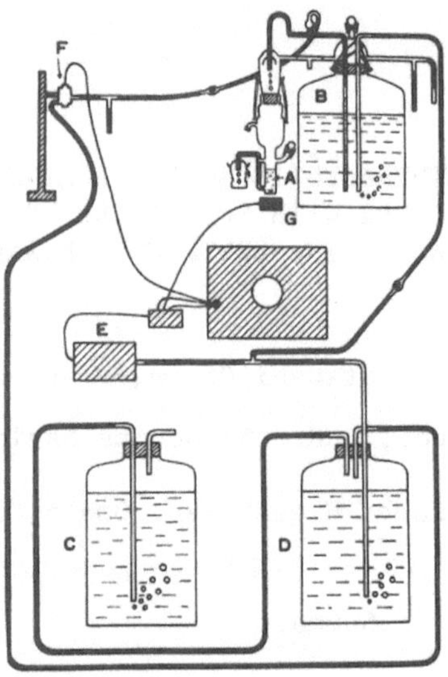

Fig. 1. Chemostat apparatus. A. Culture Tube. B. Reservoir. C and D Pressure regulaters. E. Airpump. F. Electromagnetic valve. G. Magnetic stirrer.

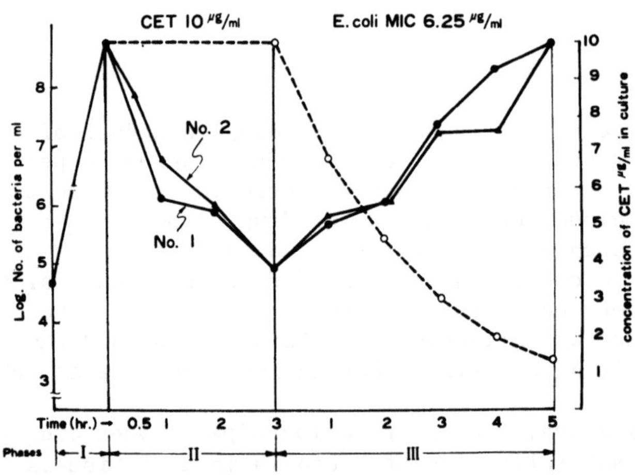

Fig. 2. Effect of 10 μg CET/ml on loss of viability and of decreasing CET concentrations on regrowth of an _E. coli_ strain with an MIC of 6.25 μg CET/ml. No.1 and No.2 represent different experiments.

Material and methods

Bacteria: Strains of Escherichia coli and Staphyloccus aureus isolated from clinical specimens were used.

Media and Antibiotics: Cephalothin (CET), Erythromycin (EM) and Kanamycin (KM) were added at the concentrations indicated in the text.

Methods: The chemostat apparatus shown Fig. 1 was used for CF culture.

Experimental conditions were as follows:

In this continuous flow culture method, Phase I can be assumed to incicate the growth of bacteria in foci of infection in absence of antibiotic, the Phase II to indicate the growth of bacteria in foci of infection in the presence of an antibiotic at 1 to 5 times of the MIC level and the Phase III to indicate the growth of bacteria in an infected host when antibiotic concentration was decreasing.

1) Phase I culture: Dilution rate is 33% per hour, and after 18 to 24 hrs at 37.C, the number of bacteria reached a maximum which was maintained thereafter. In this steady state equilibrium bacteria continued the logarithmic growth.

2) Phase II culture: After bacteria reached the steady state equilibrium, CET, EM or KM (concentration of 1.3 to 5 times of the MIC found by the oridinary stationary culture methods) was added both to the culture tube (A in Fig. 1) and to the culture fluid reservoir (B in Fig. 1). During 3 to 4 hrs incubation, samples were taken from the drop leaving the tube and number of bacteria were counted.

3) Phase III culture: Following Phase II, the culture fluid reservoir was exchanged with the other one containing the medium without a drug, and the incubation was further continued.

Relationship between the bacterial multiplication pattern and the change of antibiotic concentration in the culture tube was thus investigated by counting of the number of bacteria and measuring the drug concentration of the culture tube by cup method.

Results

In Phase II described in the previous section, there was no significant difference between the effect of CET at a concentration of 1.3 to 1.5 MIC against E. coli (Fig. 2) and that at 5 times of the MIC (Fig. 3). The cell count of from 4 to 5.10^8/ml before addition of CET decreased to 2 to 7.10^4/ml 3 hrs after CET addition (Fig. 2, 3).

The bacterial growth was observed the similar pattern, in

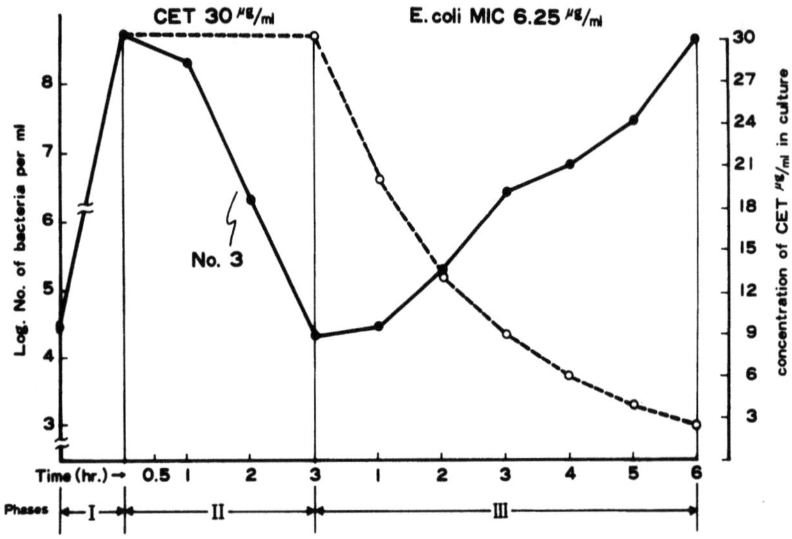

Fig. 3. Effect of 30 μg CET/ml on loss of viability and of decreasing CET concentrations on regrowth of an E. coli strain with an MIC of 6.25 μg CET/ml.

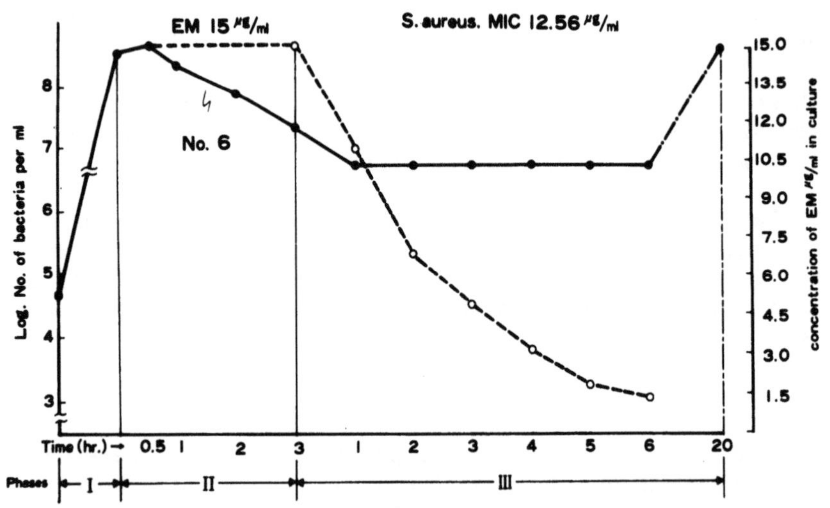

Fig. 4. Effect of 15 μg EM/ml on loss of viability and of decreasing EM concentrations on regrowth of a S. aureus strain with an MIC of 12.5 μg EM/ml.

Phase III, where CET concentration in the culture tube gradually decreased and when it was lower than the MIC regrowth of bacteria started rapidly.

In an experiment shown in Fig. 2, when CET was added at 1.3 to 1.5 times of MIC in Phase II, 4 to 5 hrs after the start of Phase III the cell count backed to the level (4.10^8/ml) at the begning of Phase II when CET was added at 5 times of MIC the recovery of the cell count in Phase III was slightly prolonged (Fig. 3).

In the case of S. aureus also as in the case of E. coli recovery of the bacteria number in Phase III was observed similar pattern.

In the studies on the effect of EM in CF culture of S. aureus, it was noted that EM at 1.2 times of the MIC gave different results from those observed with CET. In 3 to 4 hrs after additin of EM, the cell count in Phase II decreased only from 8.10^8/ml to 9.10^6/ml (Fig. 4). In addition regrowth of bacteria during Phase III was not related to the decrease of EM concentration in the culture tube, and even after complete disappearance of EM no cell increase was observed (Fig. 4).

In the studies on the effect of KM in CF culture of E. coli, it was noted that CET at 5 times and EM at 1.2 times of MIC gave different result from those observed with CET and EM. When KM was added at 3 times of the MIC, the initial cell count of 1.10^9/ml before addition of KM decreased to 4.10^5/ml in 4 hrs in Phase II (Fig. 5). However, there was a difference in Phase III, where KM concentration in the culture tube gradually decreased and regrowth of bacteria was slower than CET, after 5 hrs KM concentration was lower than the MIC, the cell count backed only to 1.10^6/ml (Fig. 5).

Conclusion

This is a model experiment which lies between in vitro and in vivo and we believe it offers a clue for analyzing the problems which have been unsolved by in vitro and in vivo experiments.

The information obtained from these experiments are summarized as follows:

1) The relationships CET concentrations and the multiplication of E. coli and S. aureus in a CF culture were observed correlation, that is when the CET concentration in culture was slightly higher than the MIC, the bacteria cell count was decreased, then the concentration was decreased than the MIC, the cell count increased rapidly. However, there was no significant difference between 5 times and 1.3 times MIC concentration in the culture.

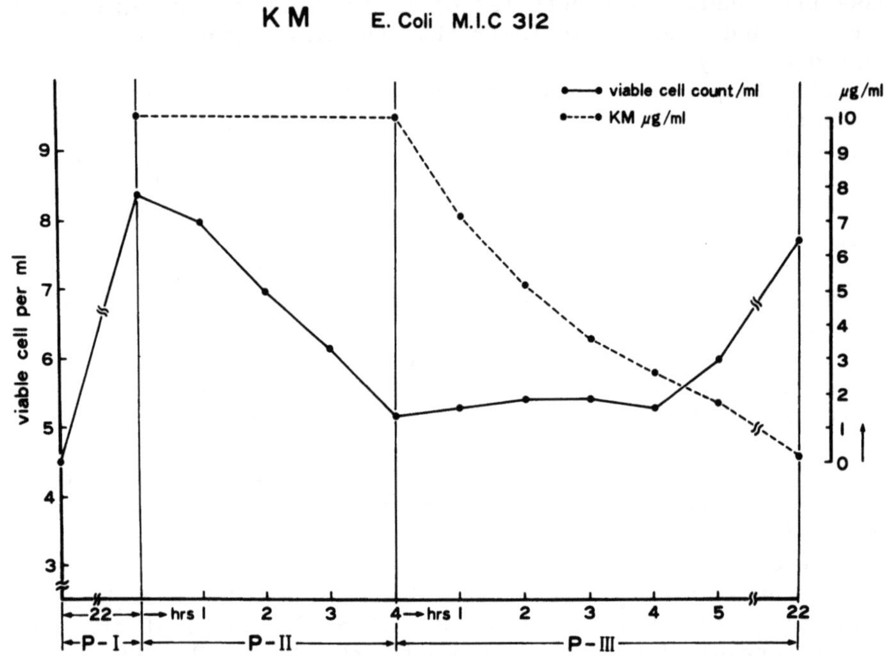

Fig. 5. Effect of 10 μg KM/ml on loss of viability and decreasing KM concentrations on growth of an E. coli strain with an MIC of 3.12 μg KM/ml.

2) In a case of EM, the relationships of EM concentration in the culture and regrowth of bacteria was not related and even after complete disappearance of EM no cell increase was observed.

3) In a case of KM, the relationship of KM concentration in the culture tube and regrowth of bacteria was observed the intermediate bacterial growth pattern, that is when KM concentration in the culture tube was 3 times MIC, the cell count was decreased similar CET, however when KM concentration in the culture tube gradually decreased and regrowth of bacteria was significant slower than CET. These difference will be mode of action of chemotherapeutic agents against bacteria growing in CF culture, that is CET act to bacterial cellwall, EM and KM to sensitive bacteria are highly affinity for their Ribosome. The defference between EM and KM will be caused by 50sRibosomal subunits and 30sRibosomal subunits respectively.

These results seems to be useful that more effective basic information for planning of a proper dosage schedule in preclinical studies.

MODE OF ACTION OF FLUCYTOSINE IN *ASPERGILLUS* SPECIES

Gerald Wagner and Smith Shadomy

Departments of Medicine and Microbiology, Medical College of Virginia, Virginia Commonwealth University, Richmond, Virginia, USA

SUMMARY

The mode of action of flucytosine (5-FC, 5-fluorocytosine) in *Aspergillus fumigatus* and *Aspergillus niger* was studied. Pyrimidines, purines and nucleosides were found to have an antagonistic effect on 5-FC activity and evidence for a common purine-pyrimidine uptake system was found. Only a small amount, 7 to 17 per cent, of 5-FC taken up by the aspergilli was incorporated in RNA and none was incorporated in DNA. DNA content of cells grown in the presence of 5-FC was from 4 to 10 times that of control cells. These data are not compatible with the scheme proposed for the mode of action of 5-FC in yeasts and it is suggested that 5-FC in the Aspergilli may inhibit DNA synthesis.

5-Fluorocytosine or 5-FC (Flucytosine; Ancobon, Roche Laboratories) has been reported to be effective in the treatment of human aspergillosis (Atkinson and Israel, 1973). However, in our laboratory mice experimentally infected with *Aspergillus fumigatus* did not respond favorably to treatment with this drug. In addition, *in vitro* determination of minimal inhibitory concentrations (MIC) of the drug for any one isolate of *Aspergillus* were seldom consistent on repeated trials even under standard test conditions. We have begun an examination of the mode of action of 5-FC in the aspergilli in an effort to explain these observations. Our results will be compared here with those obtained for the mode of action of 5-FC in *Candida albicans* (Polak and Scholer, 1973).

Initially, we examined the ability of exogenous purines, pyrimidines and some of their nucleosides to alter the MIC values for several strains of Aspergillus fumigatus and Aspergillus niger. The compounds being tested were added at a concentration of 1,000 μg/ml and the MIC of 5-FC determined by the agar dilution method. Pyrimidines and their nucleosides were found to antagonize 5-FC (Table 1). In the absence of any antagonist the MIC of 5-FC for Aspergillus fumigatus strain 4.6 was 400 μg/ml, addition of cytosine to the medium raised the MIC to a value of 4,000 μg/ml. There appear to be similar patterns of results. First, cytosine was uniformly antagonistic for 5-FC in the partially resistant strains of Aspergillus fumigatus. Second, uracil, uridine and cytosine were highly antagonistic for 5-FC with sensitive strains of Aspergillus fumigatus. Third, with sensitive strains of Aspergillus niger, deoxycytidine was found to be highly antagonistic for 5-FC.

Purines and some of their nucleosides also were antagonistic (Table 2). It is interesting to note that except for thymidine every pyrimidine and purine altered the MIC value of 5-FC for the aspergilli. The values obtained for Saccharomyces cerevisiae ATCC 9763 agree closely with those published by Polak and Scholer for the same organism (1973).

Three organisms were selected on the basis of the results of the reversal experiments for further studies. Aspergillus fumigatus strain 4.6 represented the strains of this species partially resistant to 5-FC with a MIC greater than 128 μg/ml. Aspergillus fumigatus strain 4.19 represented the susceptible strains of this species being inhibited by 0.5 μg/ml and Aspergillus niger strain 4.55 represented the susceptible strains of this particular species. The ability of purines, pyrimidines and their nucleosides to alter the total amount of radiolabeled 5-FC taken up by the selected strains of Aspergillus fumigatus and Aspergillus niger was studied in shaking broth cultures over 72 hr periods. In general, a recip-

Table 1. Antagonism of 5-Fluorocytosine by pyrimidines and some of their nucleosides

Organism		5-FC MIC, μg/ml	Cyt	Cyd	dCyd	Ura	Urd	Thyd
S. cerevisiae ATCC 9763		≤0.04	2[a]	0	0	0	0	0
A. fumigatus	4.6	400	1	-1	-1	>1	-1	0
" "	4.28	400	1	-1	-1	>1	0	0
" "	4.19	4.0	2	2	2	>3	>3	0
" "	4.33	4.0	3	1	1	3	2	0
" "	4.41	4.0	3	2	1	NG[b]	>3	1
A. niger	4.55	4.0	>3	>3	>3	>3	1	1
" "	3884	≤0.04	5	>5	5	>5	4	1

[a]Power of ten by which the MIC was altered [b]NG = no growth

Cyt = cytosine dCyd = deoxycytidine Urd = uridine

Cyd = cytidine Ura = uracil Thyd= thymidine

Table 2. Antagonism of 5-Fluorocytosine by purines and some of their nucleosides

Organism		5-FC MIC, μg/ml	Ade	Ades	Hypo	dGuas
S. cerevisiae ATCC 9763		≤0.04	2[a]	4	2	4
A. fumigatus	4.6	400	1	>1	1	>1
" "	4.28	400	1	>1	1	>1
" "	4.19	4.0	>3	>3	3	>3
" "	4.33	4.0	2	>3	3	>3
" "	4.41	4.0	3	>3	3	>3
A. niger	4.55	4.0	>3	3	>3	3
" "	3884	≤0.04	3	4	3	4

[a]Power of ten by which the MIC was altered

ade = adenine Hypo = hypoxanthine

ades = adenosine dGuas = deoxyguanosine

rocal relationship existed between the ability of a compound to alter the MIC value of 5-FC and the amount of labeled 5-FC taken up by the cells in the presence of that compound (Table 3).

We next studied the effects of incubation in the presence of 10 and 100 μg/ml of 5-FC on growth and nucleic acid content of the aspergilli. Cells were grown in liquid yeast nitrogen base supplemented with 0.5 per cent glucose with moderate shaking at 30°C. At selected time intervals the following determinations were made: cell or mycelial mass dry weight; RNA content as determined by the orcinol procedure; and, DNA content as determined by the diphenylamine procedure.

Table 3. Inhibition of uptake of 5-Fluorocytosine* purines, pyrimidines, and nucleosides

Compound	Percent Inhibition**		
	A. fumigatus 4.6	A. fumigatus 4.19	A. niger 4.55
5-FC MIC, μg/ml	400	4.0	4.0
Cytosine	95	98	94
Cytidine	0	80	0
Deoxycytidine	88	84	80
Uracil	90	97	83
Adenine	99	89	97
Hypoxanthine	99	98	83
Deoxyguanosine	91	71	56
Adenosine	40	0	90
Uridine	88	51	0
Thymidine	58	61	19

*5-Fluorocytosine-2-^{14}C

**Total uptake in absence of antagonist = 100 per cent

When grown in the absence of drug, the partially resistant *Aspergillus fumigatus* strain 4.6 attained maximum growth after 48 hrs of incubation at 30°C. Decreases in cell dry weight were seen after this time and were assumed to be due to autolysis of some hyphae. In the presence of both 10 and 100 µg/ml of 5-FC, there was an initial lag period, approximately 24 hrs long, after which growth resumed at near normal rates. Growth of *Aspergillus fumigatus* 4.19 which was susceptible to 5-FC, resembled that of the previous partially resistant organism. In the absence of drug, peak growth was reached at 64 hr. Again, in the presence of both concentrations of drug there was a prolonged lag period after which growth resumed at near normal rates. In the absence of 5-FC, growth of *Aspergillus niger* strain 4.55 attained maximum growth at 48 hr. However, unlike the strains of *Aspergillus fumigatus* tested, there was no growth in the presence of either concentration of drug during the 72 hr culture time.

Maximum RNA concentration in *Aspergillus fumigatus* strain 4.6 was observed at or just prior to the growth apex at 48 hrs and other than a shift in time, the presence of 5-FC did not greatly affect the RNA concentration. RNA concentrations in cells of *Aspergillus fumigatus* strain 4.19 exhibited a pattern similar to that seen in strain 4.6 with maximum RNA concentration occurring at 72 hrs. In general, cells grown in the presence of 5-FC had slightly higher concentrations of RNA than did the control cells.

The most dramatic effects were seen when the DNA content of the aspergilli were examined. When grown in the presence of 10 µg/ml of 5-FC, DNA content of *Aspergillus fumigatus* strain 4.6 reached a peak concentration approximately five times greater than the maximum DNA concentration in the control cells. Culturing in the presence of 100 µg/ml of drug caused DNA concentrations to increase approximately ten-fold over the control values. The same pattern was seen in *Aspergillus fumigatus* strain 4.19. In the presence of 5-FC, DNA concentrations were almost four times higher than the maximum concentration in the cells grown in the absence of drug.

When the same strains of the aspergilli are grown in the presence of radiolabeled 5-FC, 80 to 90 per cent of the labeled material disappeared from the growth medium over a 72 hr period. Preliminary studies indicated that none of the labeled compound was detected in DNA. Label was detected in RNA. However, on the basis of the total amount taken up by the cells, it is a relatively small quantity: 7 per cent in *A. fumigatus* strain 4.6 and *A. fumigatus* 4.19, and 17 per cent in *A. niger* strain 4.55. These results are quite different from those of Polak and Scholer (1973) who reported that approximately 50 per cent of the label taken up by *Candida albicans* was detected in the RNA fraction.

DISCUSSION

From our observations thus far, we would suggest the following: First, the antagonism studies indicate that the strains of *Aspergillus* may have a common relatively non-specific purine and pyrimidine uptake system. Such a system has been noted in *Neurospora crassa*. Second, the low percentages of labeled material incorporated into RNA indicate that this may not be the primary site of action. Third, inhibition of growth of the aspergilli may result from inhibition of DNA synthesis. This would occur by the metabolism of 5-FC to fluorodeoxyuridine monophosphate (FdUMP), a strong inhibitor of thymidylate synthetase. Resumption of growth may occur by enzyme alteration or simply when a significant amount of the 5-FC is bound up in FdUMP-enzyme complexes. Fourth, increased DNA concentrations seen in susceptible cells grown in the presence of 5-FC may be due to loss of metabolic control, oversynthesis, or to the stimulatory action of some fluorointermediate.

Experiments underway in our laboratory at this time have been designed to resolve these possibilities.

REFERENCES

Atkinson, W. and H.L. Israel (1973). Am. J. Med. 55, 496.
Polak, A. and Scholer, H.J. (1973). Path. Microbiol. 39, 334.

ACKNOWLEDGEMENT

This research was generously funded by a grant provided by the Brown Hazen Program of Research Corporation of America.

ACTION OF POLYENE MACROLIDE ANTIBIOTICS ON PROTOPLAST TYPE L-FORM OF E. COLI

I. Haupt, H. Thrum [x], E. Schuhmann, and R. Geuther
Zentralinstitut für Mikrobiologie und experimentelle Therapie der AdW der DDR
DDR - 69 Jena, Beuthenbergstraße 11
German Democratic Republic

Polyene macrolide antibiotics are known to exhibit biological activity against fungi and other eukarytic organisms, but not against bacteria These antibiotics cause permeability alterations in sensitive cells which lead to the loss of cytoplasmatic constituents culminating in cell death. The selective toxicity of polyene antibiotics is due to interaction with a unique component, a sterol, in the membranes of sensitive organisms. The natural resistance of bacteria on the other hand is generally explained by the absence of sterols in the bacterial cell membranes. In contrast to results of other investigators we found a real antibacterial activity with several polyene antibiotics by using the stable protoplast type L-form of E. coli W1655F$^+$ as a test organism.

Thirteen polyene macrolide antibiotics representing groups with 3 - 7 double bonds were tested. The L-form cells of E. coli were cultivated on nutrient broth extracted with ether. Growth was controlled photometrically by measurement of the extinktion at 640 nm. Antibiotics were added 2 hours after inoculation.

With respect to their antibacterial effects on stable L-form cells of E. coli the tested polyene antibiotics may be divided into three groups with decreasing activity.

Flavomycoin, flavofungin - two carbonyl conjugated polyenes -, mycotrienin, and hexaene 5001 P showed

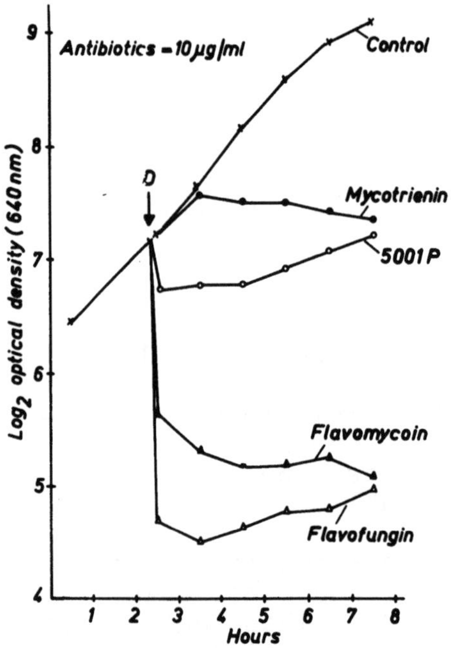

Fig. 1

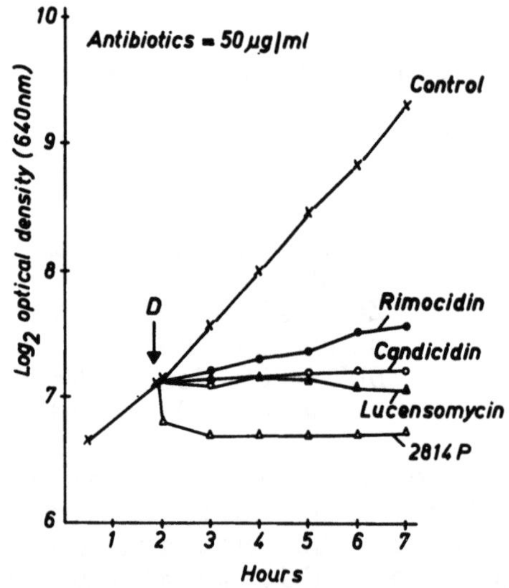

Fig. 2

Fig. 1 - 3
Effect of polyene antibiotics on the growth of the wall-less L-form cells of E. coli W1655F+.
D = drug application.

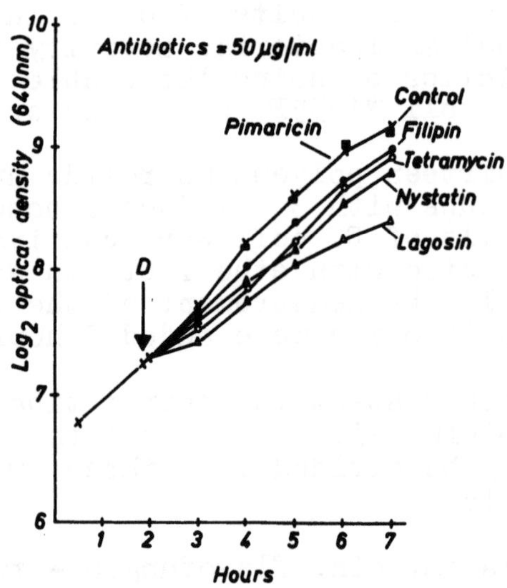

the strongest inhibition effect accompanied with lysis after addition of 10 µg/ml (Fig. 1). Among these compounds the two first mentioned antibiotics produced the most striking lytic effect. The second group including pentaene 2814 P, lucensomycin, rimocidin, and candicidin inhibited the growth of L-form cells in concentrations of 50 µg/ml to an extent of 80 - 100 % without cell lysis (Fig. 2). Members of the third group are nystatin, tetramycin, lagosin, and filipin. These antibiotics produced only slight inhibitions even at concentrations of 50 µg/ml (Fig. 3). Pimaricin showed no detectable effect.

Further experiments were done with the corresponding perhydro derivatives of eight polyene antibiotics. These compounds were prepared by catalytic hydrogenation of the original antibiotics in acetic acid using a Pt catalyst. As shown in figure 4 the perhydro derivatives of flavofungin, flavomycoin, hexaene 5001 P, and filipin had the strongest effects on the growth of the L-form cells. Generally these results correspond with those of the original antibiotics. Even low concentrations of 10 µg/ml of these compounds cause cell lysis. It is surprising that perhydrofilipin proved more effective than filipin itself.

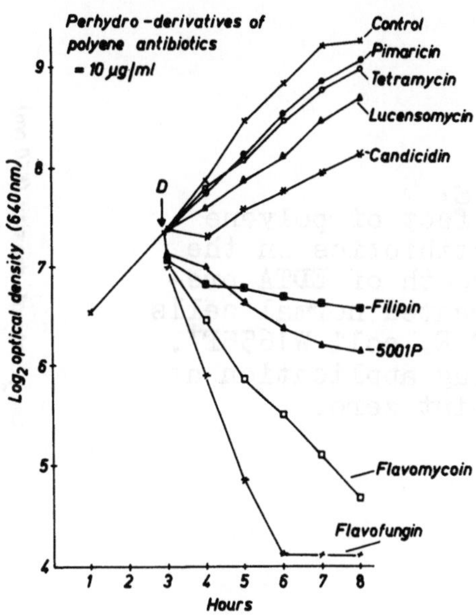

Fig. 4
Effect of perhydro derivatives of polyene antibiotics on the growth of the wall-less L-form cells of E. coli W1655F^{+}.
D = drug application.

On the other hand the perhydro derivatives of pimaricin, tetramycin, lucensomycin, and candicidin exhibited in the same concentrations only slight effects on the L-form cells. However, increasing amounts e. g. 25 µg/ml of perhydrolucensomycin and perhydrocandicidin, respectively, also produced cell lysis.

The presented results of antibacterial action of polyene macrolide antibiotics and their perhydro derivatives can hardly be interpreted on the basis of sterol hypothesis. L-form as well as normal rod cells of E. coli contain, in contrast to sensitive fungal cells, only traces of sterols. As shown in table 1 we estimated in both cell types comparable amounts of sterols. The main sterol component was identified gaschromatically as cholesterol. It is accompanied by traces of campesterol. Therefore, we conclude that the different behaviour, of normal rod form and L-form cells of E. coli W1655F+ against polyene antibiotics does not depend on differences in sterol content. It is fairly evident that the cell wall of E. coli functions as a penetration barrier.

This assumption is supported by our results with EDTA treated cells of E. coli W1655F+. We could show that

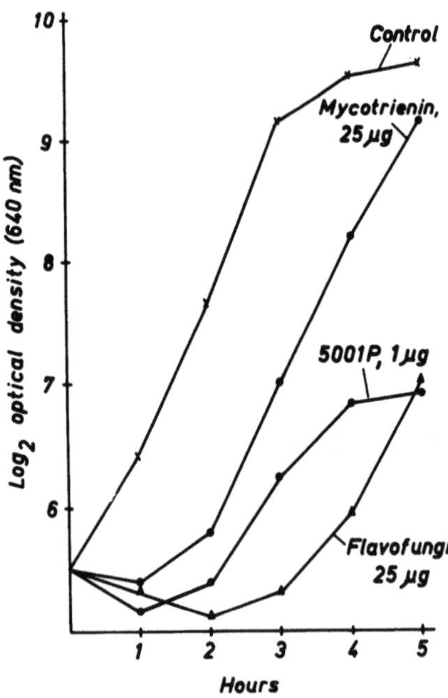

Fig. 5
Effect of polyene antibiotics on the growth of EDTA pretreated normal cells of E. coli W1655F+. Drug application at point zero.

Tab. 1. Sterol content in normal and L-form cells of E. coli W1655F^{+}

E. coli	Growth medium (μg sterol/experiment)	Dry weight g	Phospholipid-phosphate mg	Sterol content		
				μg	% of dry weight	% of phospholipidphosphate
L-form	Nutrient broth, extracted with ether (34,0)	1,3	24,5	12,5	0,00096	0,046
Normal form	Nutrient broth, extracted with ether (14,8)	1,3	13,4	6,2	0,00047	0,051
Normal form	Synthetic medium (0)	1,3	18,4	13,0	0,0010	0,071

E. coli cells can be made susceptible to polyene antibiotics by treatment with EDTA. This is demonstrated with mycotrienin, hexaene 5001 P and flavofungin. As shown in fig. 5 the sensitivity lasts for a limited time. Already one hour after EDTA treatment the cell wall defects are mostly repaired and bacteria regain insensitivity to the polyene antibiotics. Because the EDTA experiments were performed with E. coli cells grown on a sterol free synthetic medium sensibilisation induced by sterols can be excluded.

Therefore, we assume that E. coli contains target sites for polyene antibiotics and their perhydro derivatives, too. Considering the sensitivity of normal rod form and L-form cells of E. coli with extremely low sterol content the question arises again, whether sterols are really a necessary prerequisit for sensitivity against polyene antibiotics or not.

RELATIONSHIPS BETWEEN INHIBITION OF NUCLEIC ACIDS SYNTHESIS AND COMPETENCE IN B. subtilis

M.T. PEREZ-UREÑA, E. GARCIA, M. ESPINOSA, and A. PORTOLES

Inst. "Jaime Ferrán" of Microbiology.- C.S.I.C.

Joaquin Costa, 32 - Madrid, Spain

SUMMARY: The effect of four antibiotic inhibitors of nucleic acid synthesis on a stimulated competence system of B. subtilis have been studied. The most active inhibitory effect was exhibited by the drugs that inhibit the m-RNA synthesis by intercalating in the DNA (actinomycin D) or by inhibiting the RNA-polymerase (rifamycin). No effect could be observed when nalidixic acid was tested.

INTRODUCTION: Taking account of the different stages in bacterial transformation and transfection (Yasbin et al., 1972; Notani, 1974) as well as that of cell walls and membranes which represent severe barriers to the penetration of the exogenous DNA molecules, these biological systems offer several ways of elucidating the influence of some antibiotic actions at different molecular levels on the transfer and recombination of nucleic acids. Several aspects of the problem have been previously reported in bacterial transformation (Ephrati-Elizur, 1965; Ranhand and Lichstein, 1969; Nester 1964; Tomasz, 1970) and in transfection (Portolés et al. 1974; Garcia, 1974). Since, on the other hand, according to Trautner and Spatz (1973), a transfection system represents a way of studying the chemical alterations and their biological consequences on phage DNA preparations, in the present work we have become interested in determining -on a stimulating transfection system- the possible effect of four different antibiotic inhibitors of nucleic acid synthesis.

As it is known in B. subtilis SPP1 transfection several steps can be distinguished (Trautner and Spatz, 1973). So, in this system only those stages relative to the primary recombination and replication of phage DNA into the host cell can be affected. Furthermore, before the irreversible DNA binding started, possible interactions between exogenous DNA and antibiotic may occur altering the structure of the informative molecules. Consequently,three mode of actions inhibiting transfection could take place: (a) alteration of the DNA structure, (b) impairment of the template function of DNA (actinomycin, bleomycin) and (c) inhibition of enzymic processes in its synthesis (rifamycin, nalidixic acid).

MATERIALS AND METHODS: Bacteria, phage and media have been previously described (López et al., 1974).

Antibiotic and drug treatment: actinomycin D (AD) bleomycin (BL), rifamycin (RF) and nalidixic acid (NX) were used. After knowing the minimal inhibitory concentrations (MIC) (Portolés, 1960) and determining the work doses through the survival curves, drugs were added at the different times indicated in the results.

Preparation of phage DNA and transfection procedure. They were performed as usual in our laboratory (Portolés et al., 1973)

Protein synthesis was determined through ^{14}C-phenyl-alanine (^{14}C-PHE) incorporation in the bacteria.

Assay method: in this technique three main steps were followed: 1) Physiologically low competent (PLC) cells and stimulative metabolic supernatants (SMS) were obtained according to Joenje et al., (1972); 2) development of the stimulated competence of the PLC cells on SMS with and without antibiotics added at different intervals during the stimulation; and 3) sampling for transfection and protein synthesis control.

RESULTS AND DISCUSSION: On Fig. 1 survival percentages for the variable concentrations of the drugs are indicated. As can be observed RF was the most active bacterial inhibitor followed by AD, NX and BL without great differences between the last two. On this basis we selected the work doses that gave a survival of over 75%.

Normal conditions of the stimulative assays are depicted in Fig. 2. Clear differences during the ^{14}C-PHE incorporation appeared closely related to the increasing of the transfection frequencies produced by SMS.

In these conditions two kinds of inhibitory actions on nucleic acid synthesis (Gale et al., 1972) were tested. The first one included agents that impair the template function of the DNA (AD, BL) while the second one was constituted of drugs that inhibit enzymic processes involved in the DNA-synthesis (RF, NX) by different ways. The Figs. 3 and 4 show the variable actions of AD and BL respectively depending on the time of addition.

In both cases the inhibitory actions are detected in the first

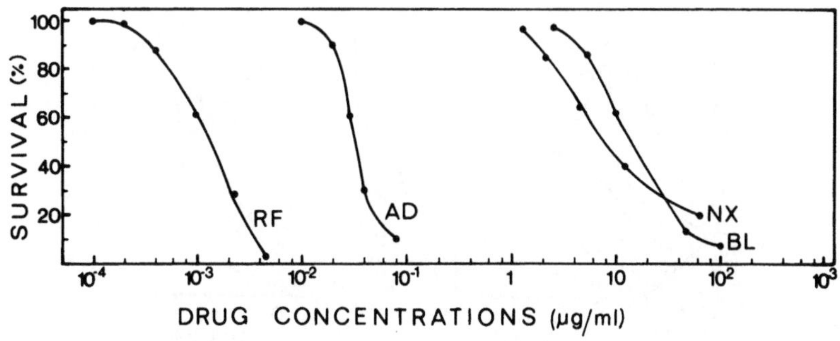

Fig. 1. Effect of the Different Antibiotics Acting on Nucleic Acid Synthesis on PLC Cells of B. subtilis.

stages of the stimulation, AD being the most effective since the influence is exhibited even though drug was added as late as 120 min.

When we tested RF and NX in the same conditions as above, a different pattern of action was observed, as indicated in Figs. 5

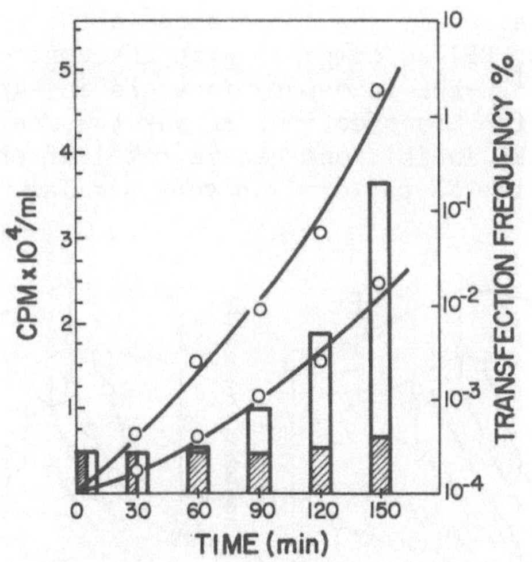

Fig. 2. Normal Conditions of Competence Stimulation Measured as Transfection Frequency and Protein Synthesis. At 0 Times PLC Cells were Suspended in SMS at an OD500=0.08 and Incubated for 150 Min. at the Times Indicated, Samples Were Tested for Transfection (▭) and Protein Synthesis (A) and Controls in Minimal Medium (▨ And B) Were Done.

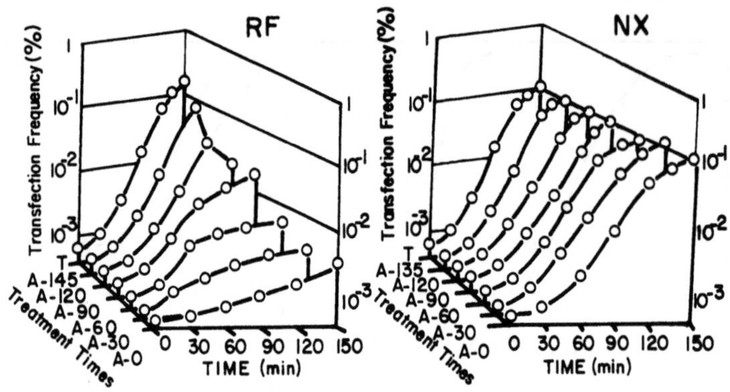

Fig. 3 and 4. Stimulation of the Competence Development in the Presence of RF and NX Added at Different Times.

and 6. The inhibitory action of RF was detected during the total time of stimulation, since the addition of the drug 5 min. before the end of the experiment was enough to produce some decrease in the transfection frequency. However, when NX was assayed, no action could be detected.

Finally, Fig. 7 summarizes the pattern of protein synthesis during the stimulation of the competence in the presence of the drugs (NX, BL, AD, RF) as compared with the control (SMS). As can be observed, the ^{14}C-PHE incorporations are in agreement with the results obtained for transfection. RF was the most active drug while the AD and BL inhibitions became total after 30 and 90 min. respectively and the NX pattern was very similar to the control.

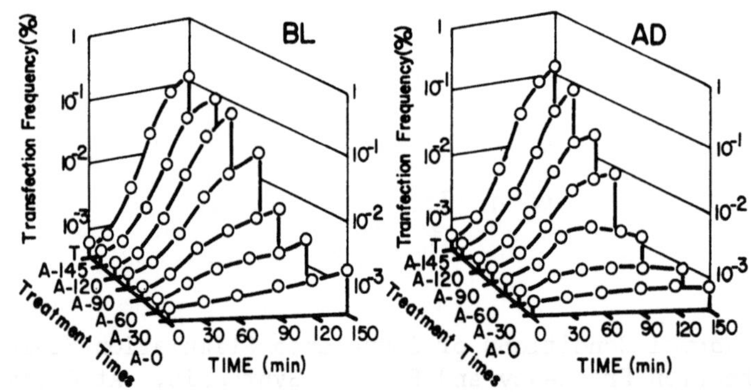

Fig. 5 and 6. Stimulation of the Competence Development in the Presence of BL and AD Added at Different Times.

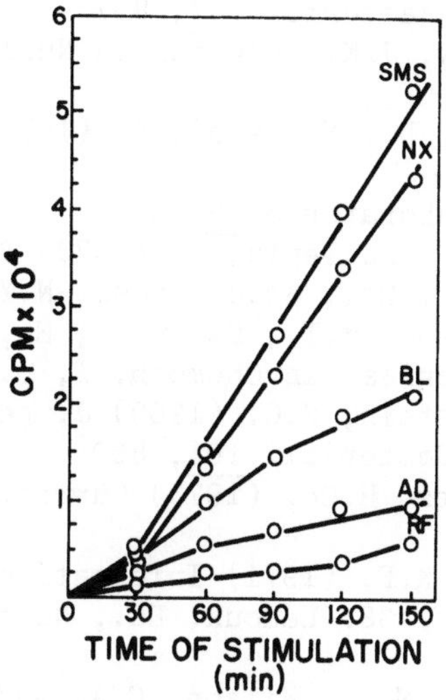

Fig. 7. ^{14}C-Phenyl-Alanine Incorporation During the Stimulated Competence Process with and without Antibiotics.

The most active drugs were those that inhibited the m-RNA synthesis by intercalating in the DNA (AD) or by inhibiting the RNA-polymerase (RF). The variable action observed, depending upon the time of the addition of BL does not have a clear explanation. The NX appears as a conflictive substance, since Wilson and Bott (1971) found an inhibitory effect on the Ø 29 transfection and Pedrini et al., (1972) claimed that this drug does not affect the bacterial transformation. Our results are in agreement with this last report, since no effect could be observed both in the transfectability and in the protein synthesis.

REFERENCES

Ephrati-Elizur, E. (1965). Biochem. Biophys. Res. Comm. 18, 103

Gale, E.F., Cundliffe, E., Reynolds, P.E., Richmond, M.H. and Waring, M.J. (1972). The Molecular Basis of Antibiotic Action, Wiley & Sons, London.

Garcia, E. (1974) Thesis Fac. Sci. Madrid.

Joenje, H., Gruber, M. and Venema, G. (1972) Biochem. Biophys. Acta 262, 189

López, R., García, E., Espinosa, M., Pérez Ureña, M.T. and Portolés, A. (1974). Progress in chemoth. I, p. 144. Daikos, Ed.

Nester, E.W. (1964) J. Bacteriol. 87, 867

Notani, N.K. and Setlow, J.K. Progress in Nucleic Acid Research, 39 (1974)

Pedrini, A.M., Geroldi, D., Falaschi, A. (1972) Mol. gen. Genet. 116, 91

Portolés, A. (1960). Laboratorio 29, 21

Portolés, A., López, R. and Tapia, A. (1973) Bacterial Transformation, p. 65 Archer, Ed., Acad. Press, N.Y.

Portolés, A., Pérez Ureña, M.T., Espinosa, M., Garcia, E. and López, R. (1974) Progress in Chemoth. I, p. 140, Daikos, Ed.

Ranhand, J.M. and Lichstein, H.C. (1969) J. gen. Microbiol. 55, 37

Tomasz, A. (1970). J. Bacteriol. 101, 860

Trautner, T.A. and Spatz, H.Ch. (1973) Current Topics Microbiol. Immunol. 62, 61

Wilson, G.A. and Bott, K.F. (1971) Informative Molecules in Biological Systems, p. 38. Ledoux, Ed., North Holland Pub Co. Amsterdam.

Yasbin, R.E., Tevethia, M.J., Wilson, G.A. and Young, F.E. (1973) Bacterial Transformation, p. 3. Archer, Ed. Acad. Press. N.Y.

^{14}C-PHENYL-ALANINE INCORPORATION IN THE PRESENCE OF VERAL ANTIBIOTICS ON B. subtilis TRANSFECTION

A. PORTOLES, M. ESPINOSA, E. GARCIA, and M.T. PEREZ-UREÑA

Inst. "Jaime Ferrân" of Microbiology. C.S.I.C.

Joaquin Costa, 32 - Madrid - Spain

SUMMARY: Using a system for competence stimulation in B. subtilis six inhibitors of protein synthesis were tested through the ^{14}C--phenyl-alanine incorporation, cell survival and competence. When a 20% mortality is produced, independently of the doses, gentamycin and lincomycin were the most active drugs. However, in absolute comparisons, tetracyclin molecules presented the maximal activity in such a sensitive biological system.

INTRODUCTION: During the competence state on bacterial transformation a "de novo" protein synthesis has been reported and its specific importance has also been detached in D. pneumoniae (Tomasz, 1970) and in B. subtilis (Tichy, 1972) as well as on a transfection system in B. subtilis (Portolês et al. 1974). The fact that those new proteins have such a specific role in the acquisition of the competence without affecting the cell growth, makes the transformation and transfection excellent biological systems to assay different antibiotic inhibitors of the ribosome function.

In the present work the particular activities of different antibiotics on the "de novo" protein synthesis and its physiological role during the competence development have been studied at drug concentrations lower than those required to inhibit the bacterial growth.

MATERIAL AND METHODS: Microorganisms. As recipient and indicator bacteria a prototrophic strain of B. subtilis (AR1T) and another B. subtilis (MCB strain) have been respectively employed. SPP1 bacteriophage was used as DNA source following the method described by Rottlander and Trautner (1970).

Antibiotics and treatments: Six different substances were used acting at the specific ribosome site indicated in Table I. Use of drugs were restricted to the stimulation periods (2.5 hr) and then removed by membrane filtration through a 0.22 μ Millipore filter. Afterwards cells were washed and resuspended either in minimal salts medium or in culture supernatants before adding DNA.

Culture media. A salt minimal medium (Bott and Wilson, 1968) (MBW) was used as a growth medium where bacteria developed competence. When the peak of the transfection frequency was reached, cells were removed by centrifugation and the supernatant used as stimulative fluid since a competence stimulation activity (CSA) is produced (Joenje et al., 1972).

Determinations of antibiotics activity. First of all, minimal inhibitory concentrations (MIC) were estimated by the twofold serial dilution technique in Penassay broth (Difco) using resazurine as rH indicator as previously described (Portolés, 1960).

Competence development. Competence levels were determined through a transfection procedure (Garcia,1974). The competence development was studied by using a biological system of stimulation similar to that described by Joenje et al. (1972).

Protein synthesis determinations. Estimation of the protein synthesis was measured as the incorporation of ^{14}C-phenyl-alanine (^{14}C-PHE) by precipitation with 10% trichloroacetic acid (TCA) during 30 min in the cold. Radiactivity of the TCA precipitable products collected in the filters was determined.

RESULTS AND DISCUSSION: After knowing the MIC values for each antibiotic the effects of different concentrations of drugs were tested. For this purpose, several cultures of physiologically low competent (PLC) cells in MBW were grown during 2.5 hr in the presence of antibiotics. At the end of this time viable cells were counted by platting, and the results appear in Fig. 1. These results show the variable activity of the six drugs tested and let us choose the work doses in which a survival of up to 75% occurred.

TABLE I. Specificities of Antibiotic Actions on Protein Synthesis at Different Ribsomal Subunits.

30 S	30 S/40 S	50 S
Streptomycin (STR)	Tetracyclin (TTC)	Lincomycin (LMC)
Gentamycin (GTM)	Doxicyclin (DXC)	Chloramphenicol (CHL)

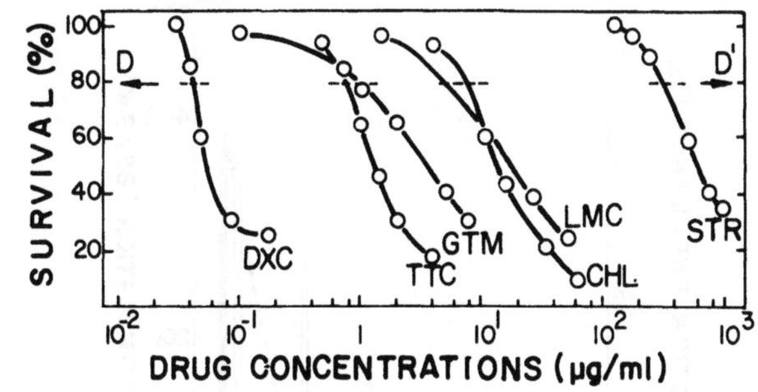

Fig. 1. Effect of the Different Antibiotic Concentrations on PLC Cells of B.subtilis.

Afterwards the basic stimulative conditions in this biological system were determined without antibiotics. PLC cells were suspended in metabolic fluid from highly competent cultures at $O.D._{500}$ = 0.08 and incubated at 37° with shaking (250 rpm). At different times, indicated in Fig. 2, samples were removed and tested for transfection to check the development of the competence stimulation. As a control, cultures on MBW were established in the same conditions. Although some small differential behaviour between both cultures appears from the 30 min., it was observed that active ratio of stimulation delayed until the 90 min.

From Table II results we can conclude that the ^{14}C-PHE incorporation and the development of the competence follows a similar pattern when the activities of the different drugs at doses producing an identical inhibitory action on the bacterial growth are separately considered. Then,when a 20% mortality is produced independently of the doses, it is possible to assume -according to data in Table II- that: i) STR, in spite of its wide variety of metabolic effects (Fitzgerald et al., 1948; Stern et al., 1966; Anand and Davis, 1960) had a lower activity on the competence levels than the other antibiotics, consequently with the light streptomycin-resistance of the AR1T strain, observed in Fig. 1. On the other hand, the protein synthesis is completely stopped at 90 min. This may be due to possible changes in the composition of the cell membrane as it was reported on S. marcescens by Bermingham et al., (1970). This phenomenon could be similar to those observed with colistin (García, 1974); ii) GTM appears as the most active drug inhibiting the bacterial competence and the ^{14}C-PHE incorporation. It may be as a consequence of a strong miscoding for a very efficient drug/ribosome ratio (Weisblum and Davies, 1968) interacting at multiple sites on the 30S ribosomes and, consequently, it affects the synthesis of the especific competence proteins; iii) TTC and DXC are classical broad-spectrum antibiotics producing an intermediate effect between the two drugs previously discussed. Possibly

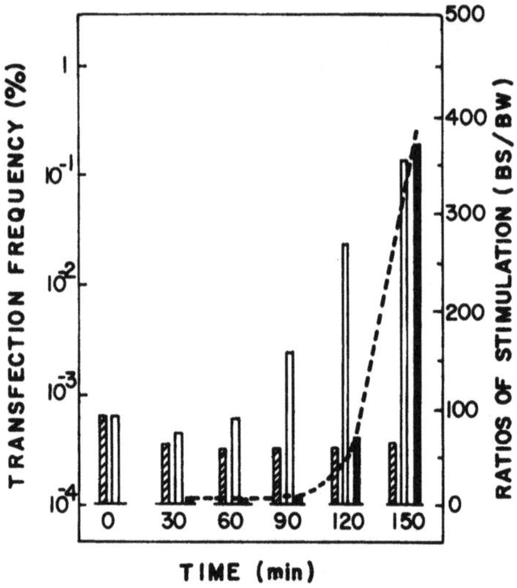

Fig. 2. Comparative Study of the Competence Development in BW Minimal Medium (▨) and in CSA Culture Supernatants (☐) as a Function on the Time. The Ratios of Stimulation and Its Variations are also Indicated (■ ---).

TABLE II. Variations in the ^{14}C-phenyl-alanine incorporation during the stimulated competence in the presence of different antibiotics.

Antibiotics and doses (µg/ml)	Transfection frequency %(a) and c.p.m. (b) values at the different observation times of: 0	30	60	90	120	150 min.
None	(a)065	095	38	20	70	105
	(b)00	48	140	260	380	512
STR 300	(a)065	070	13	32	76	81
	(b)00	039	058	059	062	062
GTM 095	(a)065	051	032	021	016	011
	(b)00	019	022	025	029	031
TTC 075	(a)065	079	14	21	25	48
	(b)00	026	042	056	063	065
DXC 0045	(a)065	078	12	19	24	49
	(b)00	024	039	055	064	069
LMC 50	(a)065	075	095	13	20	40
	(b)00	020	036	042	054	086
CHL 75	(a)065	078	15	20	29	35
	(b)00	024	038	046	075	098

(a) and (b) values represent PFU ($x10^{-8}$) and c.p.m. ($x10^{3}$) respectively

both these two substances cause a bewildering variety of effects on this biological system in which the chelating activities on Mg^{2+} ions (Albert, 1958) could produce unexpected inhibitory actions on the competence; iv) LMC after GTM is the most active inhibitor of the competence and the ^{14}C-PHE incorporation at this 20% mortality. However the inhibition of the protein synthesis begins to be less active after 2 hrs. It may be due because during this time -although slowly- longer peptide chains have been formed on which the LMC is unable to produce its inhibitory effect (Cundliffe, 1969). and v) CHL presents a relatively higher inhibitory action on the competence more than on the protein synthesis in which it may act as an analogue of phenyl-alanine (Woolley,1950). An alternative explanation for this differential behaviour could be based on the secondary inhibitory effect on the teichoic acid synthesis (Stow et al., 1971) which might affect the competence at a cell wall level.

Finally, an absolute comparison for dose unit can be established for the six antibiotics as studied in Fig. 3. A tridimensional graph summarizes the three effects considered, on the bacterial growth, protein synthesis and transfectability, calculated per drug concentrations of one ng/ml. So, in a sensitive biological system such as transfection it is possible to conclude that: i) tetracyclin molecules are the most active antibiotics inhibiting the bacterial competent state and the differences which appear

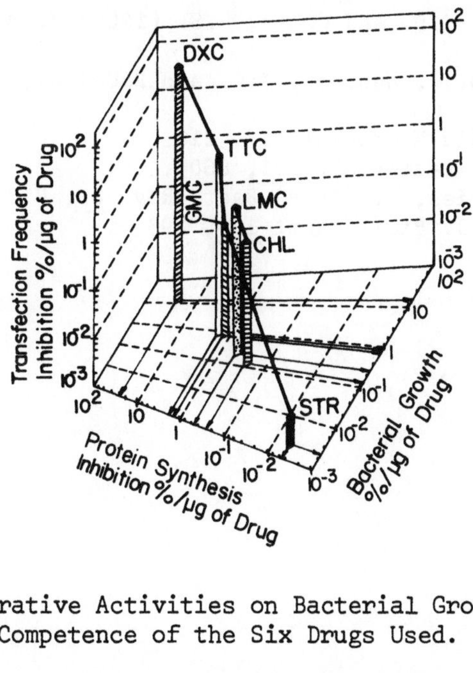

Fig. 3. Comparative Activities on Bacterial Growth, Protein Synthesis and Competence of the Six Drugs Used.

between the DXC and the TTC may be due to a permeability variation; ii) drugs as LMC and CHL acting on the 50 S ribosome subunit are proportionately more active on the transfectability than on protein synthesis; iii) when the action of two aminoglycoside molecules (GTM and STR) are comparatively observed, some marked differences of their activity can be observed corresponding to the antibiotic-resistance level; and iv) since transfection procedure, as here indicated, allows us to study antibiotic actions on the bacterial metabolisms in specially delicate conditions, it is a very useful biological system.

REFERENCES

Albert, A. (1958) Symp. Soc. Gen. Microbiol. 8, 112

Anand, N. and Davis, B.D. (1960) Nature 185, 22

Bermingham, M.A.C., Deol., B.S. and Still., J.S. (1970) Biochem. J. 119, 861

Bott, K.F. and Wilson, G.A. (1968) Bacteriol. Rev. 32, 370

Cundliffe, E. (1960) Biochem. 8, 2063

Fitzgerald, R.J., Bernheim, F. and Fitzgerald, D.B. (1948). J.Biol. Chem. 175, 195

Garcia, E. (1974). Doctorate Thesis. Fac. Sci. Madrid

Joenje, H., Gruber, M. and Venema, G. (1972) B.B.A. 262, 189

Portoles, A. (1960) Laboratorio 29, 21

Portolés, A. Pérez Ureña, M.T., Espinosa, M., Garcia, E. and Lopez, R. (1974) Progress in Chemotherapy I, p. 140 Daikos Ed.

Rottlander, E. and Trautner, T.A. (1970) Molec. Gen. Genetics 108, 47

Stern, J.L., Barner, H.D. and Cohen, S.S. (1966) J. Mol. Biol. 17, 188

Stow, M., Starkey, B.J., Hancock, I.C. and Baddiley, J. (1971) Nature 229, 56

Tichy, P. (1972) Folia Microbiol. 17, 213

Tomasz, A. (1970) J. Bacteriol. 101, 860

Weisblum, B. and Davies, J. (1968) Bact. Rev. 32, 493

Wooley, D.W. (1950) J. Biol. Chem. 185, 293

IRREVERSIBLE INACTIVATION OF RIBOSOMES BY ANTIBIOTICS

C. Coutsogeorgopoulos

Grace Cancer Drug Center, Roswell Park Memorial Institute

Buffalo, N. Y. 14263, U.S.A.

SUMMARY

The peptide bond-forming activity (as measured by the puromycin reaction) of ribosomes (E. coli) charged with poly (U) and Ac-phe-tRNA at the P-site, is abolished irreversibly by spiramycin (10^{-5}M). The rate of this inactivation is decreased by chloramphenicol (3×10^{-6}M) or lincomycin (10^{-5}M) but it is not affected by gougerotin (4×10^{-5}M). In contrast to spiramycin, sparsomycin (10^{-7}M) decreases irreversibly the activity of the ribosomal complex but does not abolish it. On the assumption that the antibiotics remain bound to the modified ribosome, these results may mean that, in contrast to previous proposals, sparsomycin and puromycin do not bind to overlapping sites whereas spiramycin and puromycin may bind to overlapping sites.

- -

According to current thinking, antibiotics which inhibit protein synthesis by acting on the ribosomes, bind to well-defined ribosomal sites (e.g. "chloramphenicol site," "puromycin site," etc.). The methods used for characterizing these sites have assumed that the antibiotic binds reversibly to the ribosomes and thus, analyses carried out by the Scatchard, the Lineweaver-Burk or the Dixon plot have been employed in order to deduce binding constants (K_I) and relative potencies (for a review see Vazquez, 1974). We have developed new methodology and have shown (Coutsogeorgopoulos et al., 1975) that certain antibiotics, which in the past have been considered to interact with the ribosome reversibly, can modify the peptide bond-forming capacity of the ribosome irreversibly. Whether this irreversible interaction requires the retention of the inhibitor on the ribosome (covalent or "tight" binding) remains to be determined.

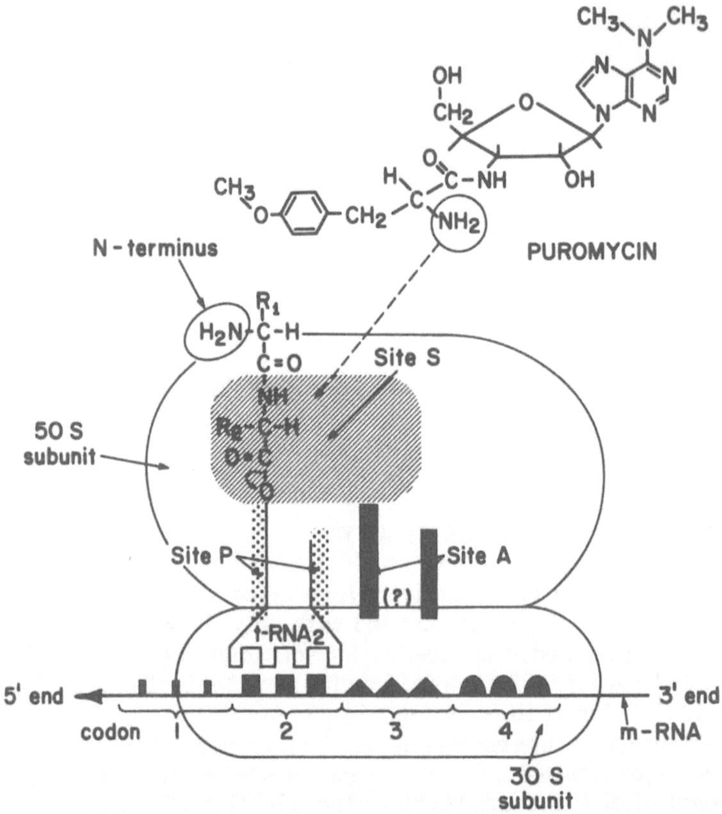

Fig. 1. Schematic representation of the peptidyl-tRNA-m-RNA-ribosome complex. The t-complex used in this study contains Ac-phe-tRNA in place of peptidyl tRNA and poly(U) as the messenger. Sites P, A, and S are defined to be present on a complex active in peptide chain elongation (Coutsogeorgopoulos, 1967). Due to the absence of a second amino acyl-tRNA on the complex shown, site-A may not exist as such. Site-S includes but is not identical to what has been called "peptidyl transferase centre" (Vazquez, 1974); in this study the t-complex has been formed in the presence of the full complement of factors and ribosomal proteins present in the ribosomal wash and may contain the peptidyl transferase in a state different from that of washed ribosomes and isolated 50S subunits.

In the model system which we have used, salt-washed ribosomes (E. coli) interact with a model peptidyl-tRNA (Ac-phe-tRNA) and poly (U) as the messenger to form a ternary complex (t-complex) in the presence of the ribosomal wash and GTP. The isolated t-complex contains the peptidyl-tRNA bound to the P-site (Fig. 1), as evidenced by the fact that it can react quantitatively with puromycin to form peptide bonds. This reaction (puromycin reaction) measures the activity of the catalytic area involved in peptide bond formation (site-S, Fig. 1). Because puromycin participates in peptide bond formation, it will be termed the substrate (S) in this discussion, whereas the term "antibiotic" will be used for the other antibiotic inhibitors. Our methodology permits us to monitor the following three reactions occurring simultaneously or in sequence. Eq. (1) represents the puromycin reaction as carried out under our conditions. The isolated t-complex (C) reacts with puromycin (S) and after Ac-phe-puromycin (P) formation, C is converted to a form (C') in which it cannot react again with S. Eq. (2) represents the irreversible interaction of an antibiotic (I_1) with C, and Eq. (3) the reversible interaction of a

$$(1) \quad C + S \underset{k_2}{\overset{k_1}{\rightleftharpoons}} CS \xrightarrow{k_3} P + C'$$

$$(2) \quad C + I_1 \underset{k_5}{\overset{k_4}{\rightleftharpoons}} CI_1 \xrightarrow{k_6} (CI_1)'$$

$$(3) \quad C + I_2 \rightleftharpoons CI_2$$

second antibiotic (I_2). In Eq. (1) puromycin (S), present in large excess over C, reacts in a pseudo-first order reaction in which S remains virtually constant and C decreases exponentially. The progress of (1) can be followed by using the differential rate equation $dP/dt = k_3S(Co-P)/(K_m + S)$ and determining the <u>initial rate</u> of the reaction, on the condition that less than 10% of the total amount of C (Co) has reacted. It can also be followed by using the integrated rate equation $\ln [Co/(Co-P)] = k_3S\,t/(K_m + S)$ and determining product (P) formed at any time (t) until more than 80% of Co has reacted (Coutsogeorgopoulos, 1973, 1974, 1975). The choice of approach for determining the progress of (1) is critical when reaction (2) occurs simultaneously with (1). At the time intervals used for determining the initial rate of (1) and depending on the values of k_6 and I_1 in relation to k_3 and S, either the reversible complex CI_1 alone, or both CI_1 and $(CI_1)'$ may have been formed. In the latter case, the use of the standard graphical kinetic analyses, which pertain to reversible inhibition (Lineweaver-Burk, Dixon, plots etc.), will lead to incorrect conclusions. On the other hand, if the integrated rate equation is used to follow the progress of (1), enough time is available to observe any change which the presence of I_1 may cause to the kinetic order or reaction (1) and which, at least in certain cases, results from an irreversible step in reaction (2). By use of this approach, antibiotics which inhibit the puromycin reaction can be placed into two groups. Sparsomycin (10^{-7} M), spiramycin (10^{-6} M), amicetin (4×10^{-5} M), and blasticidin S (5×10^{-7}M) alter the kinetic order of (1). On the other hand, chloramphenicol (3×10^{-6}M), lincomycin (10^{-5}) and gougerotin (4×10^{-5}) retain the kinetic order of (1). The antibiotics of the second group either do not form the $(CI_1)'$ complex ($k_6 = 0$) and their interaction is described simply by equation (3), or they may allow the fast formation of a complex analogous to

$(CI_1)'$ which may then react with puromycin to give P. The inhibitors of the second group (I_2) display competitive kinetics, as shown by determining the k_{obs} at various puromycin concentrations and plotting $1/k_{obs}$ vs. 1/S. This implies either that I_2 combines only with C but not with CS, or that the CI_2S complex can be formed from CS and I_2 (or from CI_2 and S) but that the CS and CI_2S complexes would then break down to form P at the same rate although the affinities of C and CI_2 for S would differ. With regard to the first group of antibiotics, which alter the kinetic order of (1), we have obtained results (Coutsogeorgopoulos et al., 1975) which suggest that when I_1 is sparsomycin (10^{-7}M), the complex $(CI_1)'$ reacts with puromycin. Assuming that sparsomycin remains bound to the modified ribosomal complex, this result suggests that sparsomycin does not block the binding of puromycin. On the other hand, when I_1 is spiramycin (10^{-5}M), the $(CI_1)'$ complex does not react with puromycin (Coutsogeorgopoulos, et al., 1975). This demonstrates that spiramycin can react after the t-complex has been formed and it does not exclude the possibility that spiramycin may block the binding of puromycin. When at fixed concentrations of sparsomycin or spiramycin and at various concentrations of puromycin reactions (1) and (2) proceed simultaneously, analysis of the initial rates by the Lineweaver-Burk plot may show competitive or mixed competitive-noncompetitive kinetics depending on whether, by the time P is measured, only the CI_1 complex has been formed or the $(CI_1)'$ complex has also been formed. On the other hand, if reaction (2) is allowed to proceed first, and after removing the excess of I_1 puromycin is then added, reaction (1) will occur only with the fraction of Co which has not been converted to $(CI_1)'$ and the graphical kinetic analysis will produce plots like those afforded by reversible noncompetitive inhibitors. Despite this similarity, the "noncompetitive" plot in the case of spiramycin indicates that since $(CI_1)'$ does not react with puromycin, reaction (1) occurs with a reduced concentration of C. In fact, if enough time is allowed for reaction (2) to proceed to completion, the activity of the t-complex towards puromycin is lost completely. On the other hand, in the case of sparsomycin the apparent noncompetitive plot results from the fact that the $(CI_1)'$ complex reacts with puromycin forming a new species $CI_1'S$ which yields P with a rate constant lower than k_3 of reaction (1). Thus, these apparent noncompetitive plots do not imply a simple reversible interaction of C with I_1 and do not allow the estimation of K_I values for spiramycin or sparsomycin.

We have also developed a new method which allows the examination of the interaction of I_1 and I_2 with C when reactions (2) and (3) occur simultaneously but independently of (1). The t-complex (C) is first adsorbed on a nitrocellulose disc in a fully active state and is then allowed to interact for a defined period of time with I_1 in the absence of puromycin (reaction 2 only) or in the absence of puromycin but in the presence of I_2 (reactions 2 and 3 simultaneously). The discs are then washed free of excess of I_1 and I_2 (Coutsogeorgopoulos et al., 1975) and puromycin is allowed to react with unmodified C (reaction 1). Using this method, we have found that chloramphenicol (3×10^{-6}M) or lincomycin (10^{-5}M) reduce the rate of inactivation of the t-complex by spiramycin (10^{-5}M), whereas gougerotin (4 x 10^{-5} or 4 x 10^{-4} M) does not; at 6.25 x 10^{-5} M puromycin, gougerotin (4 x 10^{-5} M) reduces the k_{obs} of reaction (1) by 68%.

REFERENCES

Coutsogeorgopoulos, C. (1967), Biochemistry 6, 1704.
Coutsogeorgopoulos, C. (1973), Proc. 8th Intl. Congr. Chemoth. 1, 376.
Coutsogeorgopoulos, C. (1974), Fed. Proc. U.S.A. 33, Abs. 629.
Coutsogeorgopoulos, C., Miller, J.T., and Hann, D.M. (1975), Nucleic Acids Research (in press).
Vazquez, D. (1974), F.E.B.S. Letters, 40 Suppl. 63.

THEORETICAL BASIS OF ANTIBIOTIC COMBINATIONS

M. de M. Pinto-Ribeiro

Faculty of Medicine

Lisbon University, Portugal

Antibiotic combinations inducing synergism are extremely useful while those producing antagonism are dangerous. Antibiotics can now be classified functionally as shown in Table 1.

GROUP 1 antibiotics act when the septum formation terminates division and during cytoplasmic growth, which forces the cell membrane to restructure. Bacteria without cell wall,as L-forms, are obviously resistant.

GROUP 2 strikes the permanently active cytoplasmic membrane. All phases of the bacterial cycle are therefore susceptible.

GROUP 3 has 2 different subgroups: the tetracycline subgroup leads to reversible inhibition of protein synthesis while the gentamicin subgroup alters synthesis without interruption, loading bacteria with abnormal molecules. Consequently gentamicin and allied drugs cannot act if there is no active protein synthesis. Besides, they enhance bacterial metabolism (contrasting with most other antibiotics) until exhaustion ensues.

GROUP 4 irreversibly inhibits m-RNA polymerase, quickly stopping protein synthesis. Its antibiotics will not act upon metabolically quiescent bacteria.

GROUP 5 antibiotics stop DNA synthesis (but not its precursors uptake) just after cytoplasmic growth and before division.

TABLE 1

ACTIONS OF ANTIBIOTICS

	Central Antibiotics	Mode of Action	Type of Action	Effect
Group 1	Penicillin	Inhibition of cell membrane (murein) synthesis	Phase - dependent	Cidal
Group 2	Polymyxin	Cleavage or metabolic inhibition of cytoplasmic membrane	Phase - independent	Cidal
Group 3	Tetracycline subgroup	Reversible inhibition of ribosomic protein synthesis	Phase - dependent	Static
	Gentamicin subgroup	Ribosomic miscoding producing abnormal proteins	Phase - dependent	Cidal
Group 4	Rifampicin	Irreversible inhibition of m-RNA production	Phase - dependent	Cidal
Group 5	Nalidixic acid	Irreversible inhibition of DNA replication	Phase - dependent	Cidal
Group 6	Sulphonamides Trimethoprim Nitrofurantoin	Irreversible inhibition of intermediate metabolism (folic acid synthesis, etc.)	Phase - dependent	Cidal

TABLE 2

EFFECTS OF ANTIBIOTIC COMBINATIONS

Group	Central Antibiotic	1 Penicillin	2 Polymyxin	3a Tetracycline	3b Gentamicin	4 Rifampicin	5 Nalidixic Acid	6 Sulphonamides Trimethoprim Nitrofurantoin
1	Penicillin	+/++++	+	---	++++	---	---	---
2	Polymyxin	+	+/++++	+	+	+	+	+
3a)	Tetracycline	---	+	-/++	---	+++	---	+++
3b)	Gentamicin	++++	+	---	+	---	---	---
4	Rifampicin	---	+	+++	---	+	---	++++
5	Nalidixic Acid	---	+	---	---	---	+	---
6	Sulphonamides Trimethoprim Nitrofurantoin	---	+	+++	---	++++	---	+/++++

KEY: ++++ = synergism between 2 cidal antibiotics; +++ = synergism between 1 cidal and 1 static; ++ = synergism between 2 static antibiotics; + = additive effect; --- = antagonism

GROUP 6 antibiotics specifically inhibit steps of essential metabolic pathways of the cytoplasmic pool. These irreversible changes occur during the cytoplasmic growth phase (active metabolism) and soon entail protein synthesis arrest due to lack of essential factors (folic acid, etc.).

Table 2 summarises the effects of the different antibiotic combinations upon 1 bacterial strain, provided bacteria are sensitive to both the selected antibiotics. It does not consider more complex aspects concerning mixed infections.

GROUP 1 antibiotics will act synergistically between themselves (if blocking different steps of murein biosynthesis) or additively (when affecting the same step, as penicillin and cephalosporin). They may potentiate Group 2 drugs if bacteria are resistant to these by impermeability of their cell membrane. Group 1 antibiotics are inhibited by drugs of the tetracycline subgroup and of groups 4, 5 and 6, which stop cytoplasmic growth and/or prevent division. The gentamicin subgroup enhances group 1 effects by increasing the rhythm of protein synthesis and is itself potentiated by the accelerated penetration induced by Group 1 drugs.

GROUP 2 does not alter the action of other antibiotics because the involved targets are not interdependent. They generally combine with additive effect. Synergism will occur if the cytoplasmic impermeable to the other antibiotic.

GROUP 3 - Tetracycline Subgroup drugs antagonise each other when competing for the same step of protein synthesis (as chloramphenicol, erythromicin and lincomycin). They potentiate Groups 4 and 6 (which also stop protein synthesis), and antagonise the gentamicin subgroup (needing protein synthesis) and nalidixic acid (by inhibiting DNA precursors uptake and/or metabolic processes starting division). The Gentamicin subgroup, needing protein synthesis, is antagonised by antibiotics arresting it. It inhibits Group 5, probably because the abnormal proteins counteract division, thus with-holding the target of Group 5 antibiotics.

GROUP 4 stops protein synthesis, therefore enhances the effect of Group 6 and tetracycline antibiotics, and obviously inhibits Group 1, gentamicin subgroup and Group 5 drugs.

GROUP 5 antagonises group 1 by arresting bacteria before septum formation. Besides, if Group 1 antibiotics act before those of Group 5, the affected bacteria will not go through the process inducing division. Group 5 is antagonised by Groups 3, 4 and 6, which prevent division by stopping or altering protein synthesis.

GROUP 6 antibiotics specifically block essential intermediate metabolic pathways. Combined between themselves they produce synergism : multiple blocks of the same or of different pathways will accelerate the lethal metabolic standstill. They obviously antagonise Groups 1 and 5 and the gentamicin subgroup and potentiate the antibiotics of the tetracycline subgroup and of Group 4.

Though this model of interaction between antibiotics needs further laboratorial and clinical confirmation, it has been used with good results to adapt antibiotic combinations to patients needing thorough treatment. Preference should be given to combinations involving antibiotics with cidal action, acting simultaneously (not sequentially), accelerating or intensifying the intervention of the other drug and with different mechanisms of action.

ANTIBIOTIC SENSITIVITY OF <u>HAEMOPHILUS INFLUENZAE</u>

P. Cavanagh, Sandra Kattan, R. B. Sykes

Public Health Laboratory, Stoke-on-Trent; London

Hospital Medical College; Glaxo Research Ltd., Middlesex

Consecutive sputum samples from over 1600 patients with chest conditions yielded the Haemophilus spp. which are the subject of this communication. 55% yielded significant organisms and 55% of these were Haemophilus spp. "Chronic chests" yielded 72% and "pneumonia","post-anaesthesia" and "paediatric" chests yielded 4%, 19% and 5% of our strains respectively.

Selective[1,2,3,4,5] agar containing horse blood, 5 ug/ml bacitracin and 10 ug/ml of nicotinamide adenine dinucleotide was used to recover strains from non-homogenized sputum.

Oxoid sensitivity test agar containing .25% of saponin-lysed horse blood (X factor) and 10 ug/ml of NAD (V factor) was used for both disc and plate dilution methods of sensitivity testing.

We use a 2 ug disc of ampicillin in preference to a larger disc which may give rise to spurious results. Disc tests were confirmed by MIC methods. This table shows our results:

Biotype	Total examined	Resistant to: Ampicillin	Tetracycline
H. influenzae	365	9 (2.4%)	13 (3.5%)
H. parainfluenzae	192	7	5
H. parahaemolyticus	76	1	1
H. haemolyticus	5	0	0

Ampicillin resistant strains of H. influenzae were not recovered from meningitis during the period of this investigation, but geographic variation[6] in ampicillin resistance has been reported elsewhere and although this might be due to differences in prescribing habits, the importance of resistance transfer factor should not be overlooked.

The mechanisms of ampicillin resistance in Haemophilus spp. is governed by the presence of β-lactamase[7], which destroys penicillin, ampicillin and cephalosporin. This resistance is unstable and may be transferred within the genus and also to Esch. coli and Pseudomonas spp.; the mechanism of transfer has not yet been identified.

Tetracycline resistance was examined by a scintillation technique and may be analogous to plasmid-directed tetracycline resistance in Staphylococci[8], we have not performed tetracycline transfer, but French workers have identified plasmid-controlling tetracycline resistance in one strain of H. influenzae[9].

Chloramphenicol resistance is enzymic; spectrophotometry and cross resistance to gentamycin and kanamycin suggests that this enzyme is an acetylase.

Williams and Andrews[10] reported the unsuitability of available cephalosporins in the treatment of infections caused by H. influenzae, but only 4 of an extended range (550 strains) of fresh isolates of Haemophilus spp. grew on agar containing two or more ug/ml of a new cephalosporin, cephuroxime.

To sum up, ampicillin and tetracycline, depending on the geographic location of the patient, still appear to be acceptable drugs for the treatment of exacerbations of chronic bronchitis and related conditions.

The overall proportion of resistance strains is so low in our Laboratory that we have ceased the routine disc sensitivity test.

Although the overall prevalence of ampicillin resistance might be quite low in Britain, we would support a survey of strains recovered from cases of meningitis. It is probably unnecessary to continue disc methods of sensitivity testing, except on specimens from meningitis, where it may be possible to perform direct tests on CSF containing even scanty numbers of organisms, if the capsule swelling reaction and a film stained with dilute carbol-fuchsin suggests H. influenzae as the pathogen.

In conclusion we should like to suggest that the inflexible application of protocol designed for the rationalisation and standardisation of sensitivity testing in laboratories of differing capabilities can be carried too far; the fastidious requirements of H. influenzae have led us in the first place to use a medium which is not part of any recognised protocol, and secondly to recommend a sensitivity test disc of very small drug content.

Finally, we have been led to abandon routine testing of strains by the disc method in favour of batch MIC's; Robert May, who contributed so much to the study of chronic bronchitis in this City, would certainly agree with this.

REFERENCES

1. FLEMING, A, (1929), Brit.J.exp.Path., 10, 226
2. HOVIG, B, & AANDAHL, E.H., (1969) Acta path. microbiol. scand., 77, 676
3. JARVIS, J.D. and EWINS, S.P. (1968) J. med. Lab. Technol., 25, 261
4. BABER, K.G., J. med. Lab. Technol., 26, 391
5. MAY, R., "Chemotherapy of chronic bronchitis and allied disorders"; second edition, 1972, p.99
6. WILLIAMS, J.D., ANDREWS, JENNY, & CAVANAGH, P., 13th Interscience Conference on Antimicrobial Agents and Chemotherapy; Washington, DC, Sept. 1973
7. SYKES, R.B., MATHEW, M. and O'CALLAGHAN, CYNTHIA H. (1975) J. med. Microbiol (in press)
8. SOMPOLINSKY, D., ZAIDENZAIG, Y., ZIEGLER-SCHLOMOVITZ, RUTH and ABRAMOVA, NILI, (1970) J. gen. Microbiol, 62, 351
9. DANG VAN, ANNIE, BIETH, GILDA and BOVANCHAUD, D.H. (1975) C.R.Acad.Sc.Paris, t.280, 1321
10. WILLIAMS, J.D. and ANDREWS, JENNY, (1974) Brit. med. J., i, 134

DRUG SENSITIVITY PATTERN OF GRAM-NEGATIVE ROD

Fumio Matsumoto, Yasushi Ueda, Masahisa Ohmori, and Kohya Shiba
Dept. of Internal Medicine, The Jikei University School of Medicine
3-25-8 Nishi-shinbashi, Minato-ku, Tokyo, Japan

It is well known to us all that antibiotics from the same group may differ in antimicrobial activity.

The present study was undertaken to investigate the sensitivity pattern of gram-negative rods to antibiotics from two different groups. The results are presented below.

MATERIALS AND METHODS

The gram-negative rods studied were isolates of the species E. coli, Klebsiella pneumoniae and Proteus mirabilis of 100 strains each and 150 strains of Pseudomonas, all obtained during the three-year period from 1972 to 1974 mostly from clinical specimens of urinary tract infections.

Eight cephalosporins and five aminoglycosides were tested, e.g. cephalothin (CET), cephaloridine (CER), cephalexin (CEX), cefazolin (CEZ), cephapirin (CEP), cephradin (CED), cephacetrile (CEC), ceftezole (CTZ), Kanamycin (KM), Gentomicin (GM), Dibekacin (DBK), Tobramycin (TDB) and Amikacin (AKC). The agar-plate dilution technique for antimicrobial activity testing was used to determine the minimal inhibitory concentrations (MIC) of these drugs for the gram-negative rod, employing one loopful of diluted overnight culture containing 10^6 cells per ml as an inoculum size and reading the plates after 24 hours of incubation at $37^{\circ}C$.

Selected E. coli, Klebsiella pneumonia and Proteus mirabilis strains for which MIC of greater than 100 ug/ml of a cephalosporin or Kanamycin had been observed were further tested for R-factor transfer by using them as donors and a nalidixic acid-resistant mutant E. coli K-12 ML 1410 as the recipient.

RESULT

The spectrum of activity of cephalosporins against the isolates of the three species: E. coli, Klebsiella pneumoniae and Proteus mirabilis is shown in Table 1. The MIC was greater than 50 ug/ml for 3 to 6% to 24% and 20 to 32% of the strains of these species respectively. The incidence of the organism with MIC over 50 ug/ml was low particularly for cefazolin and ceftezole.

Table 1: Sensitivity of Cephalosporins against E. coli, Klebsiella pneumoniae and Proteus mirabilis

Cephalo-	E. coli			Kl.pneumoniae			Prot.mirabilis		
sporins	=100	50	=25	=100	50	= 25	=100	50	= 25ug/ml
CET	4	0	96	18	3	79	28	2	70strains
CER	3	0	97	15	8	77	27	2	71
CEX	4	2	94	13	8	79	28	4	68
CEZ	3	0	97	12	6	82	18	2	80
CEP	4	2	94	18	6	76	28	3	69
CED	4	2	94	13	6	81	28	2	70
CEC	3	2	95	15	5	80	22	6	72
CTZ	3	1	96	12	8	80	18	4	78

The resistant patterns of E. coli and two other species isolates for which the cephalosporins exhibited MIC values 100 ug/ml or over. As shown in Table 2, with all three bacterial species, strains resistant to all the cephalosporins were most frequent, e.g. 3 out of 4 E. coli, 12 out of 18 Klebsiella pneumoniae and 18 out of 28 Proteus mirabilis strains, respectively. As the data indicate, there were a few cephalothin, cephapirin resistant strain in case of Klebsiella pneumoniae. There were resistant strains for drugs other than cefazolin and ceftezole or for those other than cefazolin, cephectrile and ceftezole in case of Proteus mirabilis. In the strains other than those resistant to all the above eight cephalosporins, none was found resistant to cefazolin or ceftezole.

Table 2: Patterns of resistance to Cephalosporins in E. coli, Klebsiella pneumoniae and Proteus mirabilis

	No. of strains					
	E.coli		Kl.pneu-moniae		Prot. mirabilis	
Sensitive : 50ug/ml	96		82		72	strains
Resistant : 100ug/ml						
CET.CEP	0	4	3	18	0	28 strains
CET.CEX.CED.CEP	1		0		0	
CET.CER.CEP.CEC	0		2		0	
CET.CER.CEX.CEP.CED.	0		0		6	
CET.CER.CEX.CEP.CED. CFC	0		1		4	
CET.CER.CEX.CEP.CED. CFC.CEZ.CTZ.	3		12		18	
Total	100		100		100	

The MIC of Kanamycin was greater than 25ug/ml only for 9 of E. coli, 12 of Klebsiella and 16 strains of Proteus respectively, thus indicating remarkable antimicrobial activity of the drug against these three species. Strains of these species inhibited by more than 25 ug/ml of four other aminoglycosides including gentamicin were remarkably infrequent, being 1 to 3% of the strains tested.

The results of experiments in which cephalosporin or kanamycin resistant strains were tested for ability to transfer R-factors are summarized in Table 3. As can be seen, 30 to 90% of cephalosporin-resistant strains proved to be capable of transferring R-factor to E. coli K-12.

Namely, 3 of the 4 E.coli strains, 11 of the 18 Klebsiella pneumoniae strains and 9 of the 28 Proteus mirabilis strains demonstrated the capacity of R-factor transfer. Similarly, 7 of the 9 Kanamycin-resistant E.coli isolated, 3 of the 6 Kelbsiella isolates and 5 of the 8 Proteus isolates also showed this capacity.

Table 3: Experimental results of R-factor transfer with E.coli, Kl.pneumoniae and Prot.mirabilis

Antibiotics	No. transferred/no. tested		
	E.coli	Kl.pneumoniae	Prot.mirabilis
CET	3/4	11/18	10/28
CER	3/3	10/15	10/27
CEX	3/3	11/13	9/28
CEZ	3/3	11/12	9/18
CEP	3/4	11/18	9/28
CED	3/4	11/13	9/28
CEC	3/3	10/15	10/22
CTZ	3/3	11/12	9/18
KM	7/9	3/6	5/8

donor: MIC = 100ug/ml, recipient: E.coli K-12 ML 1410 (Nalidixic acid resistant).

As shown in Table 4, all the strains resistant to cephalosporin or to Kanamycin were also found to be insusceptible to streptomycin, tetracycline, chloramphenicol or ampicillin and that they all had R-factor against one or more of the four drugs. None of these strains, however, was shown to possess R-factor against either cephalosporin or Kanamycin alone.

Table 4: Experimental results of R-factor transfer with E.coli, Kl.pneumoniae and Prot.mirabilis

Transferred Resistant *(SM,TC,CP,ABPC)		No. transferred/no. tested		
		E.coli	Kl.pneumonia	Prot.mirabilis
Cephalosporin R-factor	SM	3/3	6/11	8/10
	TC	3/3	3/11	6/10
	CP	3/3	3/11	6/10
	ABPC	3/3	11/11	10/10
Kanamycin R-factor	SM	7/7	3/3	5/5
	TC	7/7	2/3	4/5
	CP	7/7	2/3	4/5
	ABPC	7/7	3/3	5/5

* SM: Streptomycin, TC: Tetracycline, CP: Chloramphenicol ABPC: Ampicillin.

In the spectra of activity of gentamicin, dibekacin, tobramycin and amicacin against 150 Pseudomonas isolates, twenty strains were inhibited by more than 25 ug/ml of gentamicin, 24 strains by dibekacin, 18 strains by tobramycin and 29 strains by amikacin, respectively, thus the highest frequency being with amikacin.

The pattern of drug resistance to gentamicin and the three other antibiotics exhibited by the Pseudomonas strains is shown in Table 5.

Table 5: Patterns of resistance to Aminoglycosides in Pseudomonas aeruginosa

	No. of strains	
Sensitive: 12.5 ug/ml	110	
Resistant: 25 ug/ml		
DKB	1	
AKC	16	
DKB.TOB	1	
DKB.AKC	2	40
GM.DKB.TOB	9	
GM.DKB.AKC	3	
GM.DKB.TOB.AKC.	8	

Sixteen strains proved to be resistant to amikacin alone, the incidence being highest, while there were 9 strains resistant to gentamicin, dibekacin and tobramycin alone and 8 strains were resistant to all the four antibiotics. Furthermore, all the isolates with cross-resistant to two or three drugs proved to have resistance to debekacin and those showing cross-resistance to three drugs were resistant to gentamicin and dibekacin. A characteristic finding was that amikacin-resistant strains displayed a trend of being either devoid of cross-resistance to any other drug or cross-resistant to three other drugs.

SUMMARY

The antimicrobial activity against the E.coli, Klebsiella pneumoniae and Proteus mirabilis strains was compared among cephalosporins and aminoglycosides.

1. It was noted that the cephalosporins might be grossly divided into two groups according to their activity against these gram-negative bacilli. That is, cefazolin and ceftezole are potent anitmicrobial agents against them whilst the rest have virtually equivalent activity. It is noteworthy that a half to two-thirds strains resistant to any one cephalosporin had cross-resistance to all the remaining cephalosporins as well and, frequently, these strains were shown to possess R-factor.

2. Kanamycin is a considerably potent drug against gram-negative rods. The most Kanamycin-resistant strains were found to possess the R-factor.

3. The most active among the antipseudomonas aminoglycosides studied was tobramycin. However, resistant pseudomonas strains were most frequent against amicacin while it is noteworthy that there were amikacin-sensitive strains among the isolates resistant to gentamicin, dibekacin or tobramycin. The four antipseudomonas aminoglycosides have been observed to be classificable into groups: gentamicin, dibekacin and tobramycin in one group and amikacin alone in the other group.

PATHOGENS, ISOLATED FROM PATIENTS IN INTENSIVE CARE UNITS AND THEIR SURROUNDINGS WITH REGARD TO THEIR ANTIBIOTIC SUSCEPTIBILITY

C.Krasemann, K.Botzenhart, H.Rüden

Institute f. Med. Microbiology a. Immunology of the University, 53 Bonn, Venusberg; W.-Germany

The prevention and management of infections in intensive care units impose severe problems. One of the causes is the prevalence of highly resistant gramnegative rods, whereas on the other hand the suitable measures to prevent cross infections by medical staff and instruments are often not practised consequently enough.

We have studied the occurrence of bacteria in patients and their surroundings in 4 different intensive care units of the university hospital of Bonn in the period from July 1974 to December 1974. During this time a total of 190 patients stayed in these wards, one of which belonged to surgery, the second to neurosurgery, and the two others to non-surgical units. The patients remained on these wards up to several months.

Cerebrospinal fluid, blood, swabs from wounds, endotracheal tubes, and various other clinical materials were regularly controlled for bacterial growth. For the cultivation of bacteria sheep-blood-agar and Endo-agar were used as well as thioglycolate-broth and brain heart infusion medium. The gramnegative rods were classified according to the criteria of EDWARDS and EWING. Susceptibility tests were done by the agar diffusion method according to the prescriptions of KIRBY and BAUER, and partially by tube dilution in Mueller-Hinton-broth.

The following species, named in tab.no.1, were regularly found in all 4 wards. Klebsiella spec., Emterobacter spec., Serratia marcescens, and Proteus mirabilis were most frequently isolated from the patients. In wounds, endotracheal tubes and urinary tract infections a mixture of up to six different species of gramnegative rods was regularly detected, and frequently very

Tab.No.1

Microorganisms, isolated in 4 intensive care units

Klebsiella spec.
Enterobacter spec.
Serratia marcescens
Escherichia coli
Citrobacter freundii
Proteus mirabilis
Proteus (indolpos.)
Pseudomonas aeruginosa
Bacterium anitratum

Candida albicans

Tab. No. 2

	Ampicillin			Carbenicillin			Cephalotin			Cephazolin		
Species	sen.	m.s.	res.	sen.	m.s.	res.	sen.	m.s.	res.	sen	m.s.	res.
Klebsiella			8			8	3	1	4	3	2	3
Enterobacter		1	5	4		2			6			6
Serratia			7			7			7			7
P. mirabilis	4		3	5	1	1	3		4	3		4

	Tetracyclin			Chloramphenicol			Gentamycin		Tobramycin	
Species	sen.	m.s.	res	sen	m.s.	res.	sen.	res.	sen.	res.
Klebsiella	4		4	4		4	6	2	6	2
Enterobacter		2	4	5		1	5	1	5	1
Serratia	1	5	1	6		1	5	2	5	2
P. mirabilis	1		6	2	2	3	6	1	7	

Tab. No. 3

	Species	Tetra cyclin mcg/ml	Chloram-phenicol mcg/ml	Genta-micin mcg/ml	Tobra-micin mcg/ml	Carbeni-cillin mcg/ml	Cepha-lotin mcg/ml	Ampi-cillin mcg/ml
1.	Serratia marcescens	12,5	> 100	< 0,8	< 0,8	—	—	—
2.	Serratia marcescens	25	50	12,5	25	—	—	—
3.	Klebsiella	3,125	12,5	< 0,8	< 0,8	—	6,25	—
4.	Klebsiella	> 100	> 100	< 0,8	< 0,8	—	12,5	—
5.	Klebsiella	> 100	> 100	25	25	—	6,25	—
6.	Enterobacter	3,125	12,5	25	25	> 100	—	—
7.	Enterobacter	1,6	6,25	< 0,8	< 0,8	6,25	—	—
8.	Proteus mirabilis	100	12,5	3,125	3,125	< 0,8	12,5	< 0,8
9.	Proteus mirabilis	100	100	> 100	25	0,8	25	> 100
10.	Bacterium anitratum	1,6	6,25	< 0,8	< 0,8	< 0,8	100	50

Tab. No. 4

Microorganisms, isolated from septicemia

Species	no. of cases	starting from
Klebsiella spec.	4	urinary tract inf. (2) pneumonia (2)
Klebsiella spec. + Citr. freundii	1	unknown
Serratia marcescens	1	i.v. catheter
Escherichia coli	1	unknown
Proteus mirabilis	1	urinary tract inf.
Staphylococcus aureus	1	i.v. catheter
Candida albicans	1	unknown

resistant bacteria were associated with rather sensitive ones. In some wound infections and secretions from endotracheal tubes gram-posotive cocci such as Pneumococci, hemolytic Streptococci, Staphylococcus aureus and of course Enterococci occured together with gramnegative rods, even when the patients received antibiotics which normally should be active against thes grampositive cocci.

The resistance pattern of the most frequently isolated strains is shown in Tab.no. 2. Gentamicin and Tobramycin are effective against most of the isolated strains, and moreover Chloramphenicol is effective on 6 out of 7 strains of Serratia marcescens. However, in one ward we repeatedly isolated a strain of S.marcescens which was inhibited by a concentration of 6.25 mcg/ml Chloramphenicol only and was resistant to all other antibiotics tested.
Tab. no. 3 gives the MIC's of the various S.marcescens, Klebsiella, Enterobacter, and P.mirabilis strains which were regularly isolates in the neurosurgical ward and of the Bacterium anitratum strain responsible for a case of meningitis in the same ward. Obviously, the highly resistant strains are not able to entirely banish the more sensitive strains of the same species from one ward.

In contrary to the other infections, septicemia and meningitis were normally found to be monoinfections (i.e.caused by one species of microorganisms only). Three cases of meningitis occurred in the neurosurgical ward, 2 of which were caused by S.marcescens, 1 by B.anitratum. All 3 strains were very sensitive to Gentamicin; nevertheless, all patients died in spite of adequate chemotherapy.

The cases of septicemia are characterized in Tab.no.4. Presumably more cases of septicemia occured, judging by the symptoms, but attempts to isolate the causing agent remained without success. The outcome of life-threatening infections primarily depends on the physical state of the patients. Thus patients succumbed to pneumonia or septicemia caused by Cephalotin-sensitive Klebsiella-strains in spite of receiving adequate chemotherapy. On the other hand, one case of septicemia could be cured, which had been due to a Klebsiella strain, sensitive only to Polymyxins and invading from an indwelling bladder catheter.

One case of peritonitis deserves extra mentioning: It was caused by a Providencia stuartii strain sensitive only to 2mcg/ml Novobiocin and resistant towards all other antibiotics. This fatally ending peritonitis differs from the other infections in so far as the strain involved was not detected anywhere in the surroundings of the patient and was unable to survive in it for long under experimental conditions. This was perhaps the only case of an endogenous infection. All other infections are in all probability cross infections, since the same species with identical MIC's to different antibiotics could be isolated from several patients and their surroundings during the same period of time.

The microorganisms are frequently found on the patient's bed, on the various utensils needed for bedside care, on the ground as well as on objects frequently touched, for example on light switches, tonometer cuffs etc. Special attention is to be given to moist places, where a certain spectrum of organisms can be met with in high proportion. Frequent isolation of gramnegative rods like Ps.aeruginosa, Klebsiella and Enterobacter from moist areas is well-known. Sanitary installations and items such as wash-basins, water-taps, face cloths etc. must be taken into account. Moreover, medical instruments, medicines, and medical apparatus like ultrasonic inhalers, respirators, and dialysers are to be considerd in this respect.

A characteristic of the present investigation was the isolation of S.marcescens from supply-bottles of saline used for the preparation of injections. These bottles are not infrequently seen with pierced rubber plugs, injection-needles still stuck inside, and left standing around on the drug board of the ward. The concentration of S.marcescens found in this saline solution amounted to 100 000 cells per ml. The occurence of a case of septicemia by S.marcescens on the very same ward clearly points out the danger connected with this method of handling. Furthermore, S.marcescens was detected in tracheal swabs from various patients, which provides an easy explanation for the infection mode of the saline bottles by smear infection. However, smear infection alone cannot account for the high concentration of bacteria in the saline bottles. This must be the result of bacterial multiplication in the solution itself. It is known for some time that Ps.aeruginosa is well capable of multiplying in the quality of distilled water or saline available for use in hospitals. A systematic survey of the multiplication of various species of gramnegative bacteria in different qualities of water is given in the following table. As can be seen, S.marcescens, Ps. aeruginosa and Klebsiella-Enterobacter species have particularly low demands on nutritive substances in aqueous solutions, so that growth is to be expected in distilled water as well as in tap water and in

Tab. No. 5

	Aqua bidest.	Aqua demin.	Tap water	Mineral Salt solutions
Citrobacter	-	+/-	+	++
Enterob.aerogenes	-	+	++	+
Enterob.cloacae	+/-	-	+/-	+
E.coli	-	-	-	+
Klebs.pneumoniae	-	-	+	++
Providencia	-	-	-	+
Ps.aeruginosa	+/-	++	++	++
S.marcescens	+	++	+	++

-: Reduction of number; +/-: no change
+: Growth (10-100 fold); ++: Growth (100-1000 fold)

deionized water. An increased concentration of mineral salts, however, enables growth of allmost all species of gramnegative rods tested here. Exsiccation generally leads to rapid death of the species named. This was demonstrated by an experiment, in which smooth surfaces were infected with 6 different species in concentrations of 40 ooo to 400 000 cells and left to dry. After one day under dry conditions no viabla cells of Proteus, Serratia or Ps. aeruginosa could be found (Tab. no. 6). This however , must not always be the case, because in the presence of various protective colloids or favorable factors of some other kind even sensitive species may survive in dry environment. This is very likely whenever a strong spreading of bacteria occurs. Once cells have survived the actual process of drying, there is probably no further rapid loss in viability. In the experiment shown here, E.coli, B.anitratum as well as a strain of Klebsiella and E.aerogenes survived. Of the species discussed here, in particular Klebsiella and Enterobacter were frequently isolated from dry surfaces in the surroundings of the patient and only rarely Proteus, E.coli and Ps.aeruginosa.

Tab. No. 6

	INOCULUM (0,1 ml)	AFTER 24h. DRYING
Enterob. aerog.	$3{,}0 \times 10^5$	1150
E. coli	$2{,}0 \times 10^5$	60
Klebs. pneum. I	$3{,}0 \times 10^5$	0
Klebs. pneum. II	$1{,}0 \times 10^5$	20
Prot.	$4{,}0 \times 10^4$	0
Pseud. aerug.	$3{,}0 \times 10^5$	0
Serr. marc.	$4{,}0 \times 10^5$	0
Bac. anitr.	$2{,}5 \times 10^5$	70

The spreading of germs from one patient to the other must be prevented by adequate hygienic measures. The greatest danger of cross-infection presumably lies in the manner of nursing. The details of the necessary precautions to be taken, however, can not be discussed in this report. The cleaning of the surroundings must be carried out by means of regular desinfections during the patient's stay as well as by final desinfection after the patient's dismissal. The last table (Tab. no 7) shows which species were still found after final desinfection. The occurrence of viable bacteria after desinfection is related to their concentrations before desinfection. A further explanation for the survival of bacteria following measures undertaken to remove and kill them possibly is a wrong performance of desinfection along with adaption of bacteria to concentrations of agents considerd active against them. In most

Tab. No. 7

	washbasin - tap	washbasin - outlet	urine bottle	respirator	suction app	divers dry surfaces	nursing inst	floor
Citrobacter		I		I	I			
Enterobacter sp.		II	I		I	II	I	II
E.coli		I			III			
Klebsiella		II			I			I
Proteus sp.		I					I	
Ps. aerug.	I	III		I	I		I	
Serr. marc.		II	I		II	IIII	I	

cases, an incorrect carrying-out of desinfection is likely to be responsible for its failure, which is often inconvenienced for the cleaning staff by the interior arrangement of intensive care units. For this reason, certain objects are never desinfected at all. On the other hand, it has been described that in particular Klebsiella species were able to tolerate concentrations of desinfective agents in practice which had previously been proved bactericidal in laboratory tests. Ps. aeruginosa is able to become adapted to quaterny ammonium compounds and in some degree even to phenol. It is moreover likely that the essential concentrations are not being used as a result of wrong dosage. An investigation into this problem revealed that 50 percent of the solutions tested contained no desinfective at all or were extremly underdosed.

Hence, antimicrobial measures in intensive care units demand increased attention not only in respect to the application of antibiotics, but also preventive steps against cross-infections must be performed with special care and conscientiousness. Here, as in antibiotic therapy, controls of the success of the antimicrobial measures are essential and consist in direct bacteriological investigation of objects and materials apt to be involved in cross-infection.

IN VITRO SENSITIVITY OF 10.610 BACTERIAL STRAINS TO TRIMETHOPRIM-SULFAMETHOXAZOLE AND OTHER BACTERIAL AGENTS

C. TRUFFOT, R. BISMUTH, G. PACAUD, J. GROSSET

Laboratoire Central de Bactériologie

Hôpital Pitié-Salpêtrière (75634 PARIS)

When it started being used, the combination TS was effective against most bacterial species encountered in usual practice. This paper is a report on the changes in its spectrum of action with time, the incidence of synergy between the two components and the present position of TS as compared to large spectrum antibiotics such as ampicillin, chlortetracyclin and minocyclin.

MATERIAL AND METHODS

Material : 10.610 bacterial strains were selected from september 1970 to february 1975. This figure represents the total amount of strains isolated at the "Laboratoire Central de Bactériologie du Groupe Hospitalier Pitié-Salpêtrière" from september 1970 to june 1971, from march to september 1972, from february to june 1974 and in february 1975, to the exclusion of D. pneumoniae, N. gonorrhoeae, Acinetobacter, Citrobacter, Pseudomonas and strictly anaerobic bacteria.

Methods : the sensitivity to trimethoprim (T) alone, to sulfamethoxazole (S) alone and to the combination TS is tested by the disc method on Mueller Hinton (MH) agar for S. aureus and gram negative bacilli and on MH plus 5 % horseblood for Str. faecalis and streptococci. The inoculum contains between 10^4 and 10^5 bacteria. The amount of S and T deposited on the discs is the following : S = 23,75 mcg; T = 1,25 mcg. The strain is considered sensitive to T, S, and TS when the inhibition zone around the discs is at least 15 mm in diameter. The antibacterial activity of T is considered to be "potentiated" by S, according to previous data not yet published, whenever the inhibition diameter around the TS disc is at least 5 mm longer than the one around the T disc (TS = T + 5 mm).

The sensitivity of bacterial strains to ampicillin, chlortetracyclin and minocyclin is determined by measuring the minimal inhibitory concentration (MIC) on MH agar or on MH plus 5 % horseblood for Str. faecalis and streptococci. The antibiotic concentrations tested range from 0,06 to 128 mcg/ml. 10^4 to 10^5 bacteria are inoculated. The strains with an MIC of 4 mcg/ml or less are considered sensitive to either one of the three antibiotics, to the exclusion of S. aureus whose sensitivity to ampicillin is defined by the lack of penicillinase secretion.

RESULTS

1. The evolution of the resistance of the main bacterial species to the combination TS and to sulfonamides between 1970 and 1975 is shown in figures 1 and 2. The evolution of the resistance to the combination TS varies according to the different species.

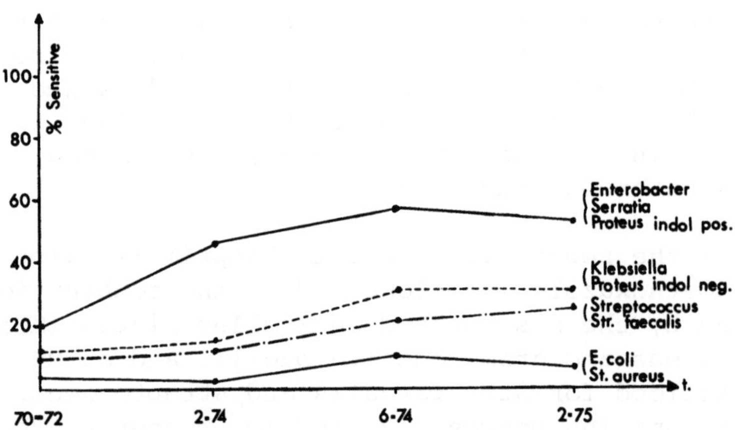

FIG. 1: EVOLUTION OF RESISTANCE TO TS

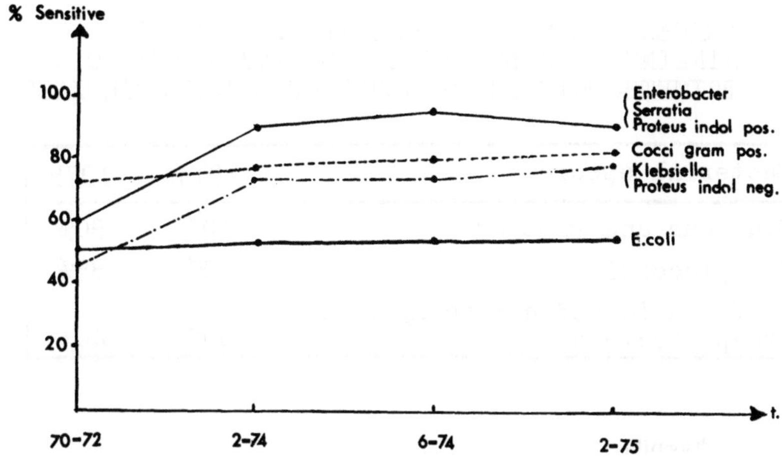

FIG. 2: EVOLUTION OF RESISTANCE TO SULPHONAMIDES

The strains of E. coli and S. aureus remain sensitive in 95 % of the cases. But the incidence of resistance increased from 10 % to 25 - 30 % for Str. faecalis, streptococci, Klebsiella and indol negative Proteus and from 20 to 60 % for indol positive Proteus, Serratia and Enterobacter. Although it was already frequent in 1970 - 1972, the resistance to sulfonamides developed concurrently with the resistance to TS. There was no increase in the incidence of resistance to sulfonamides of gram positive cocci and E. coli whereas there was an increase of 20 to 30 % in all other enterobacteriaceae.

2. The originality and advantage of the combination TS being the synergy of action between trimethoprim and sulfamethoxazole and the frequent persistence of that synergy in spite of the resistance to sulfonamides, two samples of sulfonamide resistant strains were tested as to the existence of that synergy (the 513 strains isolated in february 1974 and the 421 isolated in february 1975). Table 1 shows that the percentage of sulfonamide resistant strains whose sensitivity to trimethoprim is "potentiated" in the presence of sulfamethoxazole varies from one bacterial species to another.

TABLE 1: PERCENTAGE OF SULPHONAMIDE RESISTANT STRAINS WITH ENHANCED SUSCEPTIBILITY TO TRIMETHOPRIM IN PRESENCE OF SULPHAMETHOXAZOLE

Bacterial species	1974	1975
S.aureus and Proteus	90%	90%
Streptococci	60%	85%
St.faecalis and enterobacteria except Proteus	30%	40%

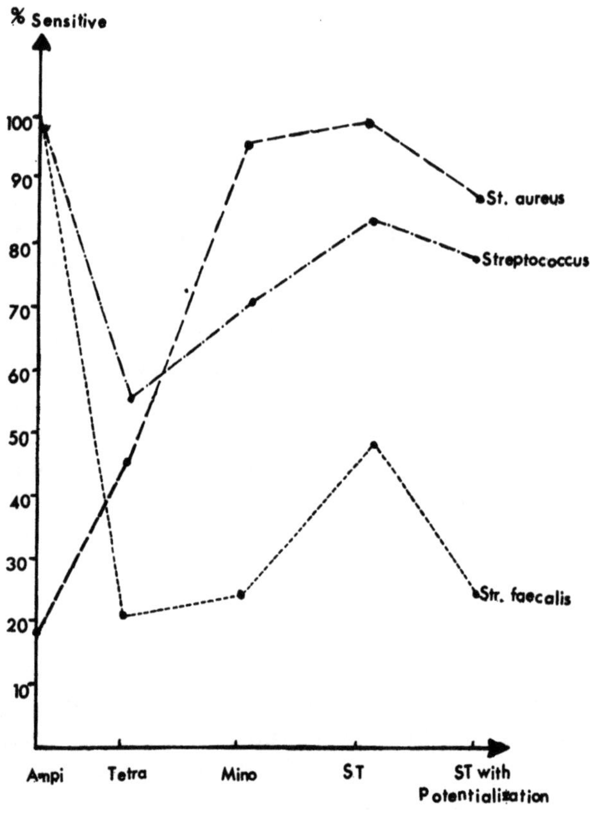

FIG. 3: PERCENTAGE OF GRAM POSITIVE COCCI SENSITIVE TO AMPICILLIN, CHLORTETRACYCLIN, MINOCYCLIN, TS AND TS WITH POTENTIATION

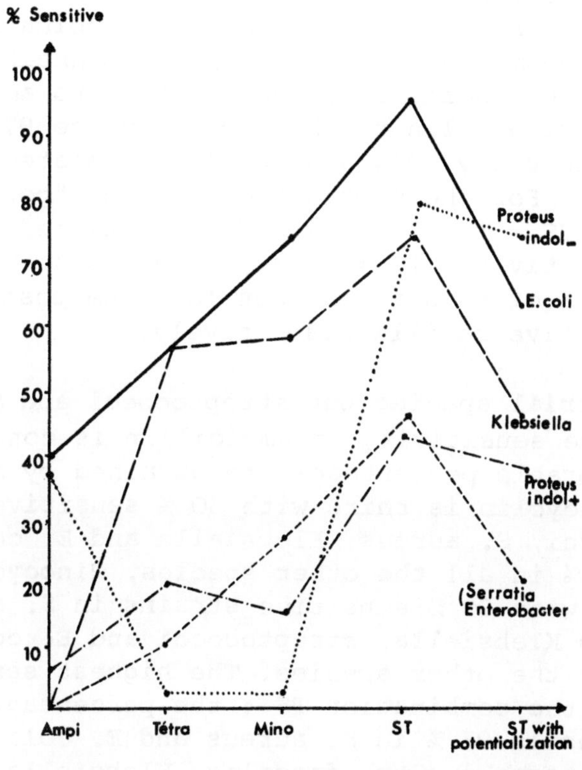

FIG. 4: PERCENTAGE OF GRAM NEGATIVE ENTEROBACTERIA SENSITIVE TO AMPICILLIN, CHLORTETRACYCLIN, MINOCYCLIN, TS AND TS WITH POTENTIATION

Three different groups of bacteria can be distinguished : those for which "potentiation" is almost constant : S. aureus and Proteus; those for which it is frequent (60 to 85 %) : streptococci; and those for which it is observed in only 30 to 40 % of the cases : Str. faecalis and enterobacteriaceae other than Proteus.

3. From a strictly bacteriological standpoint, it is possible to determine the place of the combination TS among the commonly used broad spectrum antibiotics by comparing the incidence of sensitivity to ampicillin, tetracyclin, minocyclin to that to TS on the 970 strains isolated in february 1974 and the 1023 isolated in february 1975. For the combination TS, the "potentiated" sensitivity (TS = T + 5 mm) was differentiated from the ordinary sensitivity (TS = 15 mm). Figures 3 and 4 sum up the results of this comparison for gram positive cocci and gram negative bacilli respectively.

For all bacterial species but streptococci and Str. faecalis whose sensitivity to ampicillin is constant, the less favorable percentages are obtained by ampicillin. Tetracyclin is third with 50 % sensitive strains in streptococci, S. aureus, Klebsiella and E. coli but less than 20 % in all the other species. Minocyclin comes second with 90 % sensitive strains in S. aureus, 50 to 75 % in Klebsiella, streptococci and E. coli and under 30 % in the other species. The highest sensitivity rate is with the combination TS : the percentage of sensitive strains is 95 % in S. aureus and E. coli, 70 to 80 % in streptococci, Str. faecalis, Klebsiella and indol negative Proteus and still 40 % in indol positive Proteus, Serratia and Enterobacter. If among the TS sensitive strains the only ones that are sensitive with potentiation are considered, the sensitivity rate remains superior in Proteus and equal in all the other bacterial species to that of minocyclin. It can be said therefore that the combination TS is the commonly used broad spectrum antibiotic to which bacteria are less resistant to date.

THE PREVALENCE OF AMPICILLIN, CEPHALOSPORIN AND SULPHONAMIDE RESISTANCE AMONGST URINARY TRACT PATHOGENS

J. Andrews[1], M.J. Bywater[2], A.M. Emmerson[3], C. Keane[4], D.S. Reeves[2], R. Wise[1]
1. Dudley Road Hospital, Birmingham
2. Southmead Hospital, Bristol
3. Whittington Hospital, London
4. Federated Dublin Voluntary Hospital

SUMMARY

A total of 2,031 clinical isolates of Gram negative bacilli was obtained from hospitals in 4 centres and these cultures were tested for resistance to ampicillin, cephazolin and sulphonamide.

Ampicillin and sulphonamide resistance in outpatients ranged from 15-28% of Esch. coli strains and 4-11% of Proteus mirabilis strains. Resistance to cephazolin in outpatients ranged from 0-3% of Esch. coli and 0-6% for Proteus mirabilis. Resistance patterns for Esch. coli, Proteus mirabilis and Klebsiella strains isolated from inpatients were much higher and varied widely.

These patterns are presented and the reasons for these variations discussed.

INTRODUCTION

The choice of urinary antimicrobial agents is a wide one and depends on many factors. For considerations such as dosage, route, frequency of administration, tolerance, safety, cost and efficacy against causative organisms sulphonamides have been widely used in the treatment of primary urinary tract infections. In spite of the widespread use of sulphonamides and other urinary antimicrobial agents the striking fact remains that the majority of pathogens isolated from the urinary tract in general practice patients maintain a high degree of sensitivity to the various drugs tested. For this reason most primary urinary tract infections are treated by general practitioners without recourse to laboratory studies. Nevertheless, variations in the resistance patterns do occur both in general practice and in hospital populations which emphasises the need for periodic re-assessment.

The present epidemiological study involving 4 busy clinical microbiology laboratories was constructed to provide information on the prevalence of ampicillin, cephazolin and sulphonamide resistance amongst urinary coliform bacilli as defined by standardised minimum inhibitory concentrations (M.I.C).

MATERIALS AND METHODS

Organisms were isolated from patients with symptomatic and asymptomatic urinary tract infection. The standard criteria for significant bacteriuria were followed and urinary isolates were identified according to the established techniques. Cowan and Steele (1974)[1]. Each of 4 centres in Birmingham, Bristol, Dublin and London collected 500 urinary isolates; 250 strains from inpatients and 250 strains from outpatients. Primary disc sensitivity tests were performed according to local techniques before organisms were numbered and stored on nutrient agar. All isolates were then collected together and M.I.C's determined by an agar dilution method for ampicillin, cephazolin and sulphadiazine.

Sulphonamide M.I.C's (Method as performed at Southmead). Medium Oxoid DST agar with 5% lysed horse blood. Plates were poured with sulphadiazine incorporated to give final concentrations of 2.5, 5,10,25,50,100 and 200 micrograms/ml. Inoculum Organisms were diluted in saline to a concentration of 10^3-10^4 organisms per ml. A Leec Multipoint Inoculator was used to inoculate the sulphonamide incorporated and control plates. All plates were incubated at 37°C overnight.

Ampicillin and Cephazolin M.I.C's (Method as performed at Birmingham). Medium Oxoid DST agar. Plates were poured with ampicillin or cephazolin incorporated to give final concentration of 0.06-1024 µg/ml in doubling dilutions. Inoculum Organisms were diluted to give a final count of 10^3organisms per inoculum on the plate. A Denley Multipoint Inoculator was used to inoculate the antibiotic incorporated plates and the controls. All plates were incubated at 37°C overnight and the lowest concentrated of drug which inhibited growth was recorded as the M.I.C.

RESULTS

Two thousand and thirty one organisms were examined of which 1,462 were Esch.coli (72%), 260 were Proteus mirabilis (12.8%) and 149 were Klebsiella spp. (7.3%). The prevalence of resistance of Esch. coli to sulphonamide for the 4 centres is shown in Table I.

TABLE I

SULPHONAMIDE RESISTANCE (MIC> 50μg/ML) IN 1462 URINARY ESCH. COLI

Centre	Inpatients		Outpatients	
	No.of strains	% resistant	No.of strains	% resistant
Birmingham	131	30.5	208	21.6
Bristol	171	19.3	198	17.6
Dublin	167	42.0	226	14.6
London	162	35.1	199	28.1

The resistance patterns of inpatient isolates and outpatient isolates are compared. This shows the strikingly high sulphonamide resistance to Esch. coli in Dublin inpatients (42%) compared with the very low resistance to the same organism in Bristol inpatients (19%). Esch.coli resistance to sulphonamide in outpatients in London (28%) is high compared with the other 3 centres.

Broader patterns of resistance to the 3 drugs of 1,462 Esch.coli are shown in Table II.

TABLE II

RESISTANCE PATTERNS OF 1462 ESCH.COLI ISOLATED FROM URINARY TRACT INFECTIONS

Centre	No.of strains	% of strains resistant		
		Ampicillin MIC>32μg/ml	Cephazolin MIC> 32μg/ml	Sulphonamide MIC>50μg/ml
Birmingham				
Inpatients	131	32.1	3.1	30.5
Outpatients	208	25.1	0.5	21.6
Bristol				
Inpatients	171	21.1	4.2	19.3
Outpatients	198	17.2	2.0	17.6
Dublin				
Inpatients	167	39.6	1.2	42.0
Outpatients	226	15.5	0.0	14.6
London				
Inpatients	162	23.5	6.9	35.1
Outpatients	199	19.5	3.0	28.1

This table shows the comparatively high ampicillin resistance to Esch. coli in inpatients in Dublin (40%) and Bristol (32%) and in outpatients in Bristol (25%). This table also shows the general overall low resistance (less than 7%) to cephazolin in 1,462 Esch. coli isolates.

The prevalence of resistance pattern of 260 Proteus mirabilis isolates to the 3 drugs is shown in Table III.

TABLE III

RESISTANCE PATTERNS OF 260 PROTEUS MIRABILIS ISOLATED FROM URINARY TRACT INFECTIONS

Centre	No. of strains	% of strains resistant		
		Ampicillin MIC≫32μg/ml	Cephazolin MIC≫32μg/ml	Sulphonamide MIC>50μg/ml
Birmingham				
Inpatients	48	13.6	2.3	11.3
Outpatients	18	11.2	5.6	5.6
Bristol				
Inpatients	46	4.4	0.0	8.7
Outpatients	26	3.8	0.0	3.8
Dublin				
Inpatients	36	36.2	11.1	22.2
Outpatients	18	5.6	0.0	11.2
London				
Inpatients	52	9.6	5.7	13.4
Outpatients	20	5.0	0.0	10.0

Resistance of Proteus mirabilis to ampicillin is frequently below 10% although higher levels of resistance are shown at Birmingham in both in and outpatients. Comparatively speaking, the resistance of Proteus mirabilis to ampicillin in Dublin (36%) is extremely high. This table also shows the fluctuating patterns of resistance of Proteus mirabilis to sulphonamide ranging from about 4% to 11% in outpatients to 8% to 22% in inpatients. Resistance of Proteus mirabilis to cephazolin is 11% in Dublin inpatients and 5.7% in London inpatients compared with very low resistance in Bristol and Birmingham.

The prevalence of resistance patterns of 149 Klebsiella spp. isolate to the 3 drugs is shown in Table IV.

TABLE IV
RESISTANCE PATTERNS OF 149 KLEBSIELLA SPP. ISOLATED FROM URINARY TRACT INFECTIONS

Centre	No.of strains	% of strains resistant		
		Ampicillin MIC>32μg/ml	Cephazolin MIC>32μg/ml	Sulphonamide MIC>50μg/ml.
Birmingham				
Inpatients	41	87.8	21.9	48.8
Outpatients	17	76.4	23.6	5.9
Bristol				
Inpatients	15	80.0	6.7	20.0
Outpatients	9	77.2	11.1	11.1
Dublin				
Inpatients	31	87.1	35.4	61.4
Outpatients	8	75.0	0.0	0.0
London				
Inpatients	21	95.2	14.3	33.4
Outpatients	7	71.5	0.0	0.0

Resistance of Klebsiella spp. to ampicillin is generally very high but several isolates from all 4 centres had MIC's of the order of 8 to 16μg/ml which lowered the overall resistance of Klebsiella spp. to ampicillin to approximately 86% in inpatients and 75% in outpatients when the 'cut off point' was taken at 32μg/ml or more. Resistance of Klebsiella spp. to sulphonamide alone is extremely variable with patterns of high resistance in inpatients and very low resistance in outpatients. Resistance of Klebsiella spp. to cephazolin shows a very high resistance in inpatients in Dublin (35%) and a uniformly high level of resistance in both inpatients and outpatients in Birmingham.

DISCUSSION

It is essential that the results obtained by antibiotic sensitivity tests by disc diffusion methods relate both to the M.I.C. of the antibiotic in vitro and the concentration of the antibiotic attainable at the site of the infection. In order to make a strict comparison of resistance, the M.I.C's of isolates from all centres were measured centrally by carefully standardised techniques.

Excretion of antibiotics is often rapid and very high levels are frequently obtained but failure to eradicate the causative organisms in the urinary tract may occur in spite of extremely high concentrations of the antimicrobial agent. Comparative work (Williams &

Leigh 1966) has shown that when the M.I.C. to sulphonamide exceeds 50μg/ml the success in eradicating the infecting organism from the urinary tract is poor. This level has been adopted as the 'cut off point' for resistance to sulphonamide.

Recent work with cephazolin (Rimmer, 1975) has shown that once the M.I.C. exceeds 40μg/ml clinical success is only of the order of 5%. For this reason the 'cut off point' for resistance to cephazolin has been arbitarily set at 32μg/ml or more. For ampicillin, the range of M.I.C's falls clearly into a bimodal distribution and levels at 32μg/ml or more have been accepted as the 'cut off point' for resistance to ampicillin. Using these criteria for resistance, tables have been constructed comparing the resistance patterns of Esch. coli, Proteus mirabilis and Klebsiella spp. to ampicillin cephazolin and sulphonamide.

Resistance patterns vary among different countries and variation in resistance patterns have been shown by Slocombe & Sutherland (1969), McAllister et al., (1971) and Robertson (1971) throughout the U.K. but Grüneberg and Bettleheim (1969) were able to show that the serological types of Esch. coli causing domiciliary infection varied significantly between localities only a few miles apart. We too have shown variations in resistance patterns but the majority of strains of the two most commonly isolated organisms in outpatients namely, Esch. coli and Proteus mirabilis still remain sensitive to ampicillin and sulphonamide. It is often difficult however to define outpatients since many may be simply domiciliary patients or they may be antenatal patients attending hospital outpatient clinics infrequently or they may be urological patients attending outpatient clinics having recently been discharged from hospital. Thus the results from these different centres may depend largely on the type of clinical material rather than on any geographical basis per se.

Resistance of Esch. coli and Proteus mirabilis to cephazolin is extremely low in outpatients and may well reflect the low frequency of prescription. It would seem possible that General Practitioners' prescribing habits for all infective illnesses, not only for urinary tract infections, play the major role in determining the resistance of intestinal coliforms and hence of urinary pathogens. Resistance patterns of coliforms in hospital may in part be a reflection of cross infection of organisms with or without R factors.

The resistance patterns of Esch. coli and Proteus

mirabilis to ampicillin and sulphonamide in inpatients as shown here vary widely and perhaps one of the functions of a microbiologist is to be aware of these local differences and make them known.

The resistance of Esch. coli and Proteus mirabilis to cephazolin is low in inpatients apart from 11% found in Dublin inpatients. Klebsiella spp. are generally insensitive to ampicillin but may well be sensitive to cephazolin or even sulphonamide in outpatients.

REFERENCES

COWAN, S.T., & STEEL, K.J. - Manual for the identification of Medical Bacteria - Cambridge University Press, London (1974).

GRÜNEBERG, R.N., & BETTLEHEIM, K.A. - Geographical variation in Serological types of urinary Escherichia coli. - Journal of Medical Microbiology 2 219-224 (1969).

McALLISTER, T.A., ALEXANDER, J.G., DULAKE, C., PERCIVAL, A., BOYCE,J.M.H., WORMALD, P.J., - The sensitivities of Urinary Pathogens. Postgraduate Medical Journal (September Supplement) 47: 7-14 (1971).

RIMMER, D.M.D. - Personal Communication (1975).

ROBERTSON, M.H. - A six year survey of resistance patterns of urinary tract pathogens in general practice. - Postgraduate Medical Journal 47 111 (1971).

SLOCOMBE, B., & SUTHERLAND, R. - Sensitivity of Gram negative bacilli to ampicillin after six years' clinical use - Journal of Clinical Pathology 22 644-648 (1969).

WILLIAMS, J.D., & LEIGH, D.A. - The sensitivity of organisms to sulphonamides. - The British Journal of Clinical Practice. 20: No.4 177-181 (1966).

CHANGES OF ANTIMICROBIAL SUSCEPTIBILITY OF ANAEROBIC BACTERIA FROM CLINICAL SPECIMEN

JUN OKADA, TOYOKO OGURI and NOZOMU KOSAKAI

Juntendo University School of Medicine

2-1-1 Hongo, Bunkyo-ku, Tokyo, Japan

INTRODUCTION

There has been a rather remarkable upsurge of interest in anaerobes and in the anaerobic infections in recent years. Especially Bacteroides species occupies a preeminent position in anaerobic infections, because of its frequency of isolation and its resistance to commonly used antimicrobial agents. The antimicrobial susceptibility of anaerobes against nine antibiotics has been tested for as long as ten years in our laboratory, and the changes in antibiotic patterns were observed for three periods.

The samples tested for this study included approximately nine hundred isolates of various anaerobes from clinical specimens, mainly isolated from pus and secretes, between 1965 and 1975. These strains included genera of Peptococcus-177, Peptostreptococcus-107, Veillonella-82, Clostridium-34, nonsporulating Gram-positive bacilli-145, Bacteroides-298 and Fusobacterium-28 strains.

The procedure used for the antimicrobial susceptibility testing was a modified agar plate dilution method using the Liver veal agar plate with five percent sheep blood. The plate were incubated for 48 hours(in anaerobic condition) utilyzing phosphorus method or steel wool method, and the minimal inhibitory concentrations(MIC) was defined as the lowest concentration of antibiotics which showed no growth, a barely visible hase or a single colony.

The antimicrobial agents tested are following: penicillin G, ampicillin, cephaloridine, erythromycin, josamycin, lincomycin, clindamycin, chloramphenicol, thiamphenicol and tetracycline. Among these drugs, thiamphenicol was tested for the purpose of comparison with chloramphenicol.

RESULTS

Penicillin G: For almost all isolates of the 976 strains tested against penicillin G, the MIC was less than 6.25 mcg/ml. The major exception is Bacteroides, since more than 65% of strains are resistant.

Cephaloridine: 97% of 525 strains except Bacteroides were inhibited by 6.25 mcg/ml or less of cephaloridine. But cephaloridine inhibited only 20% of the 351 strains of Bacteroides at 12.5 mcg/ml. Penicillins and cephaloridine showed little activity against Bacteroides.

Erythromycin: Erythromycin showed erratically active against most anaerobic species at the level of 12.5 mcg/ml. Only 10 to 30% of strains of Clostridia, Veillonella, Fusobacteria and Bacteroides are sensitive to 1.56 mcg/ml. At 25 mcg/ml, most anaerobes including 85% of Bacteroides, are susceptible. But a marked increase in resistant strains of 25 mcg/ml or more was observed in Bacteroides.

Josamycin: Josamycin has an anaerobic spectrum comparable to erythromycin. Bacteroides is generally sensitive, but a moderate increase in resistancy.

Lincomycin: Lincomycin showed similar activity against most anaerobes as erythromycin and josamycin, but has a little better activity than the two macrorides. About Bacteroides, a marked increase in resistancy was observed among recently isolated strains of Bacteroides.

Clindamycin: Clindamycin showed excellent activity against nearly all anaerobes. But 29 of the strains of Bacteroides were resistant of 6.25 mcg/ml, which has been used as a break point by some workers. Several studies have demonstrated that over 97% of clinical isolates are susceptible to 3.1 mcg/ml, but the result of our study indicate that 81% of strains are susceptible to 3.1 mcg/ml. Against 227 strains tested, 97.4% of of anaerobes were more sensitive to clindamycin than lincomycin.

Chloramphenicol: Chloramphenicol is active against a wide range of anaerobic bacteria but a slight increase of resistant strains was recognized in a few peptococcal strains. The majority(96.5%) of strains were suceptible to 12.5 mcg/ml of chloramphenicol.

Tetracycline: The majority of isolates, especially genera of Peptococcus, Peptostreptococcus and Bacteroides were resistant to tetracycline. At the level of 1.56 mcg/ml, our data indicate 40% of these organisms were resistant to tetracycline. Tetracycline was once regarded as the agent of choice for anaerobic infections, but now, this drug is no longer recommended as anaerobic infections.

Table 1. Percentage of Resistant Strains

GENUS	period	penicill-in G	ampi-cillin	cephalo-ridine	erythro-mycin	linco-mycin	josamycin	chloram-phenicol	tetra-cycline
Peptococcus	I	0	0	1.4	6.8	2.9		1.3	11.7
	II	5.6	2.8	3.4	5.6	8.6	7.0	9.3	10.8
	III	1.3	0	4.0	15.4	10.7	15.2	11.8	32.0
Peptostreptococcus	I	3.4	0	4.3	0	1.8		0	11.9
	II	0	0	0	0	0	0	0	40.9
	III	7.7	8.6	5.2	7.1	7.9	2.7	0	30.9
Veillonella	I	0	0	0	30.3	0		0	8.3
	II	3.0	3.0	6.4	52.9	12.5	51.5	0	12.1
	III	7.7	0	0	15.4	8.3	58.3	0	7.7
Clostridium	I	0	0	0	0	0		0	11.1
	II	15.4	15.4	18.2	15.4	23.1	14.3	0	23.1
	III	0	0	0	0	0	0	0	0
nonsporulating Gram-positive bacilli	I	0	0	0.9	0.9	3.9		1.9	10.3
	II	7.1	14.3	15.4	7.1	0	6.7	0	21.4
	III	0	0	0	3.7	3.8	4.5	0	11.1
Bacteroides	I	35.3	31.4	38.7	8.4	3.3		2.3	9.0
	II	85.4	88.7	95.7	10.4	4.2	4.0	0	42.7
	III	78.7	82.6	95.4	38.5	30.5	29.3	10.7	68.4
Fusobacterium	II	29.2	33.0	70.8	87.5	66.7	87.5	0	0
	III	0	0	20.0	80.0	20.0	100	20.0	0

(≧ 25 mcg/ml)

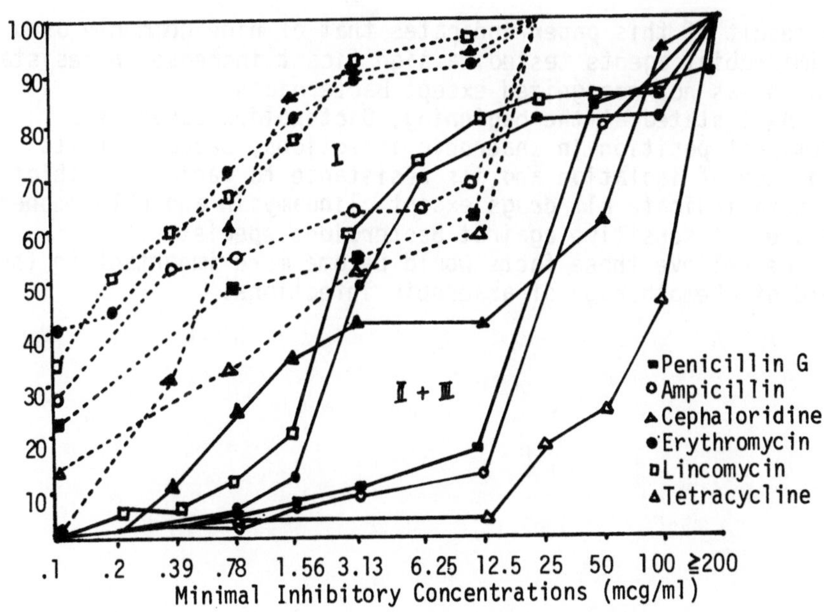

Figure 1. Cumulative percent of Bacteroides species

MIC "break point" between susceptible and resistant strains varies by antibiotics and by reporter. Table illustrates the percentage of anaerobic organisms using a break point of 12.5 mcg/ml. At the table shows, marked increase in resistant strains of Bacteroides are recognized during three periods. As I stated at the beginning, Bacteroides occupies a preeminent position in anaerobic infections, because of its frequency of isolation and its resistance to commonly used antimicrobial agents.

Figure illustrates the cumulative percent of Bacteroides species inhibited by six antibiotics, above mentioned, and the changes in susceptibilities between first period and second and third period. In the first period, 55% of strains were inhibited by 12.5 mcg/ml or less of penicillins and cephaloridine, but in the second and third period, only 20% of strains were inhibited at the level.

With erythromycin and lincomycin, more than 90% of strains were inhibited by 12.5 mcg/ml of these drugs in the first period, while in the second and third period, less than 70% of strains were inhibited.

With tetracycline, as I above mentioned, a marked increase in resistant strains was observed.

With chloramphenicol, increase in resistancy was not recognized for three periods.

CONCLUSION

The result of this paper indicates that of nine commonly used antimicrobial agents tested, a significant increase in resistant strains was not recognized except Bacteroides.

As I stated at the beginning, Bacteroides occupies a preeminent position in anaerobic infections, because of its frequency of isolation and its resistance to various antibiotics. Our data indicate all drugs except clindamycin and chloramphenicol are not sensitive against Bacteroides species.

We believe these facts would become more important in the field of chemotherapy of anaerobic infections.

BACTERICIDAL EFFECT OF CEPHALOSPORIN DERIVATIVES IN PATIENT MATERIAL CONTAINING ENTEROBACTERIACEAE RESISTANT TO AMPICILLIN

Gerhard Lebek

Inst.f.Hygiene u.Mikrobiolgie d.Universität

Bern, Friedbühlstrasse 51, CH-3008 Bern

Gram positive organisms and Neisseria strains are quite evenly influenced by all cephalosporins. Their antibacterial activity is strong against penicillinase forming and penicillinase-free Staphylococci and - especially - against Pneumococci, Neisseriae and Streptococci group A. For these resistance tests with cephalosporins is no problem. For routine sensitivity testing only one of the cephalosporin antibiotics may be considered. The same is true for the testing of Streptococci group D with reduced sensitivity.
Gram negative rods, however, differ greatly in their response towards individual cephalosporins. The resistance level cannot be foreseen (is inpredictable) and unevenly distributed for individual derivatives. For Enterobacteriaceae these differences may depend on the content of certain R-factors. Such factors may contain determinants for β-lactamases differently active against individual cephalosporin derivatives and therefore conferring to the carrier organisms different sensitivity patterns against these individual antibiotics. This is why for such germs resistance testing using one derivative only is not representative for all others.
For routine sensitivity testing it is not possible to consider at one time all available and soon to be marketed cephalosporin derivatives. Consequently the question arises whether certain derivatives might not be defined as indicator substances for all other similar

antibiotics. On the other hand β-lactamases might be classified according to the sensitivity profile of cephalosporin derivatives based on the different substrate specifities of such R-factor determined enzymes.
In order to clarify this problem we have studied the sensitivity of a selected series of ampicillin-resistant Enterobacteriaceae and Pyocyaneus strains against the available and some (possibly) soon to be marketed cephalosporins.

For the drug material we are indebted to Merck,Sharp & Dohme, Squibb, Ciba-Geigy, Lilly and Bristol Laboratories.
For the preparation of the substances to be studied the drug firms declarations of the drug activity ratio was respected.

Methods

A 37°C overnight culture of the test strains in Columbia Broth (BBL Nr.94 136,pH 7,5 ± 0,2) was diluted to 10^{-4} - 10^{-6} . 0,1 ml of this was put on agar plates (Trypticase Soy Agar, BBL Nr.11 047,pH 7,5 ± 0,2)containing rising concentrations of individual cephalosporin derivatives. After a 48h incubation at 37°C the bactericidal effect of each substance concentration was calculated from the difference in number of colonies between drug free and drug containing media. Each test was done twice, if differences in the results occurred the test was repeated once more. Only clones were used which were homogenously resistent throughout the total population and did not suffer any R-factor loss.
Of some of the tested E.coli strains the R-factor was transferred with the usual method to E.coli K12 and was tested for resistance against all the used cephalosporin derivatives.
Fig.1 shows the results of the comparative bactericidal tests for some selected ampicillin-resistant coli from patient material against 11 cephalosporin derivatives and ampicillin.
For each drug the concentration for a 50% and 100% bactericidal effects are tabulated. Certain activity profiles can be distinguished for the E.coli. The detail evaluation is not discussed here. The initial hypothesis is confirmed with the presented results, namely that testing of one cephalosporin derivative against coli alone doesn't permit to determine in the same time the activity of the other derivatives.
Cefoxitin and Cephamandole, often also Cephazolin are very active in tests with individual strains where other cephalosporin derivatives are only slightly active. These drugs,

therefore, should be tested individually. Possibly Cefoxitin or Cephamandole may be used as indicator-substances for the evaluation of β-lactamase resistent cephalosporins whereas cephalothin would have to be carried along in sensitivity testing, for the time being. Against this recommendation several arguments exist as can be derived from this table. In practice it must be found out how often such a resistance test fails.

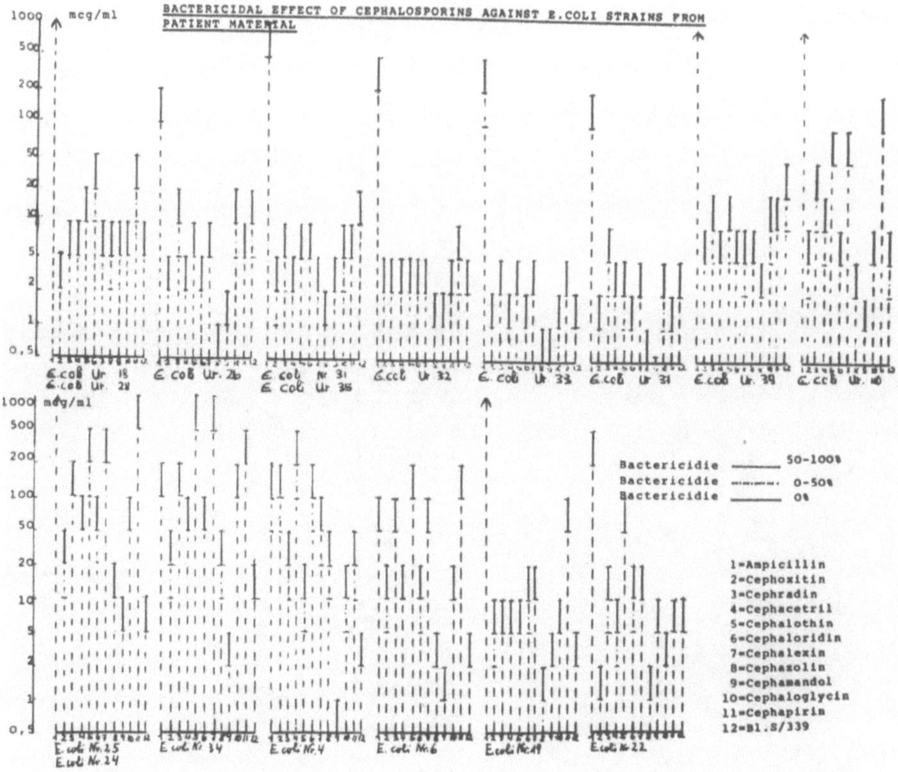

Fig.2 contains the test results for E.coli K12 as carrier of different R-factors. It can be seen that all cephalosporins are less sensitive than ampicillin against R-governed β-lactamases. In these organisms no big differences are found for the 11 tested drugs.

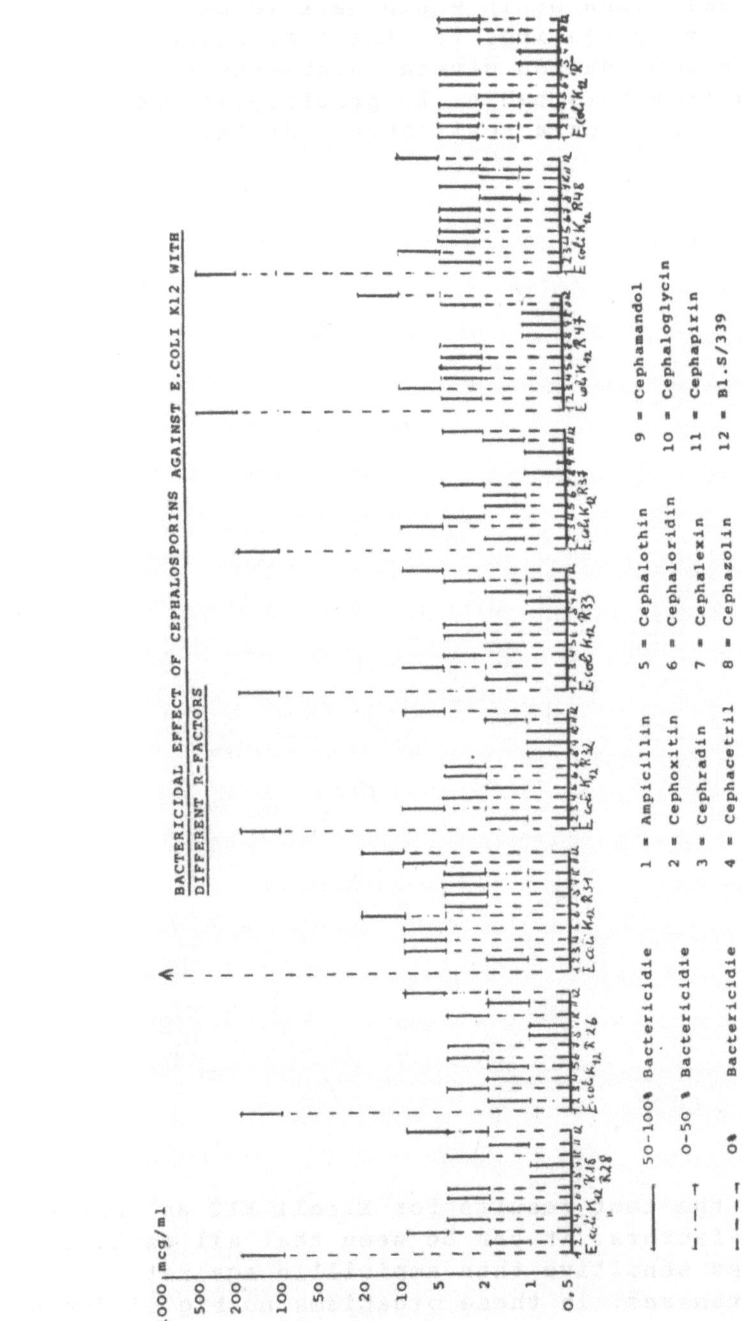
BACTERICIDAL EFFECT OF CEPHALOSPORINS AGAINST E.COLI K12 WITH DIFFERENT R-FACTORS
1000 mcg/ml
500
200
100
50
20
10
5
2
1
0.5
50-100% Bactericidie
0-50 % Bactericidie
0% Bactericidie
1 = Ampicillin
2 = Cephoxitin
3 = Cephradin
4 = Cephacetril
5 = Cephalothin
6 = Cephaloridin
7 = Cephalexin
8 = Cephazolin
9 = Cephamandol
10 = Cephaloglycin
11 = Cephapirin
12 = B1.S/339

FIGURE 2

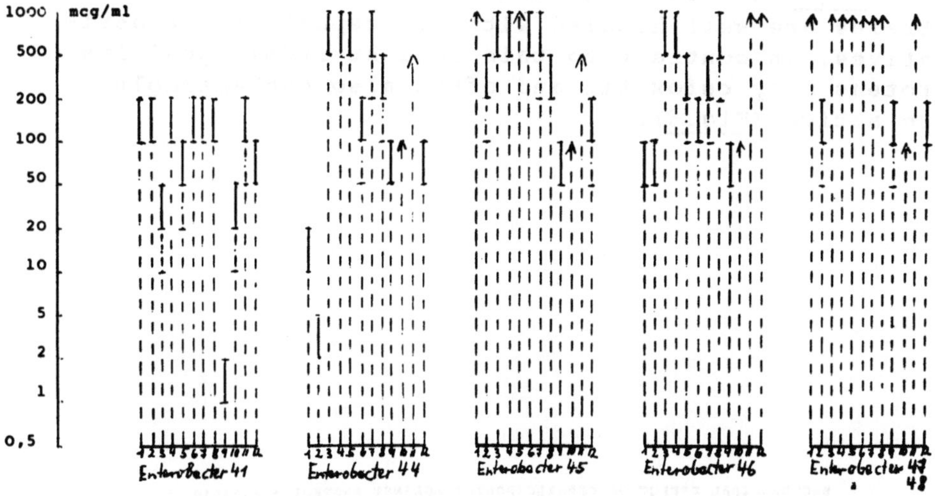

50-100% Bactericidie
0-50 % Bactericidie
0% Bactericidie

1=Ampicillin
2=Cephoxitin
3=Cephradin
4=Cephacetril
5=Cephalothin
6=Cephaloridin
7=Cephalexin
8=Cephazolin
9=Cephamandol
10=Cephaloglycin
11=Cephapirin
12=Bl.S/339

Fig.3 demonstrates the known minimal efficacy of all cephalosporins against Enterobacter strains.

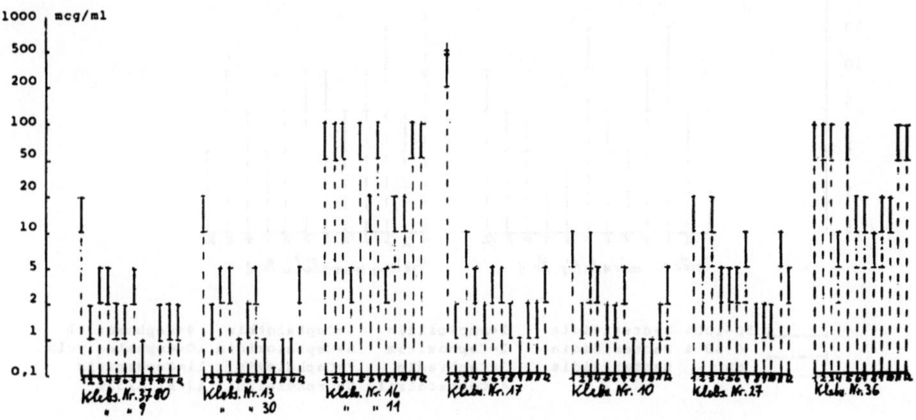

50-100% Bactericidie
0-50 % Bactericidie
0% Bactericidie

1=Ampicillin
2=Cephoxitin
3=Cephradin
4=Cephacetril
5=Cephalothin
6=Cephaloridin
7=Cephalexin
8=Cephazolin
9=Cephamandol
10=Cephaloglycin
11=Cephapirin
12=Bl.S/339

Fig.4 compiles the Klebsiella data. The selected strains show considerable differences in their potency to influence cephalosporin derivatives. No systematic rule can be elaborated.

From Fig.5 can be taken that indole negative Proteus strains are well handled with all cephalosporin derivatives. In contrast to this against indole positive Proteus only cefoxitin and often also cephamandole are active (Fig.6).

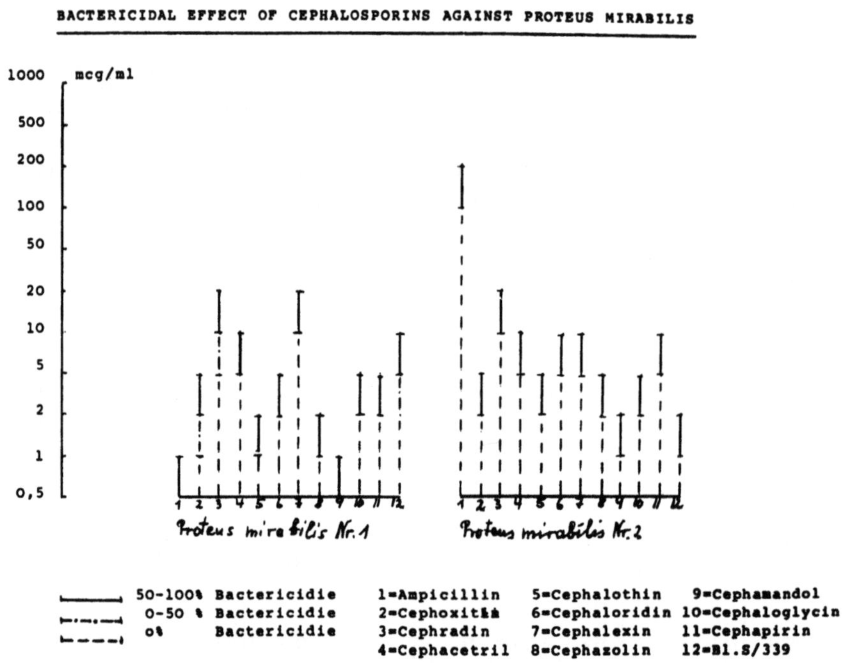

FIG. 5

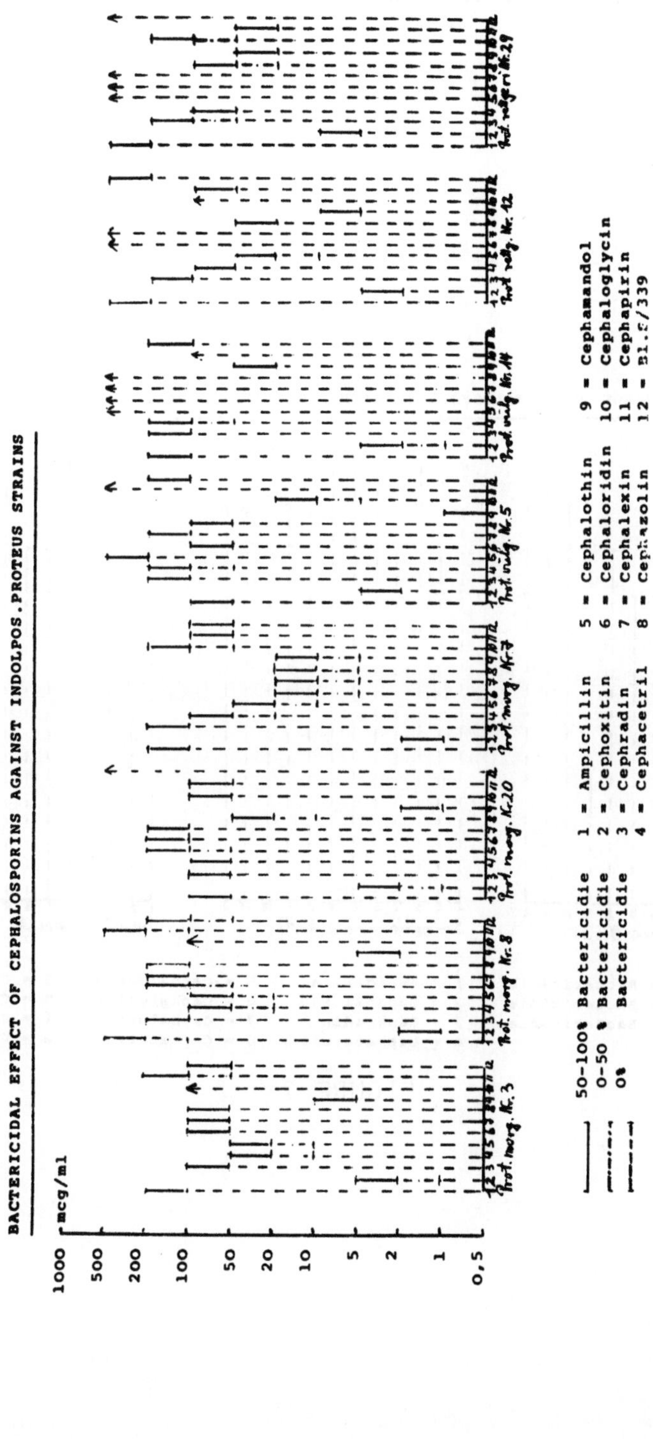
BACTERICIDAL EFFECT OF CEPHALOSPORINS AGAINST INDOLPOS.PROTEUS STRAINS
mcg/ml
1000
500
200
100
50
20
10
5
2
1
0,5
50-100% Bactericidie
0-50 % Bactericidie
0% Bactericidie
1 = Ampicillin
2 = Cephoxitin
3 = Cephradin
4 = Cephacetril
5 = Cephalothin
6 = Cephaloridin
7 = Cephalexin
8 = Cephazolin
9 = Cephamandol
10 = Cephaloglycin
11 = Cephapirin
12 = Bl.S/339

FIGURE 6

Against Serratia marcesens (Fig.7) either cefoxitin or cephamandole or no tested drug is active. Finally all tested drugs are inactive against Pseudomonas aeruginosa.

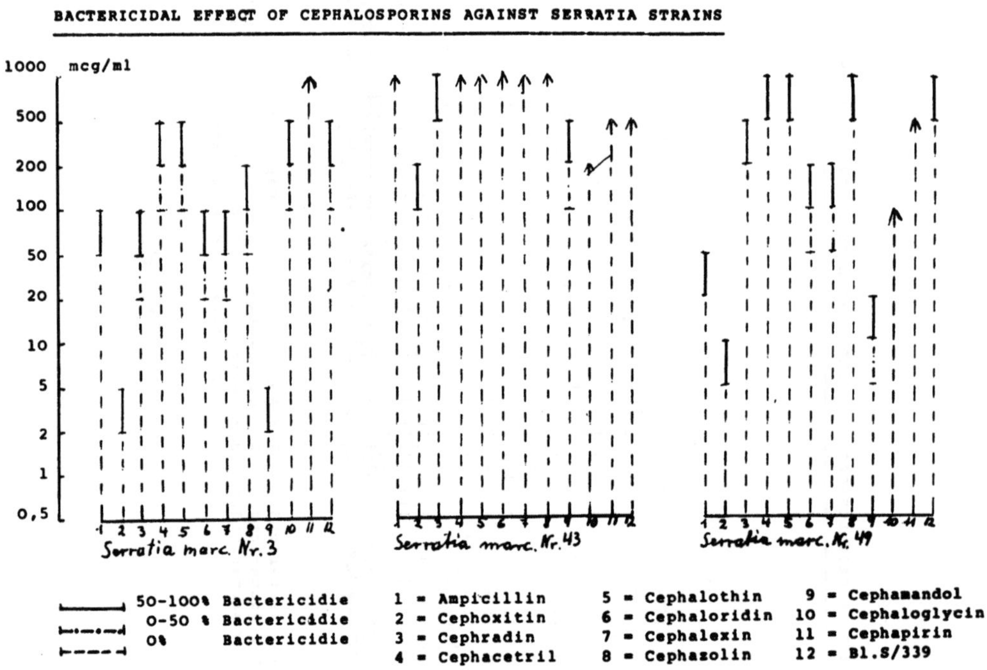

FIGURE 7

Antibacterial Activity of Rifampicin and Its Combinations Against Clinical Strains Isolated From Cases With Purulent-Inflammatory Processes

I. P. Fomina, L. N. Samoilova,
L. E. Bodunkova, S. M. Navashin

National Research Institute of
Antibiotics, Moscow, USSR

SUMMARY

The antibacterial activity of rifampicin against clinical multiresistant microorganisms the main causative agents of purulent infections especially Staphylocccus aureus including methicillin-resistant strains was much higher than that of other antibiotics. Sensitivity of gramnegative organisms (E.coli, Proteus, Pseudomonas aeruginosa) to rifampicin was moderate and it may be increased by combination of rifampicin with the antibiotics inhibiting the protein synthesis or the cell membrane functions.

The expediency of the use of rifampicin in treatment of cases with non-specific purulent-septic processes remains doubtful inspite of its broad antibacterial spectrum and high activity against most species of grampositive and gramnegative microorganisms. Possible rapid development of resistance during rifampicin therapy, moderate sensitivity of most gramnegative microbes to the antibiotic a great variety of the side effects induced by it are important restrictions to its use (Atlas and Turck 1968; McCabe and Lorian 1968; Arioli et al.1967)

Data on the study of rifampicin sensitivity to clinical strains of Staphylococcus, Proteus, Coli bacteria and Ps. aeruginosa, as well as the effect of rifampicin used in combination with other antibiotics are presented.

One hundred strains of pathogenic staphylococci isolated from patients with staphylococcal destruction of the lungs were used in the study on the antistaphylococcal activity of rifampicin. The isolates were characterized by high resistance to most antibiotics, i.e. 95 per cent of the cultures were resistant to benzylpenicillin, chloramphenicol and tetracycline, 94 per cent to erythromycin. Among the isolated 54 per cent were resistant to methicillin. The average values of the MIC of methicillin were 25 to 400 mcg/ml. No strains resistant to rifampicin were found: all of them were characterized by high sensitivity to that antibiotic. The MIC of rifampicin for both most methicillin sensitive staphylococci was 0.002 to 0.2 mcg/ml (Table 1).

Table 1

Sensitivity of 100 clinically isolated strains of Staphylococcus aureus to antibiotics

Antibiotics	Sensitive m.i.c.(mg/ml)	%	Resistant m.i.c.(mg/ml)	%
Rifampicin	0.002-0.02	100	-	-
Benzylpenicillin	0.02-0.4	5	6.2-800	95
Methicillin	1.6-6.2	46	25 -400	54
Erythromycin	0.2-0.8	6	12.5-800	94
Chloramphenicol	1.6-6.2	5	50 -200	95
Tetracycline	0.8-6.2	5	25-2000	95
Streptomycin	0.4-3.1	20	25-2000	80

Heterogenity with respect to sensitivity to rifampicin was shown. When staphylococci were grown on selective media containing 10 to 100 mcg/ml of rifampicin, the average rate of isolation of the rifampicin resistant mutants was 1.8-2x10^7 microbial bodies.

Marked heterogenity of staphylococci, Coli bacteria and Ps.aeruginosa with respect to their sensitivity to rifampicin was most pronounced on the use of the inoculum with increasing density. When the number of the microbes was 10^3 microbial bodies, the MIC of rifampicin for most of the staphylococcal strains amounted to 0.002 to 0.01 mcg/ml. However, when it was increased 10000 times, the average values of the antibiotic MIC increased up to 50-200 mcg/ml (Table 2)

Table 2

Effect of the inoculum size on the activity of rifampicin

Species	Strain No.	Minimum inhibiting concentration (mg/ml) with inocula of cells/ml			
		10^3	10^5	10^7	10^8
Staph aureus	1568 2137 2348	0.002 0.002 0.005	0.005 0.002 0.01	0.05 0.02 0.02	50 200 100
E.coli	37 265 438	12.5 12.5 6.2	12.5 25.0 12.5	50 200 25	1600 800 400
Proteus	5 15 46	3.1 6.2 12.5	6.2 6.2 12.5	6.2 200 25	800 400 1600
Ps.aeruginoas	49 1014 5843	25 50 25	50 50 25	100 100 50	200 800 100

The in vitro experiments showed a possibility of increasing the antibacterial activity of rifampicin on its combination with erythromycin, fusidin or oxacillin. The combination of rifampicin with erythromycin or oxacillin proved to be most active against multi-resistant staphyloccoci. The rate of synergism on the use of rifampicin in combination with erythromycin was 80 per cent and the MIC of erythromycin in the combination for the erythromicin resistant staphylococci decreased 31-125 times. (Table 3)

Table 3

Effect of the in vitro association of rifampicin with other antibacterial drugs on some gram-positive and gram negative microorganisms

Species	Synergism	Summation	Indiffeence	Antagonism
Staphylococcus	erythromycin	oxacillin	fusidin	-
Escherihia coli	kanamycin, polymyxin, tetracycline		ampicillin	-
Proteus			kanamycin ampicillin	-
Pseudomonas aeruginosa	tetracycline, streptomycin			-

The activity of rifampicin against the gramnegative microorganisms tested was much lower. The MIC of rifampicin for the sensitive strains of Coli bacteria. Ps. aeruginosa and Proteus ranged within 3.1-25 mcg/ml. However, the rate of isolation of the clinical strains resistant to its action was relatively low and amounted to 15, 18 and 37 per cent for E.coli, Proteus and Ps. aeruginosa respectively. Still, the rate of isolation of the action of other broad-spectrum antibiotics was high (Table 4).

Table 4

Activity of rifampicin in vitro against gram-negative clinical isolates: comparison with other antibiotics

Species	No. of strains tested	Antibiotics	m.i.c. (mg/ml)				% of resistant strains
			0.8-1.6	3.1-6.2	12.5-25	50->100	
E.Coli	80	rifampicin	-	6	62	12	15
		gentyamicin	25	55	-	-	0
		ampicillin	-	12	6	62	77.5
		tetracycline	15	2	3	60	78.7
		chloramphenicol	-	22	4	54	67.5
Proteus	50	rifampicin	-	11	30	9	18
		gentamicin	21	19	10	-	20
		ampicillin	-	22	-	28	56
		tetracycline	-	4	-	46	92
		chloramphenicol	-	12	17	21	42
Pseudomonas aeruginosa	30	rifampicin	-	-	19	11	36.6
		gentamicin	10	14	6	-	20
		ampicillin	-	-	-	30	100
		tetracycline	-	2	3	25	83.3
		chloramphenicol	-	-	3	27	90

The moderate activity of rifampicin against gramnegative organisms is usually bound to poor penetration of the antibiotic through the cell wall of coli bacteria and Proteus. To confirm this data on higher inhibitory effect of rifampicin on DNA-dependent RNA polymerase of E.coli fractions as compared to the enzyme of the intact cells are presented. (Wehrli et al. 1968)

The results of the study of the antibacterial activity of rifampicin combinations with the antibiotics inhibiting the protein synthesis, and polymyxin B may serve as an additional evidence of the postulate. The rate of synergism on the use of rifampicin combinations with kanamycin or polymyxin B with respect to coli bacteria was close. However, the MIC of polymyxin B for coli bacteria resistant to it decreased at least 200 times, up to the therapeutic concentrations, while that of kanamycin decreased 15 times and remained within the ranges higher than the therapeutic blood levels.

Table 5
Activity of rifampicin alone and in combination with other antibiotics against E. coli

Antibiotics	No. of strains tested	synergism (percentage)	mean value of mic (mg/ml) of antibiotics	mean value of mic (mg/ml) of antibiotics in combination
rifampicin +kanamycin rifampicin + kanamycin	80	74	22.3 >600	1.3+42
rifampicin +tetracycline rifampicin + tetracycline	80	61	22.3 266	3.4+110
rifampicin polymyxin I rifampicin I polymyxin	80	65	22.3 >1000	2.0+4.9

Therefore, the study of the antibacterial activity of rifampicin against clinical multiresistant strains of microorganisms, the main causative agents of purulent infections showed its high antistaphylococcal activity, which was much higher than that of other antibiotics with respect to staphylococci including strains resistant to methicillin.

Sensitivity of the above species of gramnegative organisms to rifampicin is moderate. Still it may be increased by combination of rifampicin with other drugs.

References

1. Arioli, V., Pallanza, R., Furesz, S., and Carniti, G. (1967)
2. Atlas, E., and Turck, M. (1968) J. med. Sci. 256, 247
3. McCabe, W.R. and Lorian, V., (1968) Amer. J. med. Sci. 256, 255
4. Wehrli, W., Knusel, F., Schmid, K., Staehelin M. (1968)

DYNAMICS OF METHICILLIN RESISTANT STAPHYLOCOCCI UNDER EFFECT OF ELIMINATING AGENTS

O. N. Speranskaya, I. P. Fomina,
V. S. Zueva

National Research Institute of Antibiotics
Moscow, USSR

SUMMARY

The methicillin resistant strains were isolated from 62.2 per cent of the cases with acute purulent-inflammatory processes in the lungs. High resistance levels to all widely used antibiotics, stability to the effect of heavy metal salts, as well as virulence were characteristics of methicillin resistant staphylococci. Successful elimination of the determinants of methicillin resistance from some strains and their stability in the others indicate to the dual nature of methicillin resistance in clinical staphylococcal strains.

Multiresistant staphylococci remain to be the basic causative agents of acute and chronic inflammatory processes in the respiration systems. Such staphylococci alone or in association with other microorganisms are isolated from almost two thirds of the patients especially in children hospitals, a significant part of them being methicillin resistant (MR). It was already mentioned earlier (Speranskaya et al., 1973) that the rate of isolation of such strains depended on the disease, previous antibiotic therapy and its duration. Two groups of children at the age of 20 days to 14 years suffering from the disease of the lungs and respiratory tract, i.e. children with staphylococcal destruction of the lungs in the 1st group and acute respiratory infections in the 2nd group were examined comparatively. The examination showed that MR staphylococci amounted to 62.2 per cent in the 1st group and 30 per cent in the 2nd group. No dependence of the rate of isolation of polyresistant staphylococci on the age of the patients and the period of their presence in the hospital was noted. When the

Table 1

ANTIBIOTIC RESISTANCE LEVELS OF MR AND MS STRAINS OF STAPHYLOCOCCI

	MIC mcg/ml	Pc	M	Cm	Tc	Sm	Em	Km
		%						
MS	0.05-1.0	11.1	12.4	-	12.9	4.8	25.3	11.1
	1.6-12.5	3.3	87.6	20.2	8.0	36.1	4.1	80.9
	25-50	10.0	-	32.1	35.5	8.5	30.6	-
	100	75.5	-	47.7	43.6	50.6	40.0	8.0
MR	0.05-1.0	0.96	-	-	-	5	1.0	4.0
	1.6-12.5	-	-	9.6	2.0	1.0	-	63.0
	25-50	-	2.8	20.4	9.3	1.8	1.0	10.0
	100	99.04	97.2	70.0	88.7	97.2	98.0	23.0

average period of hospitalisation was 1.5 to 2 months, multiresistant strains were isolated from all age groups during the 1st examination.

Strains of the MR staphylococci isolated from the patients in both groups were not epidemiologically connected. However, they were characterised by a similar phenotype and high resistance levels to all known antibiotics, high penicillinase activity, virulence, stability to the effect of heavy metal salts. Close phagolytic properties were characteristic of the MR strains of staphylococci. Most of the strains (69 per cent) could not be typed with the phages of the International set, 30 per cent of the strains were typed with the phages of group I (mainly 80 phage-type). One per cent of the staphylococcal strains was lyzed with the phages of groups II and III. At the same time significant differences between the MR and MS (methicillin sensitive) strains were observed, one which was the antibiotic resistance spectrum. Most of the MS strains, i.e. 74 per cent were resistant to 1 - 5 drugs, while 94 per cent of the MR strains were resistant to the effect of 5 - 9 drugs. The rate of isolation of staphylococci characterized by high resistance levels to the widely used antibiotics was higher among the MR strains than in the MS strains (Table 1). Thus, among the MR staphylococci 97 per cent of the strains were highly resistant to streptomycin, while among the MS strains only 50 per cent were resistant to the antibiotic. With respect to tetracycline the respective values were 89 and 44 per cent. As for erythromycin or kanamycin the difference was even more pronounced, i.e. 98 and 40 or 23 and 8 per cent respectively.

Children with staphylococcal destruction of the lungs were subjected to prolong antibiotic therapy with periodical changing of the drugs, such as gentamicin, lincomycin, fusidin, combinations of semisynthetic penicillins. During the treatment course repeated bacteriological examinations, i.e. at the moment of hospitalization and then every 1 - 2 weeks were performed. The repeated bacteriological examinations carried out with a purpose of studying the dynamics of the staphylococcal sensitivity to the antibiotics during the treatment course revealed in some patients definite changes in the culture sensitivity structure with appearance of additional determinants. The determinants of resistance to methicillin, oleandomycin and lincomycin were most frequent (Table 2).

To show the origin of new determinants of resistance in the above strains, they were phage typed repeatedly. Replacement of the phage type was observed in most of the strains in addition to changing of the phenotype. Changing of the staphylococcal strain belonging to a definite phage group coinciding with changing of the resistance phenotype may be evident in hospital

Table 2

DYNAMICS OF ANTIBIOTIC RESISTANCE OF HOSPITAL STRAINS OF STAPHYLOCOCCUS AUREUS

Patients	Determinants of resistance			Phage - typing patterns		
	On the 1st day after hospitalisation	On the 5th day	On the 10th day	On the 1st day after hospitalisation	On the 5th day	On the 10th day
Patient E.	Pc M Cm Tc Sm Em Om	Pc M Cm Tc Sm Em Om	Pc M Cm Tc Sm Em Om Lm	untypeable	untypeable	7 phage group III
Patient K.	Pc Cm Tc Sm Em	Pc Cm Tc Sm Em Om	Pc Cm Tc Sm Em Om M	80 phage group I	80 phage group I	47/53/77 phage group III
Patient A.	Pc Cm Tc Sm Em Om	Pc Cm Tc Sm Em Om	Pc Cm Tc Sm Em Om M Lm	80 phage group I	80 phage group I	6/54 phage group III
Patient Y.	Sm Lm	Sm Lm Pc M Cm Tc Km Em Om	Sm Lm Pc M Cm Tc Km Em Om	untypeable	untypeable	untypeable

Table 3

ELIMINATION OF METHICILLIN RESISTANCE UNDER THE ACTION OF EB AND GROWTH AT 42°C

T^o							EB			
Strain	T^o	1 passage	3 passage	10 passage	15 passage	37°C	Strain	MIC	EB 2.5mcg/ml	MIC without EB
314	37°C	800	800	200	200		314	800	1.6	1.6
	42°C	200	12.5	12.5	12.5	200				
320	37°C	800	200	200	200		405	800	12.5	800
	42°C	100	12.5	12.5	12.5	200				
351	37°C	800	200	200	200		373	1600	1.6	200
	42°C	100	12.5	12.5	12.5	200				
362	37°C	800	200	200	200		362	800	1.6	25
	42°C	100	12.5	12.5	12.5	200				

infection of the patients with new staphylococcal strains. Appearance of the determinants of resistance to macrolides during the antibiotic therapy with preservation of the intial phagolytic characteristics assumes genetic changes in the initial strain.

A possibility of elimination of the above determinants by repeated passages of the cultures, their storage, exposure to ethidium bromide (EB) and high temperature was tried during the studies on stability of methicillin resistance and investigation of the staphylococcal strains with respect to penicillinase production and penicillin resistance.

The MR strains were studied for a year with every day passages onto meat-peptone broth (MPB) media containing no methicillin. It was found that methicillin resistance was a stable character; neither determinants MR and PcR, nor capacity for penicillinase production were lost during the every day passages of the cultures or during storage as lyophilized cultures.

The main phenotypic characteristics of 25 staphylococcal strains were studied after 30 passages on MPB containing no methicillin at the temperature of 42°C. Under the above cultivation conditions, methicillin resistance decreased to the levels of the MIC corresponding to the therapeutic concentration even after 3 passages. However, further incubation at a temperature of 37°C of such cultures and the cultures subjected to repeated passages at 42°C resulted in restoration of their resistance up to the intial levels (Table 3).

Therefore, incubation it a temperature of 42°C did not result in formation of stable methicillin resistant variants. Exposure to EB in concentrations of 2.5, 5 and 10 mcg/ml resulted in stable elimination of the methicillin resistance determinants in 2 - 8 per cent among 8 strains. Strains with high initial resistance levels to methicillin (MIC 800mcg/ml) lost their methicillin resistance after exposure to EB and their MIC decreased 500 times. The elimination of methicillin resistance in these strains was stable.

As for most of the strains tested the effect of EB was transitory and restoration of methicillin resistance to the initial or lower levels was observed even after the 1st passage without exposure to EB.

Exposure to EB or high temperatures had no effect on penicillinase production and penicillin resistance.

On the basis of the studies it is possible to assume that the sites of localization of the genetic determinants of methicillin resistance in the clinical strains of staphylococci are not the same: the localization of the methicillin resistance markers may be chromosomal or extrachromosomal.

Therefore, the part of the MR strains among the multiresistant staphylococci isolated from children with acute purulent inflammatory processes in the lungs is significant. The MR strains were isolated from 62.2 per cent of the cases with acute purulent inflammatory processes in the lungs, which contradicts the literature data stating that the number of the MR strains does not exceed 30 per cent (average ranges of 0.1 - 0.2 to 20 - 40 per cent) (Benner and Kayser 1968; Parker and Hewitt 1970; Bülow 1971).

High resistance levels to all widely used antibiotics, stability to the effect of heavy metal salts, as well as virulence were characteristic of the MR staphylococci. Successful elimination of the determinants of methicillin resistance from some strains and their stability in the others indicate to the different nature of methicillin resistance in clinical staphylococcal strains.

References

1. Benner, E. J., Kayser, F. H., (1968), Lancet, 2, 741.

2. Bülow, P. (1971), Ann. N. Y. Acad. Sci., 181, 21.

3. Parker, M. T., Hewitt, J. H., (1970), Lancet, 1, 800.

4. Speranskaya O. N., Fomina I. P., Kuznetsova S. M., (1973), Antibiotics, 1, 62.

TETRACYCLINE RESISTANCE IN PNEUMOCOCCI AND GROUP A STREPTOCOCCI: A SURVEY IN THE UNITED KINGDOM

J.G. Kensit and W. Farrell

Department of Medical Microbiology, The London Hospital Medical College, London E1 2AD

SUMMARY

In a laboratory survey in 21 centres in England, Wales and Scotland 13% of pneumococci and 37% of group A streptococci were shown to be resistant to tetracycline. Resistance was commoner in isolates from hospital patients. There was a wide variation in resistance from centre to centre and it should be emphasised that advice on the use of tetracycline in any particular area must depend on local survey data.

INTRODUCTION

The incidence of tetracycline resistance among pneumococci and group A streptococci has been reported by several centres in the last few years. However, these surveys have generally been on a small scale and a larger survey on a countrywide basis was considered to be potentially valuable in illustrating the present importance of tetracycline resistance in these organisms. 21 widely spaced centres were chosen, ranging from Inverness in the north to Plymouth in the south. Most of the hospitals involved in this survey serve cities or large towns.

METHODS

Gram positive cocci showing α-haemolysis on blood agar and sensitive to Optochin (Ethyl hydrocuprein) were accepted as pneumococci. All isolates provisionally regarded as group A streptococci were formally grouped by a method involving extraction of the C-carbohydrate.

It was important to ensure that participating laboratories agreed their definitions of "sensitive" and "resistant" as applied to these organisms. Ten strains of pneumococci and 10 of group A streptococci with known minimum inhibitory concentrations of tetracycline were circulated to the laboratories involved who then examined them by disc testing as performed on routine isolates of these organisms. Results were reported to the co-ordinating centre at the London Hospital.

The survey began in the last week of January and ended in the last week of April 1975. Laboratories reported on a standard form the sensitivity of pneumococci and group A streptococci and added the following information: age and sex of the patient; category of patient, e.g. in-patient, out-patient, etc; site of the isolate, e.g. sputum, wound, etc; and whether or not tetracycline was being administered at the time a specimen was obtained.

RESULTS

A total of 1,528 pneumococci and 1,533 group A streptococci were isolated. Thirteen percent of the pneumococci and 37% of the group A streptococci were reported as resistant to tetracycline. The rate varied in pneumococci from 2% of 42 isolates in Ayr, to 32% of 145 isolates at The London Hospital. Similarly, for group A streptococci there was a wide variation from 15% of 137 isolates in High Wycombe to 70% of 43 isolates in Glasgow.

Numbers of resistant strains of pneumococci decreased from 14% of 1,203 isolates in in-patients to 11% of 192 isolates in out-patients and to 5% of 106 isolates from general practice. Group A streptococci resistant to tetracycline varied from 45% of 473 isolates from in-patients to 35% of 265 isolates from out-patients and 32% of 760 isolates from general practice.

There were significant differences in the numbers of resistant strains isolated from the respiratory tract and from non-respiratory sites. Among the pneumococci 13% of 1,310 isolates from the respiratory tract were resistant against 8% of 215 strains from non-respiratory sites. Among group A streptococci 34% of 875 isolates from the respiratory tract were resistant against 40% of 650 isolates from other sites.

DISCUSSION

This survey emphasises the wide variation throughout the country in tetracycline resistance in group A streptococci. There is a smaller variation among pneumococci, most of the centres sampled having resistance rates of 8 to 18%. Only two centres had more than 18% resistant strains.

TABLE 1

TETRACYCLINE RESISTANCE IN PNEUMOCOCCI AND GROUP A STREPTOCOCCI

Centre	Pneumococci No. of Isolates	Pneumococci % resistant to Tetracycline	Group A Streptococci No. of Isolates	Group A Streptococci % resistant to Tetracycline
Inverness	65	3	89	34
Aberdeen	58	7	224	41
Ayr	42	2	36	50
Glasgow	31	13	43	70
Edinburgh	53	13	71	23
Newcastle	47	13	53	28
York	53	9	42	17
Liverpool	38	18	7	29
Stafford	163	17	10	20
Nottingham	78	14	148	28
Birmingham	63	6	56	48
Cardiff	28	7	53	62
Epping	52	10	68	35
High Wycombe	47	4	137	15
London(St.Thomas')	198	7	135	31
" (Guy's)	22	9	38	37
" (The London)	145	32	54	39
" (U.C.H.)	85	13	82	42
Bristol	69	26	34	53
Portsmouth	32	3	79	46
Plymouth	159	8	74	49
TOTAL	1528	13	1533	37

TABLE 2

TETRACYCLINE RESISTANCE BY PATIENT CATEGORY IN PNEUMOCOCCI AND GROUP A STREPTOCOCCI

	Pneumococci		Group A Streptococci	
	No. of Isolates	% resistant to Tetracycline	No. of Isolates	% resistant to Tetracycline
In-Patients	1203	14	473	45
Out-Patients	192	11	265	35
General Practice Patients	106	5	760	32
Others	21	5	34	32
TOTAL	1527	13	1533	37

TABLE 3

RESISTANCE IN ISOLATES FROM RESPIRATORY AND NON-RESPIRATORY SITES: PNEUMOCOCCI AND GROUP A STREPTOCOCCI

	Pneumococci		Group A Streptococci	
	No. of Isolates	% resistant to Tetracycline	No. of Isolates	% resistant to Tetracycline
Respiratory	1310	13	875	34
Non-respiratory	215	8	650	40
TOTAL	1525	13	1525	36

A high level of resistance among one group of organisms is not necessarily correlated with a high level in the other group. For example, Ayr reported 2% of pneumococci resistant and 50% of group A streptococci, while Plymouth reported 8% pneumococci resistant and 49% group A streptococci. The London Hospital reported 32% of pneumococci resistant, 2½ times the national average, while only 39% of group A streptococci, a similar figure to the national average (37%). These variations are difficult to explain.

The incidence of resistance diminishes from in-patient to out-patient to G.P. patient. Numbers of pneumococci in the last group are small and are probably very highly selected. The greater percentage of resistant strains isolated in hospital presumably reflects either cross infection or an increased incidence of resistant organisms in the more severe pneumococcal infections, particularly exacerbations of chronic bronchitis, that require hospital admission. Both factors may be operative. The increase in in-patients may be related to previous courses of chemotherapy.

There are significant differences in both pneumococci and group A streptococci in the incidence of resistance in respiratory versus non-respiratory but the differences are too small to be a guide to the choice of therapy in infections of these sites.

There is a significant level of resistance among pneumococci in this country as evidenced by results from these 21 centres, but except for a few areas, tetracycline remains a reasonable drug in the initial therapy of probable pneumococcal infections in all but the most severe infections. Treatment failure caused by drug resistance must be remembered, however.

Among group A streptococci drug resistance is far commoner and, except possibly for 3 or 4 centres, it does not seem to us to be reasonable to use tetracycline as the drug of first choice in penicillin sensitive patients with probably group A streptococcal infection.

It must be emphasised that advice in any particular area about the use of tetracycline in infections caused by these organisms depends on local survey data because of the wide variation in resistance which we have shown occurs.

REFERENCES

Percival, A., Armstrong, E.C., Turner, G.C. (1969) Increase of incidence of Tetracycline resistant pneumococci in Liverpool in 1968. Lancet, 1, 998-1000.

Robertson, M.H. (1965) β-haemolytic streptococci in South West Essex with reference to tetracycline resistance. B.M.J., 2, 569-571.

Robertson, M.H. (1968) Tetracycline resistant streptococci in South West Essex: a continuing survey. B.M.J., 3, 349-350.

Robertson, M.H. (1973) Tetracycline resistant β-haemolytic streptococci in South West Essex: decline and fall. B.M.J., 4, 84-85.

LYSOGENY OF STREPTOCOCCUS PYOGENES AND TRANSDUCTION OF DRUG RESISTANCE TO TETRACYCLINE, CHLORAMPHENICOL AND MACROLIDES ANTIBIOTICS WITH PHAGES INDUCED FROM THEM

KIMIKO UBUKATA, MASATOSHI KONNO AND RYOCHI FUJII*

Department of Pediatrics, Teikyo University School of Medicine
2-11-1, Kaga, Itabashi-ku, Tokyo, Japan

It has been noticed a wider distribution of tetracycline(TC) resistant Streptococcus pyogenes throughout Japan and the emergence of chloramphenicol(CM) resistant strains. Since 1968 type T-12 strains made up the greater number and macrolides resistant strains were first noticed in 1972.

Our study on the yearly incidence of TC, CM and macrolides resistance of Streptococcus pyogenes and the mechanism of drug resistance was reported in 1973, which disclosed that 70% of streptococci isolated from clinical sources showed a complete cross resistance among all macrolides and lincomycin analogues tested. This fact can not be overlooked since our yearly consumption of those antibiotics in 1973 amounted to 126,700 Kg.

From our experiences on staphylococcal multidrug-resistance, it was quite natural to consider this rapid emergence of streptococcal drug resistance to be a result of transduction of drug resistance by their phages. The present study deals with transduction of drug resistance with phages induced from drug resistant streptococci.

Table 1 shows our method to prepare phage lysates. 114 strains of Streptococcus pyogenes isolated from throat swabs of our in- and out- patients with acute respiratory diseases from Feb. 1972 to Mar. 1974 were so treated and the phage lysates of 114 strains were spotted onto the blood agar plate culturing respective strain.

Through this cross experiment there was found only two strains eligible for recipient strain in transduction and for indicator strain to detect lysogeny(Table 2). One strain is drug sensitive and the other resistant to TC alone, both being typed as T-12.

Table 1. Preparation of Phage Lysates from Streptococcus pyogenes

Bacteria(0.5 ml) inoculated into 10 ml Todd Hewitt broth
|
Incubated with shaking for 4 hr at 37°C
|
Mitomycin C added to the culture medium(final concentration of 0.15 mcg/ml)
|
Incubated with shaking for 1 hr
|
Centrifugation for 20 min at 3,000 r.p.m.
|
Bacterial sediment suspended in 10 ml fresh TH broth
|
Centrifugation for 20 min at 3,000 r.p.m.
|
Supernatant filtered though a 0.40 μ millipore filter
|
Phage lysates

Table 2. Lytic Pattern of Phage Lysates Induced from Streptococcus pyogenes

Resistant pattern	No. of strain	Phage lysates														
		TC,CM, Mac.			TC CM	TC				CM	Sensitive strain					
		51	2	1	4	3	1	4	1*	7	16	1	1	1	1**	20
TC,CM,Mac.	51															
	2															
	1															
TC,CM	4															
TC	3															
	1															
	4															
	1(TK-4983)*	+	+		+	+	+			+	+	+	+	+		
CM	7															
Sensitive strain	16															
	1												+	+		
	1															
	1		+				+									
	1(TK-4958)**	+	+		+	+	+			+	+	+	+			
	20															

It seems that our success in inducing streptococcal prophage from donor strains came from the adoption of Todd-Hewitt culture media and the addition of mitomycin C with a final concentration to be 0.15 mcg/ml to the media. The grouping and T-typing of our strains were done with agglutination method.

As shown in Table 3, 86 out of 114 strains(75.4%) revealed to be lysogenic. Lysogeny was demonstrated in 53 out of 54 strains (98.2%) resistant to TC, CM and macrolides antibiotics. They were typed to be T-12 except one strain which was untypable. The extent of bacteriolysis is very strong with respect to the phage lysates from those strains resistant to TC, CM and macrolides. All of the strains showing double resistance to TC and CM, and single resistance to CM were typed T-12 and lysogenic. The strains resistant to TC alone, as having been noticed of its wide distribution for a long time, revealed lysogeny in less than fifty percent, so did it the sensitive strains. The extent of bacteriolysis was less marked in these cases. Lysogeny was shown in 44.7% of type T-1 and 92.0% of type T-12 strains. There is a consistency with the Zabriskie's report as to a high incidence of lysogeny among epidemic strains. It is presumed that a higher incidence of lysogeny is obtainable if we further adopt adequate indicator strains.

Eight donor strains were selected randomly from 114 strains above mentioned including five strains resistant to TC, CM and macrolides, and each one strains resistant to TC and CM singly or doubly. The two recipients were the same strains which was adopted as indicator strains for detecting lysogeny. T-typing and the MIC of various antibiotics to these strains are shown in Table 4.

Table 3. Frequency of Lysogenic Streptococcus pyogenes by T-typing

Drug resist.	No. strain	Phage plaque positive	T-1	T-12	Others *	Non Typ.
TC,CM,Mac.	54	53		52		1
TC,CM	4	4		4		
CM	7	7		7		
TC	9	4	1	3		
Sensitive	40	18	3	14	1	
Total	114	86 (75.4%)	4 (44.4%)	80 (92.0%)	1	1

Others ; T-6:2, T-11:1, T-14:1, T-22:1, T-28:8, B-3264:3

Table 4. Drug Resistance of Donors and Recipients

	Strain	TC	CM	EM	JM	CLM
Donor (T-12)	TK-4803	50	50	>100	>100	>100
	TK-4923	50	50	>100	>100	>100
	TK-4924	50	50	>100	>100	>100
	TK-4943	50	50	>100	>100	>100
	TK-4960	50	25	>100	>100	>100
	TK-4905	100	25	0.05	0.39	0.05
	TK-4917	50	3.13	0.05	0.2	0.05
	TK-4919	0.2	25	0.1	0.78	0.025
Recipient (T-12)	TK-4958	0.2	1.56	0.05	0.2	0.05
	TK-4983	50	3.13	0.05	0.39	0.05

MIC (mcg/ml)

media: HI agar + 5% defib. sheep blood, inoculum size:10^7/ml

The overnight culture of recipient cells was incubated in TH broth with shaking for 4 hr at 37°C. Then, 1 ml of the culture cells was mixed with 1 ml of phage lysate which was adjusted to yield MOI of 0.1, and the mixture was shaken for 1 hr at 37°C. After shaking, it was immediately cooled and centrifuged. The sedimented cells were washed three times with cooled TH broth to remove free phage particles. They were then spreaded on selective agar plate containing antibiotics and incubated for 48 hr or 72 hr at 37°C. The selective agar plate contained TC at 2 mcg/ml, CM at 5 mcg/ml or EM at 0.25 mcg/ml singly. The colonies that grew on the selective plate were all picked up, put to three serial culture on blood-agar plate, subjected to grouping and T-typing and finally tested sensitivity to various drugs.

Ultrathin section of a donor cell was observed under electron microscope three hours after treatment with mitomycin C. Intracellular phage particles are observable with a high electron density. Observing with negative staining of phage lysate, phage particles appear to have a regular hexagonal head and non-contractile tail with inapparent end plate. The head size is about 500 Å and the tail is about 2,400 Å.

Transduction of drug resistance into the recipient sensitive to TC, CM and macrolides was capable with phages induced from any donor strains, which is shown in Table 5. It was found that the transductants obtained were classifiable into two different groups in terms of resistant pattern. Namely, the transductants grown on TC-containing select agar plate were resistant only to TC while those grown on CM- or EM- containing agar plate were resistant to all of CM, macrolides, lincomycin and clindamycin. It should be stressed that there demonstrated a definite cross resistance among macrolides and lincomycin analogues.

Table 5. Resistant Pattern of Transductants

Donor : TC^r, CM^r, $Macrolides^r$
Recipient : TK-4958(non-resistant)

Selected drugs	Donor phage lysates				
	TK-4803	TK-4923	TK-4924	TK-4943	TK-4960
TC	TC^r(7)	TC^r(1)	TC^r(13)	TC^r(99)	TC^r(17)
CM	CM^rMac^r(5)	CM^rMac^r(9)	CM^rMac^r(13)	0	0
EM	0	CM^rMac^r(1)	CM^rMac^r(1)	CM^rMac^r(2)	0

( ):No. of transductant obtained
Phage titer/ml : 1.0~2.0 X 10^7 MOI: 0.06~0.15
Mac^r : includes resistance to lincomycin analogues

The transduction with phages induced from the strain TK-4905 resistant to both TC and CM, the strains resistant to TC(TK-4917) or CM(TK-4919) alone yielded TC and CM resistance separately(Table 6). No single case was ever experienced of the simultaneous transduction of TC, CM and macrolides resistance.

When the recipient resistant to TC alone was adopted, CM and macrolides resistance were simultaneously transduced in every case, thus resulting TC, CM and macrolides resistant transductants (Table 7).

The transductants obtained from the greatest number of donors were those resistant to TC alone : Then followed CM and macrolides resistant ones. The frequency of their occurence ranged from 10^{-6} to 10^{-7}. The resistance of the transductants to each drug tested was almost same that of the donor strains tested.

Table 6. Resistant Pattern of Transductants

Recipient : TK-4958(non-resistant)

Selected drugs	Donor phage lysates		
	TC^rCM^r	TC^r	CM^r
	TK-4905	TK-4917	TK-4919
TC	TC^r(62)	TC^r(8)	0
CM	CM^r(6)	0	CM^r(5)
EM	0	0	0

Phage titer/ml : 0.9~1.2 X 10^7, MOI : 0.05~0.09

Table 7. Resistant Pattern of Transductants

Donor: TC^r, CM^r, Macrolides^r
Recipient: TK-4983(TC^r)

Selected drugs	Donor phage lysates				
	TK-4803	TK-4923	TK-4924	TK-4943	TK-4960
CM	CM^rMac^r(4)	CM^rMac^r(15)	CM^rMac^r(4)	CM^rMac^r(7)	CM^rMac^r(1)
EM	0	CM^rMac^r(2)	0	CM^rMac^r(1)	0

Phage titer/ml : 1～2 X 10^7 MOI : 0.06～0.15

The grouping and T-typing of the transductants obtained in the recipient strain TK-4983 revealed that all of these transductants were of group A and of type T-12. However some of the transductants produced in the recipient strain TK-4958 were found not typable. From our results, it seems that there are two ways to transduce drug resistance in the Streptosoccus pyogenes. One is transduceable TC resistance alone and the other is CM resistance with or without macrolides and lincomycin analogue resistance.

The origin of multiresistant streptococcus of type T-12, now prevalent throughout Japan, is explained that CM, macrolides, lincomycin and clindamycin resistance have been transduced into the TC resistant strains.

Since the latter half of 1973, T-28 and B-3264 strains were began to be detected newly. As no drug resistance is provable among them sofar, the drug resistant pattern of group A streptococcus in Japan depends on the future epidemiology of these new type streptococcus.

LITERATURE

1) Takizawa, K., Miyamoto,Y., et al : On the drug sensitivity of hemolytic streptococci. Bull. Kanagawa Public Health Lab., 2 : 1-2, 1972(Japanese)
2) Ubukata, K., Konno, M. and Fujii, R. : Drug resistance of group A hemolytic streptococci to macrolides, lincomycin analogues, chloramphenicol and tetracycline. Shonikarinsho 26: 1451-1458, 1973(Japanese)
3) Miyamoto, Y. : Typing of group A streptococcus by agglutination method, Rinshokensa, 13: 1085-1091, 1969(Japanease)
4) Zabriskie, J. B., Read, S. E. and Fischetti, V. A.: Lysogeny in streptococci ; In streptococci and streptococcal diseases. Academic Press, 1972, New York and London. pp 99-118.

COMPARATIVE ACTIVITY OF TETRACYCLINE, MINOCYCLINE, CLOMOCYCLINE AND METHACYCLINE AGAINST GROUP A, B, C AND G β HAEMOLYTIC STREPTOCOCCI

R.Y. Cartwright and K. Korpal

St. Luke's Hospital, Guildford, Surrey, U.K.

INTRODUCTION

Tetracycline resistance in group A haemolytic streptococci was first described in the United Kingdom by Lowbury and Casan (1954).. By 1965, 44% of all β haemolytic streptococci isolated in the Institute of Laryngology and Otology, London, were resistant to tetracycline (Dadswell, 1967). Although the frequency of resistant strains declined in 1970, 28% of isolates remained tetracycline resistant (Rees, 1971).

Minocycline, a tetracycline analogue, was shown by Frisk and Tunevall, 1968, and Leigh and Simmons, 1974, to have activity against some tetracycline resistant strains of *Staphylococcus aureus*. Steigbigel, Reed and Finland, 1968, had indicated that this might apply also to group A and B haemolytic streptococci.

This study compares the activity of tetracycline, minocycline, clomocycline and methacycline against 100 strains of freshly isolated β haemolytic streptococci - 45 group A, 25 group B, 22 group C and 8 group G.

METHODS

The mean inhibitory concentrations were determined on 5% blood agar plates containing dilutions of the tetracycline analogues. The strains were grown overnight in 0.1% glucose broth which was then diluted to contain approximately 10^3/ml. colony forming units. The plates were inoculated with a multipoint bacteriophage inoculator delivering approximately 0.02 ml. fluid from each loop.

The plates were incubated for 18 hours at 37°C. The Oxford staphylococcus was inoculated on each plate as a control organism. The antigen for grouping was extracted by the autoclaving.

The possible comparative in vivo activity of the antibiotics was assessed by determining the percentage of strains which would be inhibited at the trough serum levels expected in adults taking the standard recommended dosages:

Tetracycline - 1.8 mg/L. 250 mg. 6 hrly.)
Methacycline - 1.1 mg/L. 150 mg. 6 hrly.) Steigbigel et al, 1968.
Minocycline - 2.4 mg/L. 150 mg.12 hrly.)

Clomocycline - 2.0 mg/L. 170 mg. 6 hrly. (Martin and Kliger, 1967).

RESULTS

The analogues of tetracyclines all showed greater in vitro activity against β haemolytic streptococci than the parent compound (Fig. 1.)

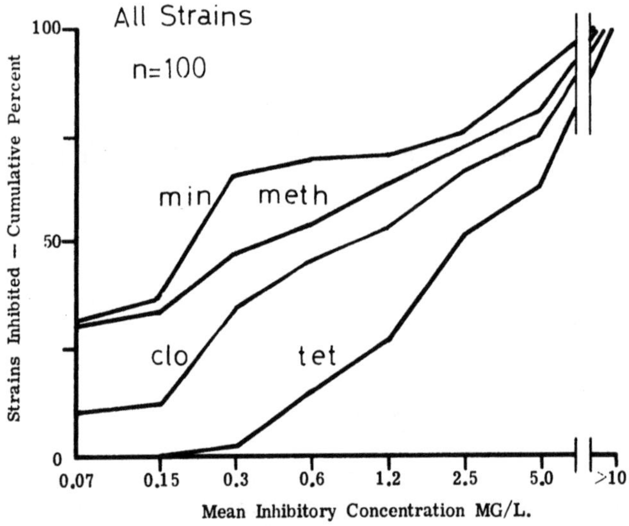

FIGURE 1 Susceptibility of all the strains tested against tetracycline (tet), minocycline (min), methacycline (meth), and clomocycline (clo).

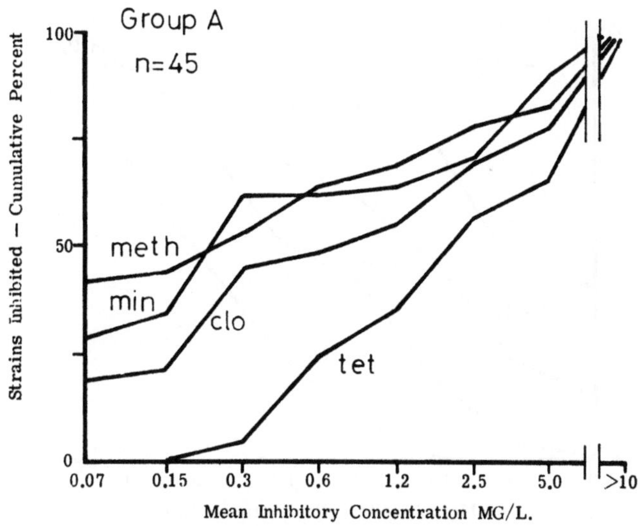

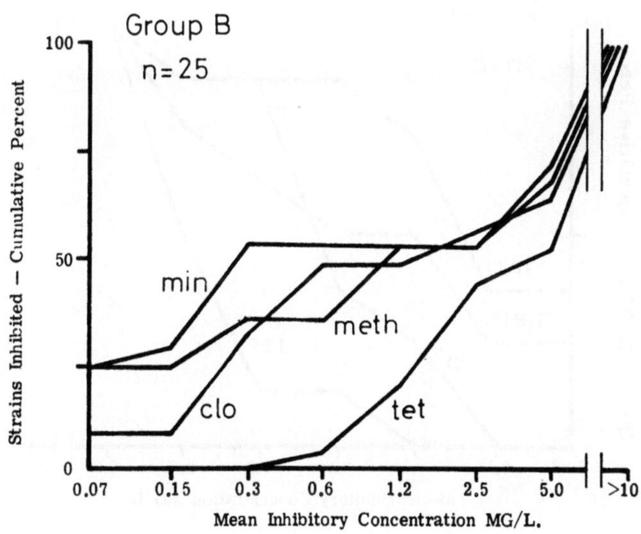

Figures 2 & 3. Susceptibility of Group A & B strains tested against tetracycline (tet), minocycline (min), methacycline (meth), and clomocycline (clo).

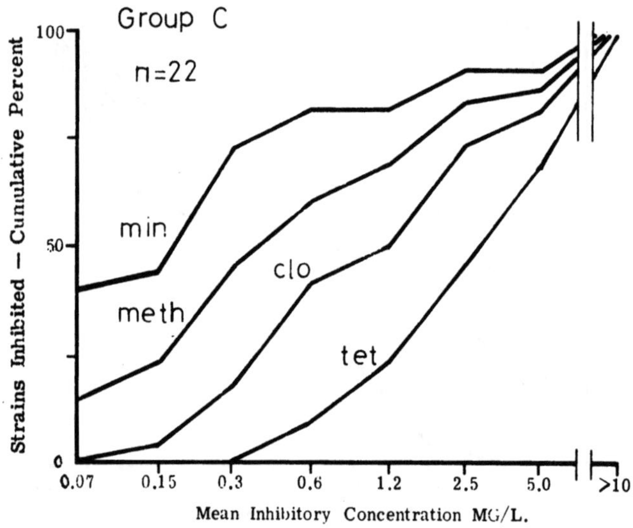

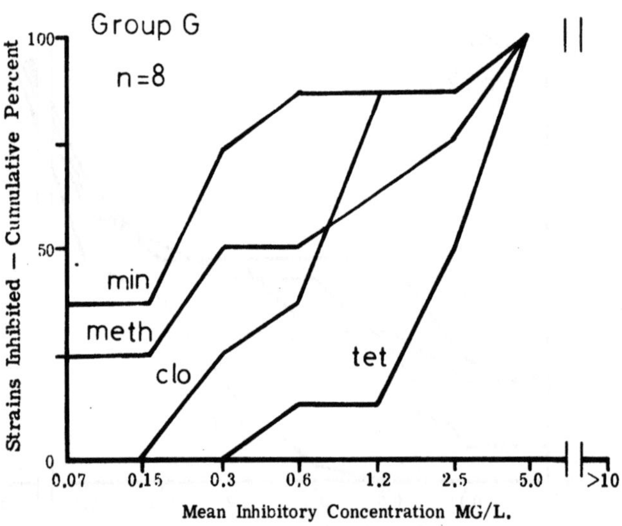

Figures 4 & 5. Susceptibility of Group C & G strains tested against tetracycline (tet), minocycline (min), methacycline (meth), and clomocycline (clo).

This difference in activity was evident in all the four streptococcal groups (Figs. 2-5).

The activity of methacycline and minocycline was similar against group A and B strains; strains in group C and G were more sensitive to minocycline than to methacycline although the number tested was fewer. Clomocycline was generally slightly less active than methacycline and minocycline but more active than tetracycline.

A bimodal pattern of resistance was most evident in group B strains against the analogues. No modal pattern was seen against tetracycline. The level of resistance for each strain was generally the same for each analogue. Four group A strains, however, with a tetracycline M.I.C's of 5 mg/L or above were sensitive to 0.07 mg/L minocycline; one group B, three group C and two group G strains had a similar sensitivity pattern. Seven of these strains were also sensitive to methacycline and six were sensitive to clomocycline at 0.6 mg/L. or less. (Table).

Only one strain was found to have greater sensitivity to tetracycline (0.3 mg/L) than minocycline (5 mg/L), methacycline (10 mg/L) and clomocycline (5 mg/L). This strain belonged to group A.

The assessment of <u>in vivo</u> activity showed that trough levels of minocycline could be expected to inhibit 73% of strains, methacycline 62%, clomocycline 62% and tetracycline 38%.

DISCUSSION

The antibacterial activity of tetracyclines is due to their ability to act against the 30S-moiety of the ribosomal A site although they may also be bound in other sites on the ribosome. To be effective they are concentrated in bacterial cells by changes in the permeability of the cell membrane. When bacterial cells first meet tetracycline there is a free passage in and out of the cell but in sensitive cells the tetracycline induces changes so that the outflow is inhibited while leaving the inflow unchanged. The resulting intracellular accumulation of tetracycline is lethal because of its inhibitory effect on protein synthesis. Resistant bacteria are unable to accumulate tetracycline - they remain permeable to its intake but are unable to prevent its loss from the cells.

Tetracycline resistance appears to be genetically determined and can be associated with R factors. (Gale, Cundliffe, Reynolds, Richmond and Waring, 1972).

The results of this study suggest that in β haemolytic streptococci more than one gene may determine resistance to tetracycline and its analogues. In the majority of strains tested

TABLE 1

Mean Inhibitory Concentrations(mg/L) of Strains showing Dissociated Resistance from Tetracycline

	Tetracycline	Minocycline	Methacycline	Clomocycline
Group A.	10.0	0.07	0.07	0.07
	10.0	0.07	0.07	0.6
	5.0	0.07	0.6	0.6
	5.0	0.07	0.6	0.3
	0.3	5.0	10.0	5.0
Group B.	5.0	0.15	1.25	2.5
Group C.	10.0	0.07	0.15	0.6
	10.0	0.07	2.5	5.0
	5.0	0.07	0.6	2.5
Group G.	10.0	0.07	0.3	0.6
	10.0	0.07	5.0	5.0

resistance was to the group of tetracyclines, in others the resistance was specific for different analogues.

The *in vitro* implications are that one analogue cannot be used for sensitivity testing against all the tetracycline group. The importance of the side chain groupings is also evident by the general pattern of susceptibility to the analogues. Weight for weight minocycline may be more effective than tetracycline because it is more able to induce a block in outgoing permeability or because a lower intracellular concentration is required to inhibit ribsomal activity. Methacycline and clomocycline occupy intermediate positions.

The possible *in vivo* activity is similar to the *in vitro* activity. This assessment is, however, on theoretical grounds and cannot be regarded as evidence of comparative clinical usefulness of tetracycline and its analogues. Both the *in vitro* results and the *in vivo* assessment suggest that tetracycline and its analogues - minocycline, methacycline and clomocycline should not be considered as first line drugs in the treatment of β haemolytic streptococcal infections. Twenty-seven out of the 100 strains tested were resistant to all these members of the tetracycline group. Resistance to penicillin was not demonstrated in any of the groups tested in this study.

SUMMARY

The *in vitro* activity of tetracycline and the analogues - minocycline, methacycline and clomocycline was tested against 100 freshly isolated strains of βhaemolytic streptococci. The analogues were all more active than tetracycline. Resistance was generally to the tetracycline group although some strains were selectively resistant to one or more of the compounds tested. The results were discussed and the potential *in vivo* activity assessed.

REFERENCES

Dadswell, J.V. J. clin. Path. 20; 641-2 (1967)
Frisk, A.R. and Tunevall, G. Antimicrob. Agents.Chemother. 335-39 (1968)
Gale, E.F., Cundliffe, E., Reynolds, P.E., Richmond, M.H. and Waring, M.J. The Molecular Basis of Antibiotic Action. John Wiley and Sons. (1972). Pp.315-321.
Leigh, D.A. and Simmons, K. Lancet 1; 1006 (1974)
Lowbury, E.J.L. and Cason, J.S. Brit. med.J. 2;914-5 (1954)
Martin, A.J. and Kliger, B.N. Clin. tr. J. 4; 721-731 (1967).
Rees, T.A. Lancet 1; 938-9 (1971)
Steigbigel, N.H., Reed, C.W. and Finland,M. Am.J.med.Sci.255;296-312 (1968)

CEPHALOSPORIN-TOBRAMYCIN ACTIVITY AGAINST ENTEROCOCCI

F.R. Fekety, B. Bruce, D. Turrell, C. Work and J. Conway

Department of Internal Medicine
University of Michigan Medical School
Ann Arbor, Michigan 48104, U.S.A.

SUMMARY

Anti-enterococcal synergism was readily demonstrable when cefazolin or cephalothin were combined with gentamicin or tobramycin, and *Str. faecalis* isolates were killed rapidly at attainable serum concentrations. The cephalosporins combined with amikacin were rarely synergistic, but ampicillin-amikacin was synergistic and bactericidal. Some of these newer combinations are worthy of further study in enterococcal infections.

INTRODUCTION

Enterococcal endocarditis is a difficult therapeutic problem because no single antibiotic is reliably bactericidal. While penicillin or vancomycin plus streptomycin or gentamicin are frequently synergistic and curative, safe alternatives are needed, particularly for allergic patients. Cephalothin plus streptomycin has been tried and found deficient (Fekety *et al.* 1966). This report compares the *in vitro* anti-enterococcal activity of cephalosporins and penicillins combined with newer aminoglycosides.

METHODS

Group D enterococci obtained from patients at the University of Michigan Medical Center were used. Susceptibility studies were done with fifteen *Str. faecalis*, one *Str. fecalis var. liquefaciens*, and four *Str. faecium* isolates in Mueller-Hinton broth using microdilution techniques (Harwick *et al.* 1968). Interactions were studied using these techniques two-dimensionally, and by study of the rate of killing using pour-plate techniques. An overnight broth culture was used; the inoculum yielded approximately 2 x 10^5 CFU/ml. Minimum bacteriostatic (MIC) and 99.9 percent bactericidal (MBC) endpoints were determined. Synergism was defined as inhibition (or killing) with less than one-half the MIC (or MBC) of two antibiotics, or fourfold inward bowing of isobolograms (Lacey, 1958), or when the rate of bactericidal action of mixtures was more than one-hundred times that of the drugs studied alone.

RESULTS

Single antibiotics. The inhibitory activity of the antibiotics is shown in Figures 1 and 2. Bactericidal curves were similar but shifted one or two dilutions higher. Gentamicin was the most active aminoglycoside. Cefazolin was more active than cephalothin, but less active than penicillin G or ampicillin. Only the latter were bactericidal at serum concentrations with more than half the isolates.

Two-dimensional studies of synergism. Synergism was frequently demonstrable when cefazolin or cephalothin were combined with tobramycin or gentamicin, and was more apparent in bactericidal tests. Figure 3 is an isobologram showing mean bactericidal action on 20 isolates with cephalothin and aminoglycosides; it indicates synergism with both. More importantly, it shows low concentrations

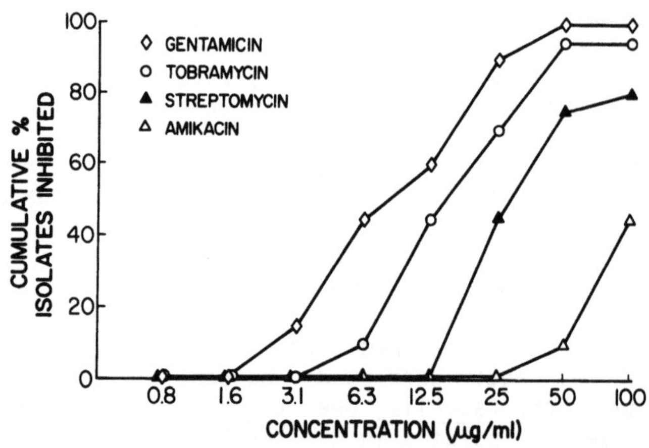

Fig. 1. Inhibition of 20 enterococci by aminoglycosides.

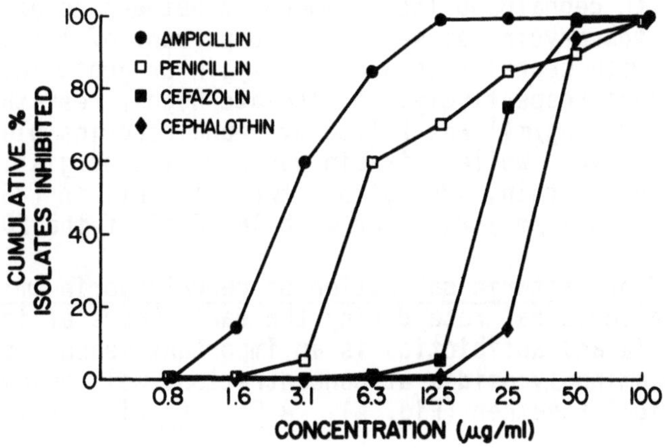

Fig. 2. Inhibition of 20 enterococci by beta-lactam antibiotics.

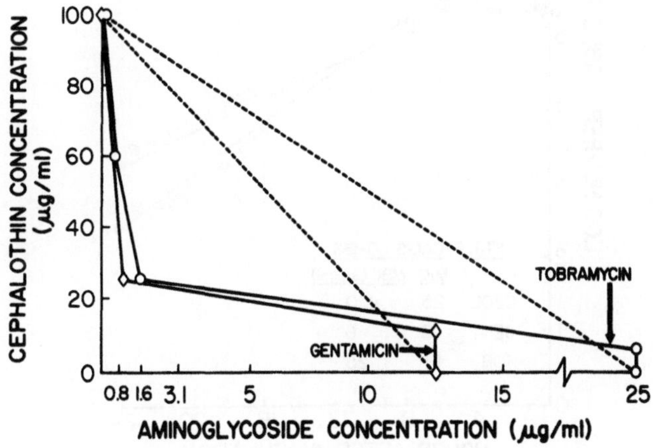

Fig. 3. Bactericidal synergism with cephalothin (20 isolates).

of aminoglycosides (1.6 μg/ml) are bactericidal in the presence of cephalothin. At least as good results were obtained with cefazolin. Gentamicin was slightly more active than tobramycin in combination with cephalosporins. Synergism between cefazolin and gentamicin or tobramycin was seen with 80 percent of isolates; the frequency with cephalothin and tobramycin or gentamicin was 75 and 65 percent respectively. An isolate highly resistant to streptomycin (2000 μg/ml) was killed by cephalosporins plus gentamicin or tobramycin. While amikacin was rarely synergistic with cefazolin or cephalothin, synergism between ampicillin (25 μg/ml) and amikacin (12.5 μg/ml) was seen with 16 (80%) of the 20 isolates.

The speed of bactericidal action of cephalosporin-aminoglycosides. The bactericidal rate during the early hours of interaction between bacteria and antibiotics is an important measure of synergism. Cefazolin and aminoglycosides at concentrations well below the MBC were bactericidal together (Fig. 4). A *Str. faecium* isolate

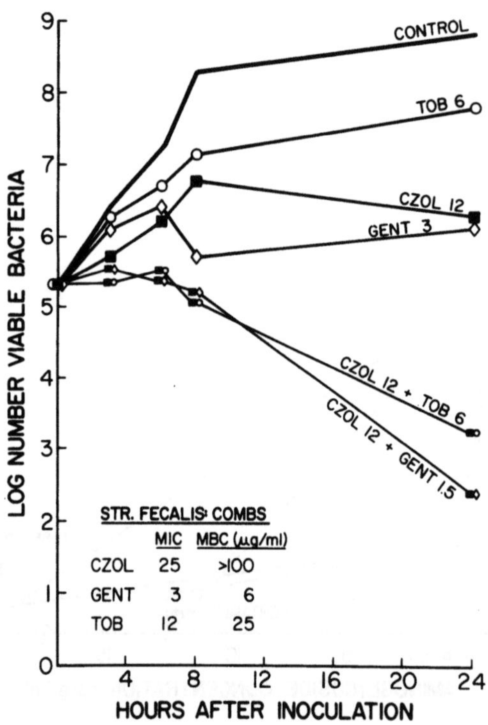

Fig. 4. Synergism in killing an enterococcus.

was killed more slowly and did not show synergism. We studied killing rates with seven Str. fecalis isolates, and confirmed in all of them the synergism demonstrated in the two-dimensional studies. Some isolates not showing synergism in two-dimensional studies did show it in killing rates. Figure 5 compares the mean bactericidal rate for cefazolin plus tobramycin with the rate for penicillin plus streptomycin with seven Str. faecalis isolates. There was no significant difference in the rates at which these two combinations killed enterococci.

DISCUSSION

These results suggest treatment of Str. faecalis infection with cephalosporins combined with gentamicin or tobramycin is worthy of further study. Even endocarditis may be curable. The serum concentrations of the aminoglycosides and cefazolin (Kirby and Regamey, 1973) needed for synergism are attainable. Synergism was demonstrated with some of our Str. faecium isolates, but preliminary observations indicate they are relatively resistant to killing.

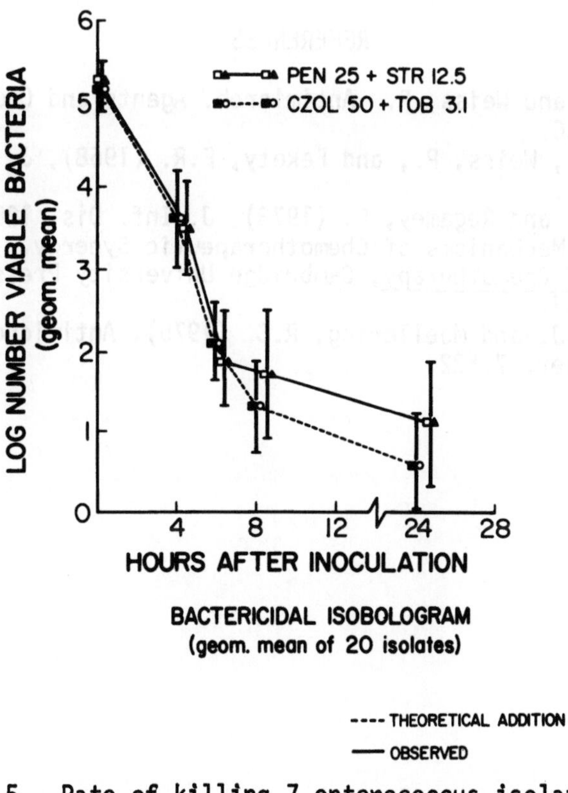

Fig. 5. Rate of killing 7 enterococcus isolates.

Others also have noted their resistance (Weinstein and Moellering, 1975). Serious infections with Str. faecium should probably not be treated with cephalosporin-aminoglycoside combinations.

Weinstein and Moellering (1975) suggested the failure of cephalothin plus streptomycin in treatment of enterococcal endocarditis may be attributable to metabolism of cephalothin to desacetylcephalothin, a relatively inactive derivative. This gives added impetus to studies with cefazolin, which is more active than cephalothin, and not deacetylated. However, cefazolin is bound to serum proteins more than cephalothin, so large doses may be required (Kirby and Regamey, 1973). Further study of these factors in animal models of enterococcal endocarditis and in infections in humans is clearly needed to establish the usefulness of these combinations.

ACKNOWLEDGEMENT

Supported by grants from the NIH (NIAID), Eli Lilly & Co., and the Bristol Laboratories.

REFERENCES

Fekety, F.R. and Weiss, P. Antimicrob. Agents and Chemotherapy-1966, p. 156.

Harwick, H.J., Weiss, P., and Fekety, F.R. (1968), J. Lab. Clin. Med. 72:511.

Kirby, W.M.M. and Regamey, C. (1973), J. Inf. Dis. 128:S341.

Lacey, B.W. Mechanisms of Chemotherapeutic Synergy. In The Strategy of Chemotherapy, Cambridge University Press, London, 1958, p. 247.

Weinstein, A.J. and Moellering, R.C. (1975), Antimicrob. Agents and Chemother. 7:522.

GENTAMICIN RESISTANT GRAM-NEGATIVE-BACILLI AT THE GERIATRIC HOSPITAL

TAKASHI INAMATSU, KOJI NAKAUCHI, and KAORU SHIMADA

THE TOKYO METROPOLITAN GERIATRIC HOSPITAL

35-2 SAKAE CHO ITABASHI KU TOKYO JAPAN

In recent years, the importance of gram-negative-bacilli has been emphasized as a cause of nosocomial infection. Since almost all these bacilli, especially Pseudomonas aeruginosa, Proteus sp., and Providence are susceptible to gentamicin, this drug has been widely used on many patients, despite of its potent oto and renal toxicity. However since recently, bacteria resistant to GM have been reported from several parts of the world. Many of these bacteria were isolated in the Burn Unit of hospitals, and the isolation of these bacilli seems to be associated with the route and dose of GM administration.

During the past two years, we have isolated many strains of gram-negative-bacilli which were resistant to GM, at the TOKYO METROPOLITAN GERIATRIC HOSPITAL, where urinary tract infection, respiratory tract infection, and decubital ulcers have been the major infections.

The present study has been made as an attempt (1) to demonstrate the incidence of GM resistant GNB, (2) to analyse the backgrounds of their isolation, and(3) to determine the activity of nine aminoglycoside antibiotics against these GM resistant strains.

INCIDENCE OF GM RESISTANT GNB.

During the past two years from 1973 to 1974, 214 strains of GM resistant gram-negative-bacilli were isolated from 201 specimens in our clinical bacteriology laboratory. These bacteria showed no inhibitory zones around the 10μg gentamicin disks placed on sensitivity test agar plate. When we discard the strains isolated repeatedly from the same specimens of the same patient, the number

Table 1. Species and source of GM resistant gram-negative-bacilli

Species \ Source	Urine	PUS	Sputum	blood	total
Pseud.	15	15	6	1	37
Provid.	13	22	1	0	36
Pr. rett.	2	12	0	0	14
Pr. vulg.	2	2	0	0	4
Pr. mirr.	1	1	1	0	3
Pr. morg.	1	1	0	0	2
Klebsiella	4	0	0	0	4
E. coli	3	0	0	1	4
Citrobact.	7	0	0	0	7
Alcaligenes	2	6	3	0	11
Others	4	1	0	0	5
total	54	60	11	2	127

of GM resistant GNB were 127 strains. The details are shown in Table 1.Many of them were isolated from urine and pus specimens, especially from decubital ulcers. The incidence of GM resistant GNB is about 2.9% in urine, 9.6% in pus, 1.2% in sputum, and 0.3% in blood. The incidence of each species of GM resistant GNB are as follows. Pseudomonas aeruginosa, 4.4%. Providence, 52.3%. Proteus rett., 8.2%. Proteus vulg., 4.7%. Proteus morg., 2.6%. Proteus mirab., 0.4%. Klebsiella,0.4%. E. coli, 0.3%. Citrobacter, 21.3%. Alcaligenes, 11.3%.

It is interesting to note that Pseudomonas, Providence, and Proteus sp. are the major bacteria resistant to gentamicin. Indeed, more than half of Providence are resistant to GM, and many of them were isolated from pus and urine specimens.

ROUTES OF GM ADMINISTRATION

Clinical records were reviewed with respect to route of GM administration. The results are shown in Table 2. Topical usage of GM such as application of GM ointment or solution on the decubital ulcers tends to yield GM resistant strains. GM resistant bacilli were isolated from the urine of patients, who received GM, irrespective of the route of administration. The reason for this may be that large amounts of GM is excreted in the urine. These

Table 2. Routes of GM administration and GM resistant GNB isolation

route \ isolated specimen	pus	urine	sputum
Systemic	1	11※	4
Systemic + Topical	23	15	—
Topical	23	10	—
no Use	3	7	3

※ TOB was used on 2 cases.

data indicate that exposure to high concentrations of GM at the infection area offers a good oppotunity to yield GM resistant strains.

ACTIVITIES OF 9 AMINOGLYCOSIDES AGAINST GM RESISTANT GNB

We determined the minimal inhibitory concentrations of nine aminoglycosides against 62 gentamicin resistant strains. The antibiotics studied were gentamicin, amikacin, deoxykanamycin B, tobramycin, kanamycin, streptomycin, aminodeoxykanamycin, lividomycin, and vistamycin. The test was performed by the agar dilution procedure using Sensitivity Test Agar (NISSUI Co.). An aliquot of a 10^{-2} dilution of the over night culture was inoculated on the plate.

Table 3 shows the susceptibility patterns of these GM resistant bacilli. The 22 strains were resistant to all these nine aminoglycosides. The 36 strains were susceptible only to amikacin. All these bacilli could for convenience be divided into 6 groups. However, the species in each group could be further divided depending on MIC levels and susceptibility to antibiotics other than aminoglycosides.

Fig. 1 and 2 show the cumulative percentages of susceptibility to Pseudomonas aeruginosa and Providence. Amikacins excellent action against GM resistant Pseudomonas aeruginosa and Providence is remarkable. Amikacin also shows excellent effect on GM resistant Proteus species.

Since an intramuscular injection of 500mg of amikacin shows up in blood at a level of more than 20μg/ml, it is reasonable to expect a therapeutic efficacy of amikacin to the infections of these gentamicin resistant gram-negative-bacilli.

Table 3. Susceptibility patterns of GM resistant bacilli to 9 aminoglycosides.
- : Resistant (MIC ≧ 12.5 μg/ml)
+ : Susceptible

GM	−	−	−	−	−	−	Susceptibility pattern
Amikacin	−	+	+	+	+	+	
DKB	−	−	−	−	−	+	
TOB	−	−	−	−	−	−	
KM	−	−	+	−	+	−	
SM	−	−	−	−	+	−	
AKM	−	−	−	−	−	+	
Livido	−	−	−	+	−	+	
VSM	−	−	−	−	−	+	
Pseudo.	8	13	0	1	0	0	No. of strains
Provid.	3	16	1	0	0	0	
Pr. rett	3	6	0	0	0	0	
Others	8	1	0	0	1	1	
total	22	36	1	1	1	1	

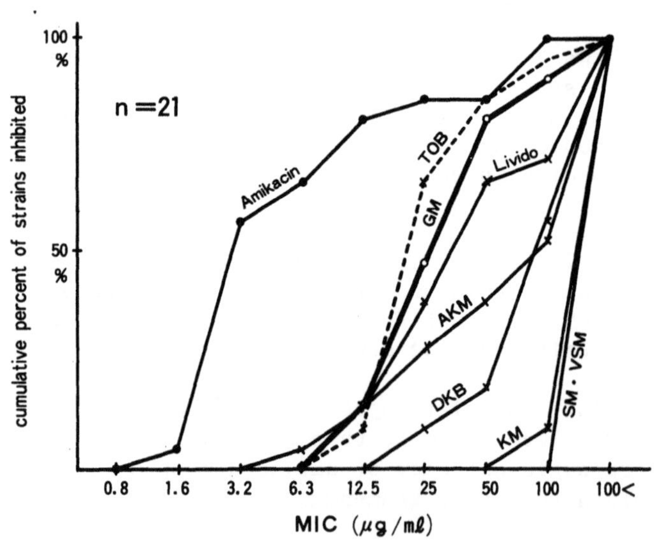

Fig. 1. Susceptibility of GM resistant Pseudomonas aeruginosa to 9 aminoglycosides.

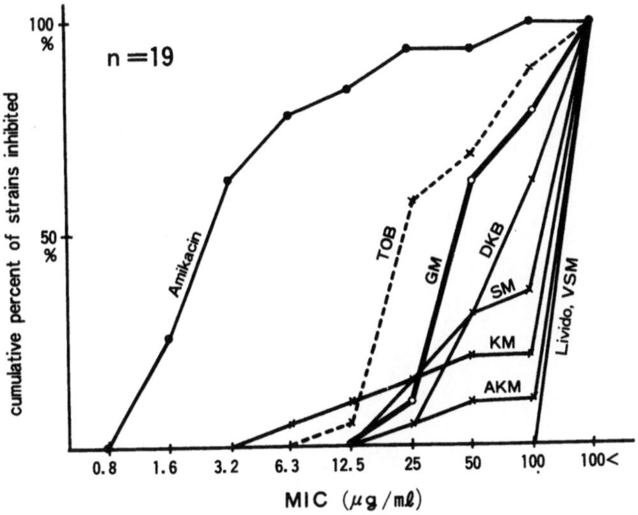

Fig. 2. Susceptibility of GM resistant Providence to 9 aminoglycosides.

R FACTOR MEDIATED GM RESISTANCE

We studied on several strains of GM resistant gram-negative-bacilli, whether their resistance to GM were transferable or not. In one of the 9 strains of Pseudomonas studied, the resistance was transfered to Pseudomonas M-1 strain. The frequency of transfer was about 10^{-6} The resistance to GM, TOB, and deoxykanamycin B was transfered concomitantly.

We also tried to transfer the GM resistance of some strains of Providence and Proteus species to some recipient strains. However, our trial were unsuccessful.

TOPICAL CHEMOPROPHYLAXIS IN SURGERY

A.V. Pollock
Scarborough Hospital
Scarborough, Yorkshire

Sepsis remains, in spite of 30 years of antibiotics, an important cause of illness and death. Figures are hard to come by, but the Report of the Public Health Laboratory Service (1960) on 2836 general surgical operations revealed clinical wound sepsis in 384 (13.5 per cent). In seven series reported from this hospital totalling 3761 operations, sepsis occurred in 513 (13.6 per cent). The incidence of infection in sutured surgical wounds is probably no less now than it was 40 years ago and it is only within the last few years that random controlled trials have yielded information of clinical value for its prevention.

The idea that the healing of a wound depends on the skill and knowledge of the surgeon is as old as surgery itself, and was not discouraged by the profession until Pare, who said "I dressed him and God healed him".

Chemoprophylaxis has, therefore, an ancient lineage. An early reference is that "...a certain Samaritan...went to him, and bound up his wounds, pouring in oil and win." (Luke X, 33). In most old texts, however, it is difficult to distinguish between chemicals which were used for the arrest of haemorrhage (and this included the boiling oil of elder for which Pare was forced to substitute a "digestive medicament" made of oil of roses, turpentine and yolks of eggs) and those, mostly magical, reputed to heal all wounds. To this day the emblem of the Royal Society of Medicine is the plant Vervain or "all heal".

It was Louis Pasteur's researches on bacteria which prompted Lister (1867) to introduce a carbolic spray and carbolic soaking of instruments and dressings. He reported that "...during the last nine months not a single instance of pyaemia, hospital gangrene or erysipelas has occurred in (my wards)." By the end of the nineteenth century the role of bacteria in wound sepsis had been generally accepted and asepsis had displaced chemical antisepsis for routine surgery.

The battles of the first World War caused the most appalling wounds. They were heavily contaminated with the soil of Flanders and it was not long before the principles of aseptic surgery had to be modified in the light of experience. Excision and delayed primary suture became the order of the day, and numerous chemicals were employed as adjuncts to this regimen. These included iodine, potassium permanganate, phenol, flavine, brilliant green and BIPP (bismuth iodiform paraffin paste), but the most favoured was the Carrell-Dakin hypochlorite solution (Hughes and Banks, 1918).

Twenty-five years later (Memoranda, 1944) the recommended method was the use of 5-15g of sulphanilamide or sulphathiazole dusted into the wound, and even the addition - if it were available - of 500 to 2,000 units of penicillin for each gram of sulphanomide.

Surgeons continued after the second World War to use sulphanamides and antibiotics for the topical chemoprophylaxis of wound sepsis, but a true assessment of their role had to await the development of controlled clinical trials. One of the first of these was of topical ampicillin in colon surgery (Nash and Hugh, 1967) and since then there have been numerous reports of adequately controlled trials of ampicillin (Rickett and Jackson, 1969; Andersen et al., 1972; Bates et al., 1974) and other antibiotics - kanamycin (Moylan and Brockenbrough, 1968), tetracycline (Longland et al., 1971), streptomycin and penicillin (Kronborg and Zachariae, 1973) and cephaloridine (Evans et al., 1974).

Wound sepsis is defined as the discharge of pus from a sutured surgical incision. A clearer understanding of its causes and prevention is gained by separating primary sepsis (where the initial discharge from a previously dry wound is of pus(from secondary sepsis (which results from invasion by pathogenic organisms of a wound which is already discharging a substance other than pus). The best example of secondary sepsis is that which develops in a burn. The initial discharge from a burned surface is of sterile serum. The subsequent colonisation and sepsis results from auto- or cross infection and its prevention depends on totally different principles from that of primary sepsis.

In a series of 3173 operations we have found the rate of secondary wound sepsis entirely uninfluenced by topical chemoprophylaxis at the time of surgery (Table 1). In clean wounds, in patients unprotected by an effective topical antibiotic, there were 32 instances of secondary sepsis in 816 operations (3.9

Table 1. Incidence of secondary sepsis in 3173 surgical wounds

	With Cephaloridine		Without Cephaloridine	
	total operations	number septic (per cent)	total operations	number septic (per cent)
Clean operations	734	23 (3.1)	816	32 (3.9)
Contaminated operations	821	34 (4.1)	802	25 (3.1)

Table 2. 249 Potentially contaminated operations: correlation between operative infection and primary wound sepsis.

	total operations	Primary sepsis (per cent)	Significance of difference chi^2	P
Operation swab sterile	75	7 (9)	7.3	<0.01
Operation swab infected	147	36 (24)		

per cent). In each case a discharging haematoma, a lymph fistula or ischaemic necrosis of skin edges became contaminated in the environment of a crowded, multi-bedded ward. Compared with this incidence, 23 out of 734 wounds protected by cephaloridine (3.1 per cent) developed secondary infection of a sterile discharge.

In potentially contaminated operations (involving incision into a hollow muscular viscus) the secondary sepsis rate without an efficient topical antibiotic at the time of operation was 25 out of 802 (3.1 per cent) compared with 34 out of 821 (4.1 per cent) when cephaloridine had been used. These differences are not significant. The prophylaxis of secondary wound sepsis, therefore, depends on the prevention of any discharge from a wound, and secondly, if the wound discharges the maintenance of a sterile atmosphere in its neighbourhood.

Our own studies on the chemoprophylaxis of wound sepsis have centred on the prevention of the primary type. The work we have done on the prevention of wound haematomas and we have shown (Arnot et al., 1975) that diathermy haemostasis gives significantly better results than ligature.

As well as distinguishing between primary and secondary sepsis, we have adopted other definitions: a clean wound is one in which there is no potential for endogenous contamination during operation and a potentially contaminated wound is one involving incision or excision of an infected lesion or a potentially infected hollow muscular viscus. Clinically we have recognised that the more heavily contaminated a wound is, the more likely is primary sepsis to occur. We have, therefore, put wounds for colonic surgery and perforated appendicitis into a separate category.

In recent trials we have refined this classification by dividing the potentially contaminated operations into those in which organisms are grown from swabs taken from the viscus or the subcutaneous tissue during operation and those in which these swabs are sterile. The incidence of primary sepsis is significantly lower when the operation swab is sterile, but still remains higher than that of primary sepsis in totally clean operations (Table 2). This is no doubt due to the occasional case in which a contaminating organism is not grown owing to a failure of bacteriological technique. We have not made any attempt to study the size of the inoculum of the contaminant but it seems clear, and our clinical results bear this out, that primary sepsis is more likely to develop after a large inoculum of pathogenic organisms than after a small one.

Apart from endogenous contamination from incision into a hollow viscus, there are several other ways in which a wound may become contaminated during surgery. In pre-Listerian days infection was usually exogenous, due

Table 3. 2491 operations: factors which may influence the wound sepsis rate

		Total operations	Primary sepsis (per cent)	Significance of difference chi²	P	Secondary sepsis (per cent)	Significance of difference chi²	P
Age	under 60	1247	94 (7.2)	10.49	<0.01	41 (3.2)	14.98	<0.001
	over 60	1194	131 (11.0)			77 (6.4)		
Build	obese	319	50 (15.7)	19.64	<0.001	17 (5.3)	0.28	>0.50
	not obese	2172	175 (8.1)			101 (4.7)		

to dirty hands and instruments. The revolution in surgical technique in the last quarter of the nineteenth century almost abolished this source. The introduction of rubber gloves by William Hasted was, of course, entirely fortuitous and the Goodyear Rubber Company made the first ones for him not for the prevention of wound contamination but for the protection of the delicate hands of a favourite nurse from the effects of the mercuric lotion in use at that time (Proskauer, 1968).

Another possible exogenous source of wound contamination is the atmosphere in the operating theatre. It has been repeatedly shown that agar plates exposed during operations will grow micro-organisms which have settled there either from droplets or from the air (Davidson et al., 1971). An enormous amount of money has been spent all over the world to try and stop this contamination. Methods have ranged from Lister's carbolic spray to positive pressure ventialtion, ultraviolet irradiation and the use of tents to ensure sterile air. None of these methods has been the subject of a controlled clinical trial, and the little evidence that we have suggests that kitchen table surgery is just as unlikely to be followed by wound sepsis as is that in the most complicated operating theatre (Seropian and Reynolds, 1969).

In 1964, the National Research Council appointed a committee to investigate the influence of ultraviolet irradiation of the operating room (Report, 1964) and the conclusion reached was that, whereas it was quite feasible to reduce contamination in this way, the rate of wound sepsis was not significantly influeced. Most studies have been consecutive - for instance Blowers et al. (1955) reported a fall in the wound infection rate from 10.9 to 3.9 per cent following modification of the theatre ventilation. Charnley and Eftekhar (1969) reported a fall in wound sepsis rate in orthopaedic operations from 8.9 per cent to 1.3 per cent after the introduction of a high air flow operating enclosure

One must be critical of reports which attribute an improvement in results to the introduction of some new technique when these studies are uncontrolled by a concurrent study of patients treated in the previously accepted way. In our own trials we have reported widely divergent rates of wound sepsis in clean operations in control cases in different years ranging from 2.9 per cent in 1971 to 1.2 per cent in 1974. These have occurred without any change in factors known to influence exogenous contamination.

As far as general surgical operations are concerned, bacterial contamination resulting in wound sepsis arises almost entirely from endogenous sources. There are two avenues of infection: first, the deposit of bacteria into the wound during surgery from a contaminated viscus or infected lesion, and secondly the seeding of blood-or lymph-borne organisms into a locus minoris resistentiae -

commonly a haematoma at the site of operation. The latter is rare, but may be the explanation of the occasional case of primary sepsis after a clean operation.

Davidson et al (1971) reported a multiple regression analysis of 14 factors which they thought might be related to the incidence of wound sepsis, and concluded that five were important: a potentially contaminated operation, the presence of bacteria in the wound at the end of the operation, nursing of patients in old-fashioned multi-bedded wards, old age and an operation lasting more than one hour. As far as primary sepsis is concerned we have confirmed the first two factors and the importance of age (Table 3) and have also found obesity to have an effect (this is defined as a thickness of subcutaneous fat - measured during operation - of 2.5 cm or more). In addition the site of operation has an influence, and we have not had a single case of primary wound sepsis in clean head and neck operations.

The prophylaxis of primary wound sepsis can be considered in three parts. In the first place, operations are conducted in strictly aseptic conditions. Instruments, swabs and nonabsorbable sutures are autoclaved, the theatre is ventilated in such a way that the air pressure is higher over the operating table than elsewhere, and the surgeon's gown and gloves are sterile. Personnel with obvious sepsis do not enter the operating room.

Secondly, every effort is made to minimise endogenous contamination during surgery. In colonic operations in particular, although it is impossible to sterilise the faeces, a great deal can be done to cut down the size of the bacterial inoculum by operating on a dry empty bowel in which the bacterial flora has been reduced by a combination of appropriate antibiotics. We showed some years ago that the use of a sterile adhesive plastic drape (Jackson et al. 1971) had no influence on the rate of wound sepsis. Newer methods have been introduced, in particular a plastic wound isolator, but we have not had the opportunity to put these to the test.

Finally, we attempt to minimise the effects of bacterial contamination by the use of an effective topical antibiotic.

Because of the dangers of encouragement of resistant strains of bacteria by the widespread use of antibiotics (Lancet, 1975) there have been attempts to re-introduce chemoprophylaxis by substances which are not used for systemic treatment. The results of most of these trials have been disappointing. A mixture of polymixin, bacitracin and neomycin sprayed into the wound (Jackson et al., 1971) proved ineffective and although Gilmore et al. (1973) claimed good results in a trial of povidone-iodine, this substance was found by Pollock and Evans (1975) to be considerably less effective than topical cephaloridine.

Four years ago, having demonstrated a clear advantage of a three-dose regimen of cephaloridine parenterally in the prophylaxis of wound sepsis (Evans and Pollock, 1973) we tested the topical application of this antibiotic (Evans et al., 1974) and again showed a considerable and significant reduction in the wound sepsis rate over untreated controls (Table 4). Ethical considerations have, thereafter, enjoined the use of cephaloridine and we have tested it against other topical agents. These have included gentamicin (Pollock and Rosenberg, 1974), povidone-iodine (Pollock and Evans, 1975) and framycetin (Pollock and Evans, 1975). None of these substances has proved superior to cephaloridine which remains our standard prophylactic regimen.

One gram of powder is dissolved in 2 ml of water and instilled into wounds before insertion of skin stitches. Its influence in clean wounds is slight, but in contaminated wounds the rate of sepsis has been halved.

Antibiotic Resistance

The year-by-year monitoring of bacteria for their antibiotic sensitivity is an enormous task for which only a computer is really adequate, and this is what Goodwin (1975) is doing at Northwick Park Hospital.

We have, in our own district general hospital, scrutinised a ten per cent random sample of bacteriological reports in 1971 and 1974 and have discovered a highly significant increase in the number of strains of organisms resistant to 2 micrograms of ampicillin between those two years in the genera Staphylococcus, Escherichia and Proteus. There has been no significant increase in resistance to cephaloridine. On the contrary, in organisms recovered from out-patients we found the reverse - an increase in the percentage sensitive to cephaloridine in 1974 compared with 1971. This work will be published in detail elsewhere.

The plasmids which confer antibiotic resistance to bacteria are widespread in the human and animal kingdom. There are five main types of beta-lactamase plasmids amongst gram-negative bacteria, and each type produces several different enzymes (Richmond and Sykes, 1973). The fact that we have not yet encountered a high incidence of cephaloridine-resistant strains of enterobacteria must not induce complacency, and we will continue to monitor the hospital bacterial population. Whether a single dose of cephaloridine helps to select bacteria carrying a resistant plasmid or not is a matter for conjecture. However, criticism must be levelled at the widespread and indiscriminate use of potent antibiotics for the treatment of minor and self-limiting diseases.

We are satisfied that it is, at present, in the best interests of patients undergoing surgery involving the possibility of bacterial contamination for us to continue to use prophylactic cephaloridine, but we will continue to search for alternatives. We are investigating in a random controlled trial the relative efficacy of cephaloridine and ampicillin, and it is hoped to assess the addition of lincomycin - to which Bacteroides species are sensitive - as these organisms may play an important part in wound sepsis after colonic surgery (Leigh, 1975). The genera Pseudomonas and Enterobacter are also resistant to cephaloridine and it may be that future policy will demand not two but three or four antibiotics for the topical prophylaxis of wound sepsis.

REFERENCES

Andersen, B., Korner, B. and Ostergaard, A.H. (1972). Topcial ampicillin against wound infection after colorectal surgery. Annals of Surgery, 176, 129-132.

Arnot, R.S., Evans, Mary and Pollock, A.V. (1975). The influence of two methods of haemostasis on the rate of wound sepsis: a random controlled trial of ligature and diathermy. British Journal of Surgery (in press)

Bates, T., Down, R.H.L., Houghton, M.C.V. and Lloyd, G.J. (1974). Topical ampicillin in the prevention of wound infection after appendicectomy. British Journal of Surgery, 61, 489-492.

Blowers, R., Mason, G.A., Wallace, K.R. and Walton, M. (1955). Control of wound infection in a thoracic surgery unit. The Lancet, 2, 786-794.

Charnley, J. and Eftekhar, N. (1969). Postoperative infection in total prosthetic replacement arthroplasty of the hip joint with special reference to the bacterial content of the air of the operating room. British Journal of Surgery, 56, 641-649.

Davidson, A.I.G., Clark, C. and Smith, G. (1971). A bacteriological study of the immediate environment of a surgical wound. British Journal of Surgery, 58, 326-333.

Evans, Christine and Pollock, A.V. (1973). The reduction of srugical wound infections by prophylactic parenteral cephaloridine. British Journal of Surgery, 60, 434-437.

Evans, Christine, Pollock, A.V. and Rosenberg, I.L. (1974). The reduction of surgical wound infections by topical cephaloridine: a controlled clinical trial. British Journal of Surgery, 61, 133-135.

Gilmore, O.J.A., Martin, T.D.M. and Fletcher, B.N. (1973). Prevention of wound infection after appendicectomy. The Lancet, 1, 220-222.

Goodwin, C.S. (1975). Antibiotic sensitivities of bacteria isolated at Northwick Park Hospital 1974-5. Journal of Antimicrobial Chemotherapy - supplement (in press).

Hughes, B. and Banks, H.S. (1918). War surgery from firing line to base. Balliere, Tindall and Cox (London).

Jackson, D.W., Pollock, A.V. and Tindal, D.S. (1971). The value of a plastic adhesive drape in the prevention of wound infection: a controlled trial. British Journal of Surgery, 58, 340-342.

Jackson, D.W., Pollock, A.V. and Tindal, D.S. (1971). The effect of an antibiotic spray in the prevention of wound infection. British Journal of Surgery, 58, 565-566.

Kronborg, O. and Zachariae, F. (1973). Topical use of penicillin-streptomycin in the prophylaxis of wound infection after gastric operations. Acta Chirugica Scandinavica - Supplement, 433, 188-190.

Lancet, The (1975). Transposons and antibiotic resistance, 1, 1411-1413.

Leigh, D.A. (1975). Wound infections due to Bacteroides fragilis following intestinal surgery. British Journal of Surgery, 62, 375-378.

Lister, J. (1867). On the antiseptic principle in the practice of surgery. British Medical Journal, 3, 246-248.

Longland, C.J., Gray, J.G., Lees, W. and Garrett, J.A.M. (1971). The prevention of infection in appendicectomy wounds. British Journal of Surgery, 58, 117-119.

Memoranda mainly based on experience in the present war (1944). A field surgery pocket book. The War Office, (London).

Moylan, J.A. and Brockenbrough, E.C, (1968). Antibiotic wound irrigation in the prevention of surgical wound infection. Surgical Forum, 19, 66-67.

Nash, A.G. and Hugh, T.B. (1967). Topcial ampicillin and wound infection in colon surgery. British Medical Journal, 1, 471-472.

Pollock, A.V. and Evans, Mary (1975). Povidone-iodine for the control of surgical wound infection: a controlled clinical trial against cephaloridine. British Journal of Surgery, 62, 292-294.

Pollock, A.V. andEvans, Mary (1975). The prophylaxis of surgical wound sepsis with cephaloridine: experiences in 2491 general surgical operations and reportina a controlled clinical trial against framycetin. Journal of Antimicrobial Chemotherapy - Supplement (in press).

Pollock, A.V. and Rosenberg, I.L. (1974). Cephaloridine and gentamicin in the prophylaxis of surgical wound infection. British Medical Journal, 2, 558-559.

Proskauer, C. (1958). Development and use of the rubber glove in surgery. Journal of the History of Medicine, 13, 373-381.

Report of an Ad Hoc Committee of the Committee on Trauma, Division of Medical Sciences, National Academy of Sciences - National Research Council (1964). Postoperative wound infections: the influence of ultraviolet irradiation of the operating room and of various other factors. Annals of Surgery - Supplement, 160, 1-192.

Report of the Public Health Laboratory Service (1960). Incidence of surgical wound infection in England and Wales, The Lancet, 2, 659-663.

Richmond, M.H. and Sykes, R.B. (1973). The beta-lactamases of gram-negative bacteria and their possible physiological role. In: Advances in Microbial Physiology, 9, 31-88. Academic Press (New York and London).

Rickett, J.W.S. and Jackson, B.T. (1969). Topical ampicillin in the appendicectomy wound: report of a double blind trial. British Medical Journal, 4, 206-207.

Seropian, R. and Reynolds, B.M. (1969). The importance of airborne contamination as a factor in postoperative wound infection. Archives of Surgery, 98, 654-658.

TOPICAL CHEMOTHERAPY AND PROPHYLAXIS IN THERMAL INJURY

Robert B. Lindberg, B.A. Pruitt, Jr. and A.D. Mason, Jr.

U.S. Army Institute of Surgical Research

Fort Sam, Houston, Texas, U.S.A.

SUMMARY

Definition of burn wound sepsis and development of animal models for reproducing lethal burn wound infection have made possible development of effective agents for control of wound infection and sepsis. Silver nitrate 0.5%, Sulfamylon and silver sulfadiazene are presently principal agents shown to be effective topical agents. Trade-off of level of effectiveness against side effects determines selection of agent. Monitoring criteria are essential if topical therapy is to be used safely.

Topical applications for burns were described even before the time of Hippocrates, who recommended covering burns with white wax and lard (Lewis, et al., 1970). A vast array of treatments have been recommended; their very number suggests their ineffectiveness. Only understanding pathology and the role of infection in burn wounds permitted rational therapy to be evolved (Teplitz and Moncrief, 1964). Teplitz' description of burn wound sepsis (BWS) was a landmark in characterizing burn wound infection. Quantitative bacteriology revealed the tremendous load of bacteria imposed on the burn victim. Since systemic antibiotics do not, in the main, diffuse effectively through devascularized burn tissue, only topical antibacterial agents can control this potentially lethal proliferation. Severely burned patients are immunologically deficient, and the bacterial load may reach 10^8 organisms per gram of tissue. Since kilograms of tissue may be involved, this mass of bacteria can be a grave problem. Total body surface involved in potentially retrievable burns lies between 30% and 60% of body surface; above 60% of total body surface, survival despite effective wound bacteriostasis is not common. An effective topical therapeutic agent should reduce the bacterial load, yield a viable wound which permits skin graft, and should protect the granulating wound through the skin-grafting stage. Moncrief (1968) described the optimal topical agent as being non-toxic, readily absorbed in effective concentrations, and free of binding in purulent exudate or tissue.

In the past decade, major topical formulations have emerged: silver nitrate (Moyer et al., 1965), Sulfamylon (Lindberg, R.B. et al., 1965; Moncrief, et al., 1966); silver sulfadiazene (Fox, 1968); gentamicin 0.1% (Stone, 1971); and Betadine(R) (Georgiade and Harris, 1972). Only silver nitrate and Sulfamylon, both introduced in 1965, have been statistically documented as effective. Silver sulfadiazene is also widely used. The status of the other two agents is as yet equivocal.

Techniques and criteria for assessing different agents have varied so widely that direct comparison is not possible. Microbiologic and pathologic criteria of Sulfamylon plus statistical assessment of its effect on a large sample of patients make it the most complete illustration of validation of a topical agent for burns. A 10-second scald burn on rats, Pseudomonas-infected, gave a model of BWS (Walker and Mason, 1968). A water-dispersible gel, composed of stearyl and cetyl alcohols, was used to bring experimental agents in contact with the burn surface, which had been seeded 24 hours earlier with 10^8 cells of a young Ps. aeruginosa culture. Burn wound sepsis resulted; bacterial counts up to 10^8 and 10^9 per gram of subcutaneous tissue, perivascular cuffing and extension into viable subcutaneous tissue occurred, with progressive thrombosis and death of adjacent tissue. Challenge strains of Ps. aeruginosa ranging from 90% to 100% lethal were selected, and stored frozen at -70°C to preserve virulence. Bacterial counts in human BWS reached 10^8 per gram of tissue, as they did in the rat model. Sulfamylon, a methylated sulfonamide, selected for detailed study after promising results on preliminary screening, exhibited *in vitro* inhibiting action for Pseudomonas from 0.09% to 0.6%, with a median inhibitory level of 0.156%. This drug is very soluble; it diffused rapidly through agar and through excised burn eschar. Treatment of burned seeded rats with various dilutions of Sulfamylon in aqueous gel were tried; treatment with 15 gms of 10% Sulfamylon per Kg of rat, twice daily for 10 days, gave 100% survival with completely lethal challenge strains. Bacterial counts in burns of treated animals were 10^4/gm of tissue; in untreated animals, counts were 10^8/gm. When 10% Sulfamylon cream was tried on human burns, the same difference in counts between treated and untreated was found. All patients admitted starting in 1965 were treated with Sulfamylon;

immediately a drop in BWS from 70% of fatal burns to less than 10% occurred. When BWS did occur in a Sulfamylon-treated patient, wound counts were at the level seen in untreated BWS; the disease when it occurred was unaltered. Prior to use of Sulfamylon, Ps. aeruginosa was predominant in tissues of 70% of fatal burns; after its use, only 9% of fatal burns showed Pseudomonas predominant.

At first, Sulfamylon HCl was used; when hyperchloremic acidosis due to HCl absorption was recognized, Sulfamylon acetate was made and tested. Although it is slightly less active in vitro and in vivo than the hydrochloride, elimination of the chloride ion outweighed this difference. An 11.1% suspension of acetate was equivalent in molarity to 10% Sulfamylon.

No increase in in vitro resistance of Pseudomonas to Sulfamylon has occurred since 1965. Over an 8-year period, mean sensitivity of over 1,500 strains was 0.131%. No problem of resistant forms has occurred.

The ultimate criterion of a topical treatment of burns is comparative mortality. Large numbers are needed to have comparable groups, since age, extent of burn, time admitted and associated injuries can all eliminate a patient from comparison. Since 1950, in the ISR, 1,064 patients received conventional treatment up to 1963 and 782 were treated with Sulfamylon from 1964 through 1967. Probit analysis of 6 groups of patients, divided 0-14, 15-40 and 40 + years, was done. Table 1 shows the results. A significant rise in survival occurred in treated patients, greatest in children and less in older groups. Crude mortality, a more common expression, is shown in Table 2. This data, extending through 1970, showed a continued striking improvement in Sulfamylon-treated burns up to the 60% range.

Side effects are not unexpected in strenuous chemotherapy. Separation of eschar is delayed by Sulfamylon, since bacterial growth, a major factor in this separation, is suppressed (Pruitt, 1970). Hypersensitivity, as a maculopapular rash, occurs in 5% to 10% of patients (Pruitt and Curreri, 1971). It is usually controlable with antihistamines plus a 1- to 2-day interruption in treatment. Acid-base changes are the main adverse side effect of Sulfamylon (Asch et al., 1970). Carbonic anhydrase is inhibited, and resulting bicarbonate diuresis may lower serum bicarbonate. Patients with respiratory alkalosis and pulmonary complications may then shift to an acidosis. Blood gasses and pH must be monitored; acidosis can be treated with bicarbonate and respiratory support. Hyperventilation, possibly due to direct sulfonamide stimulation, may occur early (Bader and Bader, 1965). Patients with respiratory impairment who develop acid-base distrubance must be removed from Sulfamylon, although when the condition is corrected, treatment can be resumed.

Table 1. Probit analysis of burn mortality in patients with conventional treatment (1950-1963) and with topical chemotherapy (1964-1967).

Year	Age		
	0 - 14 LD 50	15 - 40 LD 50	40 + LD 50
1950-1963	35.8 (32.2-40.1)*	49.1 (46-52.6)	30.4 (25.6-36.8)
1964-1967	52.8 (48 - 59.5)	59 (56-62.6)	37.2 (30.5-46.5)

*( ) 95% confidence limits of LD 50

Table 2. Burn mortality rate on all admissions

Year	% Burn				
	0 - 30	30 - 40	40 - 50	50 - 60	60 - 100
1962-1963	4.3	44.4	61.1	78.3	89.1
1964-1970	2,0	12.6	23.1	41.0	79.5

At 17 to 20 days post burn, topical treatment and hydrotherapy present a separating eschar, and facilitation of this separation, if safely done, is desirable. A new technique, using 5% Sulfamylon soaks has been used. This maintains bacteriologic control of the wound during the period when adherent non-viable tissue precludes grafting, and debridement is facilitated. The 5% solution is not as inhibitory as the 10% cream, and not more than 20% of body surface is entrusted to the soaks at one time. Discomfort, which can be severe on second degree burn with Sulfamylon, is absent with 5% soaks.

Monitoring of burn wounds by biopsy, for histology and bacteriology, is needed with all burn topical therapy of large burns (Curreri, et al., 1969). BWS may be heralded by high count of bacteria, masses of bacteria seen, inflammation at live-dead interface, and perivascular infiltration. Intensive systemic and sub eschar antibiotic infusions, and even surgical ablation of tissue involved may be required in life-threatening BWS.

Silver nitrate, 0.5%, in compresses is widely used to control burn infection. Only this and Sulfamylon have been statistically documented (Monafo and Moyer, 1965). The method is said to reduce mortality over pre-silver nitrate periods, but this data has not been analyzed statistically (Hartford and Zefferin, 1972). Animal models are not technically feasible for assessing silver-nitrate in control of experimental BWS. Surface colony counts are reduced in patients, but biopsies of burn wounds reveal high bacterial counts (10^5) from the second week onward. Carrier rates of Pseudomonas have been reported as lowered. Burn wound debridement, from the twice daily dressing change, is a major benefit of the method, although secondary eschar formation due to silver precipitation of protein is a hazard. Little silver penetrates the burn since fixation by Cl^- ion is prompt. The dressing is essentially distilled water, and Na^+, K^+ and Ca^{++} are leached from the wound, where Cl^- is also fixed. Methemoglobinemia has been reported (Polk, 1966). Monitoring and replacement of electrolyte is required. The technique is essentially a barrier to colonization and works best in burns treated very early. Late Pseudomonas sepsis may occur, as well as Clostridial myositis (Monafo, et al., 1966). The major problem is logistical: silver staining of linens, bed, floor and the environment is unavoidable. The method has, however, received wide acceptance.

Trial of other silver salts more suitable for incorporation in aqueous gels was prompted by silver nitrate success. Silver lactate and silver allantoiate were reported as effective, but little data is available. Silver sulfadiazene (Fox, 1968) has received wide acceptance. It is an insoluble complex prepared by mixing equal volumes of $AgNO_3$ and sodium sulfadiazene. It is dispersed in 1% suspension in an aqueous gel, after the precipitate has been finely ground to ensure particles will contact the wound, since it is insoluble and non-diffusing. It breaks down to release Ag^+ ions, which are promptly precipitated, and sulfadiazene which is absorbed and excreted. Both fractions exert antibacterial effect, although sulfadiazene which is absorbed and excreted. Both fractions exert antibacterial effect, although sulfadiazene blood levels are low. The compound does not cause acid-base disturbance, electrolyte alteration, nor methemoglobinemia. Staining due to silver is minimal. It must be applied assiduously to assure contact with the wound (Fox, et al., 1969), and is often supported with fine mesh gauze. At least daily treatments are adviseable. The drug has been used in conjunction with trimethoprim in combined therapy with favourable effect (Lowbury, 1970). Tissue bacterial count data has not been reported. Its use in some treatment centers has been followed by emergence of Enterobacter cloacae as a tissue-invasive opportunist, where this enteric form had previously been inconspicuous. Statistical assessment of improved mortality with silver sulfadiazene has not yet appeared. Since it appeared after silver nitrate and Sulfamylon had been shown to be effective against previously unportected burns, comparison is now to be made between two or more effective agents. Differences in survival rates are not apt to be large. The same problem in evaluation is present with topical gentamicin and polyvinyl-pyrrolidone-iodine.

Gentamicin, a widely used aminoglycoside was described by Stone as useful in either ointment or cream base in 0.1% concentration in control of Pseudomonas in burns (Stone, 1971). The material is applied in a manner similar to that used with Sulfamylon. Little absorption occurs, but success in control of patients who have escaped control by one of the other antibacterial agents has been described (Hummel, et al., 1970). The method has given rise to rapid incursion of gentamicin-resistant strains of Ps. aeruginosa, which have spread throughout hospital wards. Gentamicin may be an appropriate topical agent if used selectively, with close observation for emergence of resistant forms. Wound monitoring by biopsy is needed. There have been no significant side effects reported with gentamicin 0.1% cream.

Betadine(R), a polyvinyl-pyrrolidone-iodine mixture, is designed for disinfection of surfaces with iodine. It can be applied to burn surfaces as a soak or in a water dispersible gel (Copeland, 1972). It has some ability to penetrate eschar, but this activity is subject to the binding action of iodine by protein. A significant amount of iodine is absorbed; relationship of this iodine to thyroid function in the severely stressed patient remains to be assessed. Recommended procedure involves several applications daily; the effect is short-lived. Ultimate usefulness of Betadine(R) on burns remains to be seen.

A detailed comparison of Sulfamylon, silver-sulfadiazene and gentamicin 0.1% cream was made in our laboratory, with 5 challenge strains of

Table 3. Effect of Sulfamylon, Silver-sulfadiazene, and Gentamicin Cream on experimental Pseudomonas Burn Wound Sepsis in Rats

Treatment	Infecting Strain of Ps.aeruginosa and % surviving				
	12.4.4	8.28.3	3.24.5	4.18.9	VA-134
Sulfamylon 10%	89%	82%	43%	32%	25%
Silver-sulfadiazene	80%	71%	22%	14%	11%
0.1% Gentamicin	68%	32%	8%	7%	8%
Untreated Control	16%	3%	1%	3%	2%

Percent lethality shown is cumulative effect on 8 to 10 sequential experiments on groups of 5 to 7 animals each: a total of 40 to 70 animals with each strain.

Treatment: 1 x / da for 10 days. Survivors are animals still alive after 21 days post-seeding treatment begun 24 hours post-seeding.

Ps.aeruginosa of ascending virulence used. All of these were sensitive to the drugs compared. Treatment was made only once daily, which lowered the efficacy of Sulfamylon below its optimal twice daily application. Results are summarized in Table 3. With less virulent strains, Sulfamylon and silver sulfadiazene was less than half as effective as Sulfamylon. Gentamicin 0.1% was minimally effective except with the least virulent Pseudomonas strain. Betadine was tested using up to 3 applications per day; no survival in burned seeded rats occurred. This formulation was not, in the animal model that closely simulates Pseudomonas BWS, an effective one.

In modern burn therapy, effective topical agents make possible control of Pseudomonas BWS, the reduction of wound colonization by other species, and a significant improvement in survival of the severely burned over results obtained in the pre-topical therapy era. Infection by other opportunists has increased as Pseudomonas came under control: Staphylococcus aureus, Klebsiella, Enterobacter, Providencia, Candida, and Fungi have been involved in epidemic outbreaks of varying duration. Lethal wound sepsis may occur but has not been as well defined as is that with Pseudomonas. Topical therapy is not a sole answer to burn wound management, but the effective agents now available open the way to further progress in healing severe burns.

REFERENCES

Asch, M.J., White, M.G. and Pruitt, B.A. Jr. (1970). Ann. Surg., 172, 946.

Bader, M.Z. and Bader, R.A. (1965). Am.J.Med., 38, 165.

Copeland, C.E. (1972). Therapeutic Adv. and New Clin. Implications, In: Symposium Univ. Miami School Med., Miami, Florida.

Curreri, P.W., Shuck, J.M., Flemma, R.J., Lindberg, R.B. and Pruitt, B.A.Jr. (1969). Surg. Forum, 20, 506.

Fox, C.L., Rappole, B.W. and Stanford, J.W. (1969). S.G. + O., 128, 1021.

Fox, C.L. (1968). Arch. Surg., 96, 184.

Georgiade, N.G. and Harris, W.A. (1972). Therapeutic Adv. and New Clin. Implications, In: Symposium Univ. Miami School of Med., Miami, Florida.

Hartford, E.E. and Zefferin, S.E. (1972). J. Trauma, 9, 682.

Hummel, R.P., MacMillan, B.G. and Altemeier, W.A. (1970). Ann. Surg., 172, 370.

Lewis, S.R., Lynch, J.B., Blocker, T.G.Jr., Doyle, D.E. and Larson, D.L. (1970). Trans. 3rd Intl. Cong. Res. Burns, Prague, Hans Huber, Bern, p.11.

Lindberg, R.B., Moncrief, J.A., Switzer, W.E., Order, S.E. and Mills, W. (1965). J. Trauma, 5, 601.
Lowbury, E.J.L. (1970). Trans. 3rd Intl. Cong. Res. Burns, Prague, . Hans Huber, Bern., p. 138.
Monafo, W.W. and Moyer, C.A. (1965). Arch. Surg. 91, 200.
Monafo, W.W., Brenton, L., Gravens, D.L., Kempson, R. and Moyer, C.A. (1966). Arch. Surg. 92, 212.
Moncrief, J.A., Lindberg, R.B., Switzer, W.E., Pruitt, B.A. Jr. (1966). J. Trauma, 6, 907.
Moncrief, J.A. (1968). Surgery, 63, 862.
Moyer, C.A., Brentano, L., Gravens, D.L. and Morgraf, H.W. (1965). Arch. Surg., 90, 312.
Polk, H.G. Jr. (1966). Ann. Surg., 164, 753.
Pruitt, B.A. Jr. (1970). Surgery, 68, 412.
Pruitt, B.A. Jr. and Curreri, P.W. (1971). Arch. Surg., 103, 461.
Stone, H.H. (1971). J. Pediof. Surg., 3, 3.
Stone, H.H. and Kolb, L.D. (1971). J. Trauma, 11, 386.
Teplitz, C., Davis, D. and Moncrief, J.A. (1964). J. Surg. Res., 4, 200.
Walker, H.L. and Mason, A.D. (1968). J. Trauma, 8, 1049.

ANTIMICROBIAL APPLICATIONS FOR PROPHYLAXIS IN THE NEWBORN

HEXACHLOROPHANE

W.A.Gillespie, Beryl D.Corner, D.Burman, V.G.Alder

University of Bristol and Bristol Maternity Hospital

Bristol, U.K.

In this paper we deal only with hexachlorophane, preparations of which have been applied to the skin of newborn infants for the past 25 years, to prevent staphylococcal infection (Farquharson et al., 1952). The value of hexachlorophane as a prophylactic became clear soon after its introduction, and reductions of sepsis were reported by several authors (Simpson et al., 1960; Corner et al., 1960; Gluck and Wood, 1961; Pleuckhahn and Banks, 1963). The extent of these reductions may not always be appreciated by younger doctors and nurses who do not remember the outbreaks of sepsis that sometimes resulted in closure of maternity hospital nurseries, with neonatal impetigo, abscesses and occasionally septicaemia in the infants, and breast abscesses in mothers. The low incidence of these infections in recent years may be partly attributable to earlier discharge from hospital and improved nursing; but undoubtedly much of the improvement was due to hexachlorophane. The prophylactic value of hexachlorophane was re-confirmed by the increases in staphylococcal sepsis recently reported when hexachlorophane was withdrawn from use (Ayliffe et al., 1972; Alexander and Pitkewicz, 1973; Dixon et al., 1973; De Souza et al., 1975).

The reason why hexachlorophane worked so well is explained by the epidemiology of staphylococci in newborn nurseries (Gillespie et al., 1958; Baber et al., 1967). These organisms often colonise the umbilical cord stump, the skin (especially flexures) and the nose, within a few days of birth. In the absence of prophylaxis, the staphylococci sometimes multiplied quickly in these sites and were transferred to other infants, chiefly by the hands of the staff. A proportion of the infants, usually the heavily colonised ones, developed septic lesions and some of their mothers developed breast abscesses. The colonising staphylococci, being superficial, were easily reduced in number by applying hexachlorophane to the skin and umbilicus and this brought a reduction of sepsis.

The obvious prophylactic value of hexachlorophane led to its widespread use, and indeed over-use, not only in hospitals but also in domiciliary practice. Although it was known that hexachlorophane could be toxic when ingested, the risk of toxicity was at first ignored. However, recent demonstrations that in some circumstances toxic quantities of hexachlorophane would be absorbed through the skin, have caused much concern (Curley et al., 1971). Brain damage has been caused by bathing children with extensive burns or skin eruptions, in hexachlorophane solutions (Pleuckhahn, 1973). There is a greater risk of toxicity in premature infants. Kopelman (1973) demonstrated rather high blood concentrations of hexachlorophane in low birth weight infants washed with the disinfectant. Shuman et al. (1974) found an association between repeated bathing in undiluted pHisoHex and brain damage in premature infants, especially those under 1,400 gm. birth weight. There was also a well-publicised, though as yet incompletely documented catastrophe in France, when several infants were fatally poisoned, apparently by absorption from a dusting powder that contained a vast excess of hexachlorophane due to a mistake in formulation. For legal reasons, full information is not yet available about this disaster. Absorption through the skin has also been shown experimentally in monkeys; the toxic blood concentration appeared to be about 1 μg per ml in monkeys treated for 90 days (Hart, 1971).

There is no doubt, therefore, that hexachlorophane can be dangerously toxic if it is misused. However, it must be emphasised that the only clear records of harm done by hexachlorophane absorption in humans were when emulsions were applied to burned or damaged skin, and to low birth weight infants; or when grossly excessive quantities were used, as is alleged to have happened in France. There has been no harm recorded in vast numbers of normal infants that have been treated with hexachlorophane in many hospitals, in several countries (Pleuckhahn, 1973). This is in fact a remarkable safety record. Even so, hexachlorophane is dangerous if misused. It is therefore important to decide how, and with what precautions, hexachlorophane should be used, in order to enjoy its benefits without risk.

Our experience with hexachlorophane has been limited to its use in dusting powder containing 0.33 per cent ("Ster-zac"). We introduced this method in 1957 because paediatricians in Bristol preferred dry skin care to frequent bathing. After sealing the cord stump at birth with a plastic film, the trunk and flexures are dusted with "Ster-zac". Subsequently the umbilical and napkin areas are dusted when a napkin is changed during the infant's stay in hospital, normally about 1 week. The whole trunk is powdered all over, particularly the flexures, once daily. We calculate that the amount of actual hexachlorophane placed on the skin is less than 5 mg daily. This would be much less than with a liquid soap or emulsion containing 3 per cent of the drug. The powder has also been used on many low birth weight babies, who stayed in hospital for longer periods. Hexachlorophane used in this way has never been shown to cause harm, but in order to assess its safety margin, we studied the blood concentrations in normal and in low birth weight infants. The analyses were performed at the Huntingdon Research Centre by the method of Porcaro et al. (1969), modified for the Perkin Elmer F11 gas/liquid chromatograph. The blank value was between 0.00 and 0.02 μg per ml. Two heparinised blood samples were taken from all infants studied. The first was from the umbilical cord at birth, as a baseline. The second was taken by heel prick at 8 days when the Guthrie test was performed. We realised that capillary blood from a heel prick was liable to contamination by hexachlorophane on the skin, and that even a minute contamination might increase the apparent blood levels of hexachlorophane; but it was not justifiable to submit the infants to venepuncture. In fact, in our first series (Alder et al., 1972) some blood samples gave falsely high values, probably due to contamination from the skin or environment, though none approached the presumed toxic level of 1 μg per ml. We also demonstrated that a false result could arise from absorption from the blood of a mother who had used toilet preparations containing hexachlorophane (Gillespie et al., 1974). These findings demonstrate that great care is needed to avoid error when measuring very small concentrations of hexachlorophane in blood.

In subsequent investigations we took greater care to avoid contamination from the skin and environment (Gillespie et al., 1974). In 1973 another group of normal infants was investigated. In 1974/75 a third group of normal infants was studied, and at the same time, a group of low birth weight infants, whose weights ranged from 1.18 Kg to 2.49 Kg (median 2.29 Kg). All infants had normal skin. Table 1 shows the blood hexachlorophane concentrations at birth and 8 days.

Some of the low birth weight infants were treated for longer periods, to prevent staphylococcal sepsis while they stayed in hospital. None were treated beyond the 49th day, but blood (also required for haemoglobin estimation) was again taken from 5 of them after the treatment had stopped for at least 38 days (Table 2).

Table 1

Hexachlorophane in blood of normal and low birth weight infants treated with "Ster-zac" powder, at birth and at 8 days

Series	Hexachlorophane (μg per ml)	Age 0 days	Age 8 days
Normal infants 1973 (Gillespie et al., 1974)	No. of samples:	21	16
	Range	< 0.001-0.104	< 0.001-0.166
	Mean	0.032	0.066
Normal infants 1974/75	No. of samples:	19	19
	Range	< 0.001-0.021	0.006-0.272
	Mean	*	0.102
Low birth weight infants 1974/75	No. of samples:	18	18
	Range	< 0.001-0.030	0.018-0.296
	Mean	0.005	0.158

* 11 cases less than the experimental blank.

To summarise our results in 35 normal infants and 18 low birth weight infants: There was an appreciable increase in blood hexachlorophane concentration at 8 days compared with the level at birth before treatment commenced. But in no case did the concentration rise to one-third of the level reported as toxic in monkeys treated for 90 days. Furthermore, in a preliminary series of 15 infants not reported here (Alder et al., 1972), no blood concentration reached the toxic level though some were slightly, though erroneously high due to contamination from the skin and the environment.

The blood hexachlorophane concentrations in the few low birth weight infants studied during treatment for periods up to 49 days remained satisfactorily low, though the numbers were too small for many conclusions to be drawn. However, there was no evidence of accumulation of hexachlorophane in the blood of these infants.

DISCUSSION AND CONCLUSIONS

The powder method of using hexachlorophane, which has been highly effective in reducing staphylococcal sepsis in infants, and consequently in mothers, has been used on many thousands of infants without harm. The blood hexachlorophane concentrations reported here support this opinion. All remained well below the presumed

Table 2

Hexachlorophane in blood of low birth weight infants during and after treatment with "Ster-zac" powder

	Age (days)				
	0	8	17-24	32-49	87-100 (treatment finished)
No. of specimens	18	18	8	3	5
Hexachlorophane µg per ml					
Range	< 0.001 - 0.030	0.018 - 0.296	0.056 - 0.302	0.034 - 0.084	0.011 - 0.105
Median	0.003	0.135	0.124	0.050	0.019

toxic level derived from experiments in monkeys. An even greater number of normal infants have been treated, in other centres, with hexachlorophane emulsions and solutions. Pleuckhahn and Banks (1972) and Pleuckhahn (1973) found no evidence of harm in a thorough survey of more than 24,000 infants treated with the emulsion. At the same time, despite this impressive record of safety and efficiency, it is certain that hexachlorophane is dangerous if misused. It should not be used on burned or excoriated skin. Catalano (1975) reviews the evidence that hexachlorophane is dangerous as a topical agent applied to an injured epidermis. Hexachlorophane should be used on infants only under medical supervision. Normally, it need not be used for more than a week.

We believe that hexachlorophane powder may be used with care on low birth weight babies (and with special care on those under 1,400 gm), if the paediatrician is satisfied that the skin is normal and that the risk of staphylococcal sepsis would be serious in the absence of prophylaxis.

We conclude that hexachlorophane should continue in use under medical supervision for preventing neonatal sepsis, but with more stringent precautions than have sometimes been observed, until a still safer and equally effective agent becomes available.

We thank Mr. C.Harris of Hough, Hoseason and Co.Ltd. and Mr. T.Taylor of Huntingdon Research Centre for their advice, and analytical work. We thank Mrs. J.Lockyer for technical help.

REFERENCES

Alder, V.G., Burman, D., Corner, B.D. and Gillespie, W.A. (1972). Lancet, ii, 384.

Alexander, G.M.C. and Pitkewicz, J.S. (1973). Pediatrics, 51, 360.

Ayliffe, G.A.J., Brightwell, K.M., Ball, P.M. and Derrington, M.M. (1972). Lancet, ii, 479.

Baber, K.G., Corner, B.D., Duncan, E.H.L., Eades, S.M., Gillespie, W.A. and Walker, S.C.B. (1967). J.Hyg., Camb., 65, 381.

Catalano, P.M. (1975). Arch.Dermatol., 111, 250.

Corner, B.D., Crowther, S.T. and Eades, S.M. (1960). Br.med.J., i, 1927.

Curley, A., Hawk, R.E., Kimbrough, R.D., Nathenson, G., Finberg, L. (1971). Lancet, ii, 296.

De Souza, S.W., Lewis, D.M., Allen, L., Thomason, F. (1975). Lancet, i, 860.

Dixon, R.E., Kaslow, R.A., Mallison, G.F. and Bennett, J.V. (1973). Pediatrics, 51, 413.

Farquharson, D.D., Penny, S.F., Edwards, H.E. and Barr, E. (1952). Canad.med.Ass.J., 67, 247.

Gillespie, W.A., Corner, B.D., Burman, D. and Alder, V.G. (1974). J.Hyg., Camb., 73, 311.

Gillespie, W.A., Simpson, K. and Tozer, R.C. (1958). Lancet, ii, 1075.

Gluck, L. and Wood, H.F. (1961). New Engl.J.Med., 265, 1177.

Hart, E.R. (1971). Report submitted to Sterling-Winthrop Research Institute by Bionetics Research Laboratories, Dec. 3 (cited by Pleuckhahn, 1973).

Kopelman, A.E. (1973). J.Pediat., 82, 972.

Pleuckhahn, V.D. (1973). Med.J.Aust., i, 93.

Pleuckhahn, V.D. and Banks, J. (1963). Med.J.Aust., ii, 519.

Pleuckhahn, V.D. and Banks, J. (1972). Med.J.Aust., i, 897.

Porcaro, B.J., Shubiak, P. and Manowitz, M. (1969). J.pharm.Sci., 58, 251.

Shuman, R.M., Leech, R.W., Alvord, E.C., Jr. (1974). Pediatrics, 54, 689.

Simpson, K., Tozer, R.C. and Gillespie, W.A. (1960). Br.med.J., i, 315.

"CHLORHEXIDINE: ATTEMPTS TO DETECT PERCUTANEOUS ABSORPTION IN MAN"

D. E. Case, J. McAinsh, A. Rushton and M. J. Winrow

Imperial Chemical Industries Ltd., Pharmaceuticals Div.,

Alderley Park, P.O. Box 25, Macclesfield, Cheshire, U.K.

Chlorhexidine is a very effective and widely used antiseptic first marketed in the U.K. in 1953 under the trade name 'Hibitane'*. It is a strong base which is now extensively formulated as the water-soluble salt formed with 1,5-D-gluconolactone. The name chlorhexidine has an unfortunate resemblance to that of hexachlorophane, but the physical, chemical and antibacterial[1] properties of the two compounds are quite different (Fig. 1).

Chlorhexidine has been in clinical use for over two decades and has been used as a disinfectant in preoperative skin preparation, as a hand disinfectant, in the management of wounds and burns, as an obstetric cream, in ear nose and throat surgery, bladder irrigation, and oral hygiene (Fig. 2).

Interest in chlorhexidine as a useful antiplaque agent[2] was stimulated by Löe and Rindom Schiott in 1970[3,4] and applications of its use as a skin antiseptic are proliferating. Very many publications by our Chairman, Dr. Lowbury, extending over the last decade have commented on this latter application in considerable depth[5-13].

In the course of the last twenty two years, clinical use of chlorhexidine in these multitudinous applications has resulted in the identification of only one adverse reaction of any consequence; the compound should not be instilled directly into the middle ear, as deafness may follow. In this respect chlorhexidine appears to be no different to other antiseptics.

In the light of this experience it may seem strange to consider now, in detail, the percutaneous absorption of the

Hexachlorophene

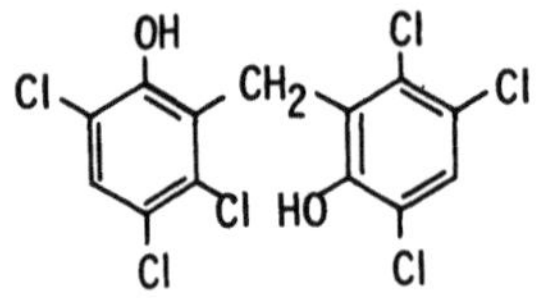

chlorinated phenol
weak acid
formulated as free phenol

Chlorhexidine

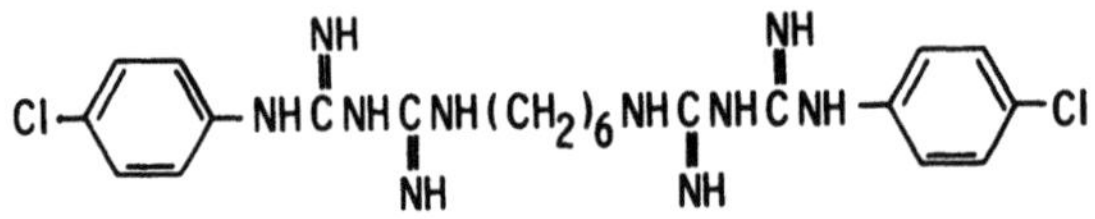

biguanide
strong base
formulated as water-soluble salts

Figure 1

'Naseptin' nasal antiseptic	1959
'Hibiscrub' surgical hand cleanser	1971
'Hibitane' acetate	1954
'Hibitane' 5% concentrate	1957
'Hibitane' gluconate 20% solution	1958
'Hibitane' hydrochloride	1957
'Hibitane' antiseptic cream	1954
'Hibitane' antiseptic lozenges	1956
'Hibitane' obstetric cream	1954
'Savlon' hospital concentrate	1956
'Savlon' liquid antiseptic	1955
'Savlon Babycare' lotion	1970-1971
'Savlon Babycare' talc	1970-1971
'Hibispray' 1-5	1970
'Mimospray' aerosol	1964
'Mimospray' body talc	1970
'Mimospray' liquid	1970
'Mimettes' feminine hygiene	1970
'Footsy' deodorant spray for feet	1972

Figure 2. Products Available Containing Chlorhexidine

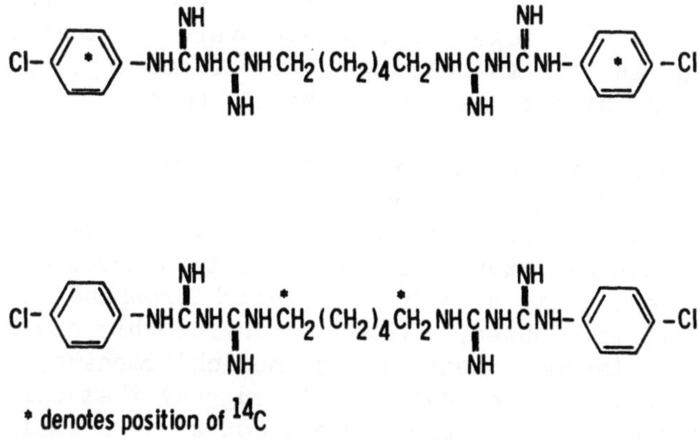

Figure 3. ^{14}C-Labelled Chlorhexidine Preparations

Species	Dose (mg/kg)	Labelled Form [a]	% Dose in urine [b]
Rat	5	R	0.4
Rat	50 [c]	R	0.4
Rat	50 [c]	R	0.7
Rat	5	C	0.2
Rat	4	C	0.7
Mouse	27	R	7.2
Mouse	8	R	3.7
Dog	50	R	1.0
Dog	5	R	0.7
Dog	5	R	0.8
Dog	5	C	0.2
Dog	0.05	R	0.9
Marmoset	7	R	1.3
Marmoset	7	R	0.4
Rhesus Monkey	6	R	1.2
Human	0.07	R	0.3
Human	Mouth rinse	R	0.4
Human	0.7	C	0.2

a: R = ring labelled; C = chain labelled
b: Mean total recovery for all experiments = 96.9% $\pm$ 3.8 (2 x SE)
c: Followed 50 mg/kg for 6 months

Figure 4. Urinary Elimination of Chlorhexidine after Oral Administration

compound. However, the reports of hexachlorophane absorption and its consequences [15-17], together with our awareness that the use of chlorhexidine in skin antisepsis was proliferating, prompted a number of studies which I shall describe in summary.

First, however, it should be clearly understood that the context in which percutaneous absorption of chlorhexidine is considered is quite different to that relating to hexachlorophane. Professor Gillespie has made it quite clear that despite its record of efficacy, it is certain that hexachlorophane is dangerously toxic if misused. There is considerable cause to question the percutaneous absorption of hexachlorophane. On the other hand, there is no such evidence to suggest that chlorhexidine is a toxic agent even if it were to be absorbed to a small extent through skin.

It is not possible at this time to review adequately the different methods available for assessing percutaneous absorption [18-20]. However, it may be fair to comment that in the pharmaceutical company there is some reluctance to pursue in vitro or in situ model systems when the whole animal study can be attempted. When man is the relevant animal and human studies are possible then they must be the primary objective.

Two different ^{14}C-labelled forms of chlorhexidine have been in use in our laboratories and contain ^{14}C in either the aromatic ring systems or in the aliphatic carbon chain of the molecule. (Fig. 3). In addition we have a glc electron capture method for chlorhexidine based upon degradation to p-chloraniline. The limit of detection for this method is 0.01-0.05 µg/ml.

In various animal and human studies it has been found that when administered orally, chlorhexidine is poorly absorbed from the gastrointestinal tract. Very small fractions of oral doses are excreted in urine (Fig. 4) and biliary excretion is minimal[21]. The fate of the two different radiolabelled forms is apparently identical suggesting that extensive metabolism does not occur[21].

In our first study to assess percutaneous absorption in man chlorhexidine digluconate was applied, either as a 5% aqueous solution or a 4% formulated handwash, to 50 square centimetres of the forearm skin of five adult male subjects. In each case, the chlorhexidine preparation, containing 18 µCi of ^{14}C, was left on the skin for three hours under a non-occluding guard.

Residual material was then recovered from the skin and the amount of chlorhexidine absorbed was determined by measuring levels of total radioactivity in urine and faeces collected up to ten days, and by measuring levels in whole blood samples withdrawn during this period.

Of all the faecal samples, just two, each one from a different subject, contained detectable ^{14}C-levels. These were less than twice the background count rate, were very close to the limits of detection, and represented less than 0.009% of the applied dose (Fig. 5).

None of the urine samples from any of the five subjects contained any detectable level of radioactivity at any time. None of the blood samples contained any detectable level of radioactivity, the limit of detection being of the order of 0.005 μg/ml (Fig. 5).

In this study we used very precise and sensitive methods to attempt to detect absorption and we concluded that percutaneous absorption of chlorhexidine from intact human skin is extraordinarily low.

However, in order to use conditions more comparable to those in general practice we undertook a second study in which 15 clinically healthy adults, 8 female and 7 male, used chlorhexidine in a hand-scrub regimen. All subjects, who had intact hand and forearm skin, carried out the hand scrubbing regime five times a day, five days each week, for three weeks. The hands and forearms were scrubbed with a bristle brush for three minutes with 5 ml of 'Hibiclens'*, a 4% chlorhexidine gluconate preparation. Nails were cleaned with a disposable cleaner, the hands and forearms rinsed with water and then finally washed for three minutes, again using 5 ml of 'Hibiclens'*.

Venous blood samples were withdrawn on days 0, 5, 12, 16 and 19 from the antecubital fossa which had been protected by an elasticated polythene cover during the washing procedures. Samples were withdrawn half an hour after handscrubbing, after one, three or five scrubbing procedures, and assayed by the glc method. No detectable level of chlorhexidine or chlorhexidine-derived material was found in any of the samples from any of the fifteen subjects.

Again, the conclusion drawn was that under the conditions of this study no detectable degree of absorption had occurred. However, to take the investigation one stage further, the same kind of procedure was followed in theatre staff.

This third study involved 25 staff in three hospitals, who had been regular users of 'Hibiscrub'* for at least six months as a preoperative antiseptic for hand disinfection. On average the preparation had been used 5 times a day, washing for one minute with 5 ml of the 5% digluconate preparation, rinsing with water and repeating the wash for a further two minutes. Blood samples were withdrawn from these subjects one to two hours after handscrubbing. No detectable levels of chlorhexidine could be detected in any of

Subject	1	2	3	4	5
Formulation	Aqueous	Aqueous	Hibiclens	Hibiclens	Hibiclens
Applied ^{14}C (µCi)	16	22	18	16	18
% dose recovered	93	81	97	98	96
Max. blood levels	ND[a]	ND	ND	ND	ND
% dose in urine	ND[b]	ND	ND	ND	ND
% dose in faeces	ND[c]	< 0.009	ND	< 0.009	ND

ND : Not detectable

a : Limit of detection for blood = 0.005 µg/ml
b : Limit of detection for urine = 0.02 % dose per day
c : Limit of detection for faeces = 0.006 % dose per day

Figure 5. Percutaneous Absorption Study with ^{14}C-Chlorhexidine

the samples; the limit of detection for the analytical method was 0.01 μg/ml.

The conclusion to be drawn from all these studies is that percutaneous absorption of chlorhexidine from intact human skin must be absolutely minimal.

This data for chlorhexidine is quite different to that for hexachlorophane, since Feldman and Maibach reported[22] that 3.1% of topically applied radiolabelled hexachlorophane penetrated intact human skin. In operating room personnel, Butcher[23] showed a mean blood level of 0.20 μg/ml after use of a hexachlorophane detergent, and 0.06 μg/ml after use of a hexachlorophane soap. Further work quoted by Lockhart[17] involved detection of mean blood levels of 0.07, 0.20 and 0.10 μg/ml hexachlorophane in volunteers taking part in chronic hand washing, face washing and surgical scrub-up studies, respectively.

In contrast to these results, our studies with chlorhexidine indicate that this compound is absorbed through intact human skin to an extraordinarily small degree, if at all. We believe that this behaviour is entirely consistent with the properties of the chlorhexidine molecule which tends to be bound to proteinaceous material and is possibly largely retained in the stratum corneum of the epidermis; the definitive evidence is, however, not yet available.

It should be remarked clearly at this point, that had percutaneous absorption of chlorhexidine been shown to occur to some extent, there would be no logical cause to anticipate adverse reaction.

Two lifespan studies in rats, in which chlorhexidine was given daily in drinking water at high dose levels, monitored clinically and followed by full histological evaluation, failed to indicate any tumourogenic effect or other toxic sign. In the second study, blood and tissue levels were monitored at periods over two years; levels in some tissues, notably the liver and kidney, were well above limits of detection and indicated that absorption from the gastroinestinal tract had occurred without any associated adverse reaction. The oral LD_{50} of chlorhexidine in rats is in excess of 3000 mg/kg and the intravenous LD_{50} 21 mg/kg. Studies involving rhesus monkeys in which neonates were bathed in a chlorhexidine digluconate solution daily for the first ninety days of their lifetime, presented no evidence whatsoever of local intolerance or systemic toxicity.

These and other animal studies, together with very extended clinical experience with chlorhexidine in man, suggest that this compound is remarkably free of any adverse reaction, even when administered chronically under conditions where it is known to give rise to appreciable blood and tissue levels.

Having established, furthermore, that percutaneous absorption in man is absolutely minimal it must be concluded that chlorhexidine, in the light of our present knowledge, is a remarkably satisfactory agent for use in skin antisepsis.

*: 'Hibitane', 'Hibiscrub', and 'Hibiclens' are Trade Marks, the property of Imperial Chemical Industries Ltd.

References

1. Hennessey, T.D., J. periodont. Res., 8, Suppl. 12, 61 (1973).
2. Journal of Periodontal Research, 8, Supplement 12 (1973).
3. Lőe, H. and Rindom Schiott, C., in "Dental Plaque" Ed. W. D. McHugh, E. and S. Livingstone, Edinburgh,. 247 (1970).
4. Lőe, H. and Rindom Schiott, C., J. periodont. Res., 5, 79 (1970).
5. Lowbury, E.J.L. and Lilly, H.A., Brit. med. J., 1, 1445 (1960).
6. Lowbury, E.J.L., Lilly, H.A. and Bull, J.P., Brit. med. J., 2, 1039 (1960).
7. Lowbury, E.J.L., J. Clin. Pathol., 14, 85 (1961).
8. Lowbury, E.J.L., Lilly, H.A. and Bull, J.P., Brit. med. J., 1, 1251 (1963).
9. idem, ibid, 2, 230 (1964).
10. idem, ibid, 2, 531, (1964).
11. Lowbury, E.J.L. and Lilly, H.A., Brit. med. J., 1, 510 (1973).
12. Lowbury, E.J.L., Lilly, H.A., and Ayliffe, G.A.J., Brit. med J. 4, 369 (1974).
13. Lilly, H.A. and Lowbury, E.J.L., Brit. med. J., 4, 372 (1974).
14. Lowbury, E.J.L. and Lilly, H.A., Br. J. Surg., 61, 19 (1974).
15. Curley, A., Hawk, R.E., Kimbrough, R.D., Nathenson, G. and Finberg, L., Lancet, 2, 296 (1971).
16. Kimbrough, R.D., Pediatrics, 51, 391 (1973).
17. Lockhart, J.D., Pediatrics, 50, 229 (1972).
18. Idson, B. in "Topics in Medicinal Chemistry", Vol. 4, Interscience (1971).
19. Scheuplein, R.J. and Blant, I.H., Phys. Rev., 51, No. 4, 702 (1971).
20. Katz, M. and Poulsen, B.J. in "Handbook of Experimental Pharmacology", 28, Part 1, 103 ( ).
21. Winrow, M.J., J. periodont, Res., 8, Suppl. 12, 45 (1973).
22. Feldman, R.J. and Maibach, H.I., J. Invest. Dermatol., 54, 399 (1970).
23. Butcher, H.R., Gravens, D.L., Ballinger, W.F., Dewar, N.E., Ledlie, E.F. and Barthel, W.F., Arch. Surgery, 107, 70 (1973).

THE DISINFECTION OF THE HANDS - Quantitative Aspects

M. Rotter, H. Mittermayer, W. Koller, G. Wewalka

Hygiene-Institute of the University
Kinderspitalg.15 A-1095 Vienna
Austria (Dir.:Prof.Dr.H.Flamm)

In the early days of microbiology the Viennese gynecologist SEMMELWEIS (1847) was the first to prove that the hands may act as very efficient vehicles for microbes on their way from one person or place to an other. He and in this country Lord LISTER demonstrated convincingly that disinfection procedures may block this way of transmission and, by this, can cause a remarkable decrease of infection rates in the hospital environment. From this time on, the disinfection of the hands has become a routine procedure not only in the medical field but also in other branches. However, except for the finding that non-contamination is even better than disinfection, only details - though very important ones - have been added to our knowledge since then. One of the most important details was the finding that the skin harbours two different kinds of microbial flora. The one being physiologically associated with the normal skin is, with regard to its composition and quantity, very difficult to influence by ablution or even by disinfection procedures. It is called the resident flora and consists mainly of grampositive organisms as Staph.epidermidis and some species of corynebacteria. The other kind of flora, the transient, is represented by any kind of microbe which is deposited on the skin. Usually, it can not gain a foothold on the healthy skin as it cannot multiply there and often it is even eliminated very quickly. It is readily removeable by cleaning and disinfection procedures. Consequently, one distinguishes, at least in German-speaking countries, strictly between the so-called "surgical" and "hygienic" disinfections of the hands. Is the former directed against both, the transient and the resident flora, so in contrast, the latter aims solely at the removal and inactivation of the transient flora without regard to the normal saprophytes of the skin. In addition, the "surgical" disinfection is required to possess a remanent action in order to suppress microbes released under the gloves during operation. This property is not necessarily required of procedures intended for the "hygienic" disinfection.

Despite of great efforts, the quantitative evaluation of the efficiency of a disinfection procedure remains still to be problematic. In this context, it is imperative to realize that not the performance of a certaindisinfectant per se has to be evaluated but the efficiency of a whole procedure including the disinfectant under the conditions of action.

As we have recently investigated several questions concerning some quantitative aspects of the "hygienic" disinfection of the hands it might be of interest to report on some of our results.

Today, we can not assess the efficacy of a disinfection procedure in terms of its influence on the infection rates as SEMMELWEIS did. Today, we have to use some other parameters like the number of viable bacteria that can be recovered from the hands before and after the standardized use of the procedure to be tested. In order to provide experimentally a controled situation which in practice would require a "hygienic" disinfection of the hands the model of the artificially contaminated hands may be used. In our experiments, the test persons immersed their hands for a few seconds into a suspension of E.coli. After drying, the number of viable bacteria can be determined which the hands are able to release. This number may, now, be compared with the counts that are received after a certain disinfection procedure in order to assess its "degermining" power. We call the bacterial counts recovered from the hands before the treatment "pre-values" and those after it "post-values". Both of them may be related to each other, mathematically. We do this by dividing the pre-values of each test person by the corresponding post-values and call the resulting values"reduction-factors".

The germs can be recovered from the hands in many ways. We investigated the suitability of 4 methods:

(1) A modification of the basin-method as described by PRICE in which the test persons wash their hands in a series of basins each containing 2000 ml of sterile water.

(2) The plastic-bag-method by GASCHEN:The contaminated hands are immersed into plastic bags each containing 100 ml of liquid wherein they are rinsed for 5 min by the rhythmic compression exerted on the bags from outside by an assistant.

(3) The finger tip-method as described in the guidelines of the German Society of Hygiene and Microbiology was performed by rubbing the finger tips during 1 min aggainst the bottom of a petri-dish that contained 10 ml of liquid.

(4) The glass cup-Method by STORY was executed by pressing a glass cylinder against the palm or the back of the hand. The cylinder was then filled with 10 ml liquid, and the area of skin inside the cylinder was rubbed vigorously for 2 min with a glass rod.The viable counts in all fluids were estimated and corrected for the different volumes.

The finger tip-method proved to be not only the most simple procedure for recovering bacteria from the hands but also the most effective as it yields counts very well comparable to those of the basin and the plastic bag-method despite of the much smaller skin area exposed (Fig.1).Hence, only this method was used in the following investigations.

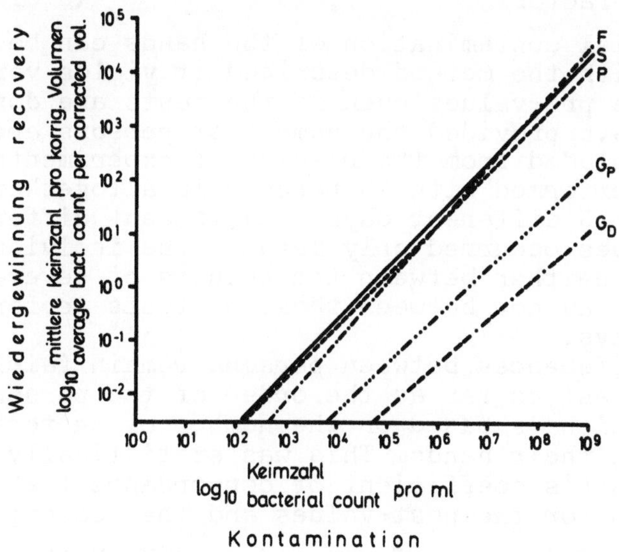

Figure 1. Comparison of several recovery methods. F=Finger tip, S=Basin, P=Plastic bag, G-Glasscylinder-method.

For the performance of tests evaluating disinfection procedures it is convenient to know that per ml rinsing fluid from the finger tips the pre-values can be expected to be constantly c. 2,7 $\log_{10}$-steps below the viable count of the contamination fluid (Tab.1).

Median values of viable counts (N=10)

Contamination fluid	Rinsing fluid (Pre-values)	Δ
$10^{8,85}$/ml	$10^{6,17}$/ml	$10^{2,68}$

An interesting finding was the fact that the counts derived from right and left hands correlated significantly. This is true for pre- and post-values and therefore also for the reduction-factors (Tab.2) From this follows that the bacterial counts of both hands of a person must not be regarded as being independent samples which fact has to be considered in statistical tests.

Correlation factors (PEARSON) r between the viable counts of right and left hands (N=10)

	r	p
Pre-values	0,874	<0,001
Post-values	0,751	<0,05
Reduction factors	0,828	<0,01

The artificial contamination of the hands can be done such that with the method described it yields very well reproducible pre-values even if the tests are done on different days provided the same test persons are used. This is concluded from the results of experiments which have been performed with 10 persons in altogether 15 tests, 3 per day on 5 different days. Significant differences of the pre-values occurred only between the individual test persons but neither between the results of several tests at the same day nor between those of tests performed at different days.

The differences between persons remain fairly constant, at least as far as the order of the persons is concerned which is based on the number of bacteria they release from their hands. This was statistically confirmed by KENDALL's coefficient of concordance (Tab.3) and is true also for the post-values and the reduction-factors.

Kendall's Coefficients of Concordance (W),N=10, K=15

	W	p
Pre-values	0,4919	≪0,001
Post-values	0,3222	≪0,001
Reduction-factors	0,3066	≪0,001

Furthermore, it can be demonstrated that this order of the persons is still the same even after a period of two months. This indicates that within a certain range the results are dependent on some individual factors. Thus, under similar conditions the hands of some persons will always release for instance more bacteria into the rinsing fluid than those of others. As this applies also to the reduction-factors which represent a measure for the "degermining" power of a disinfection procedure the results of an experiment may be influenced by the composition of the test population, to a certain degree.

In other experiments the kinetics of the release of test bacteria from the contaminated hands was studied under various conditions. Summarizing the results (Fig.2) it can be shown that with rubbing the finger tips repetitively in a series of petri-dishes, as described for the finger tip-method, the strongest release of bacteria as expressed by reduction factors takes place in the first two successive petri-dishes. During the later sequences the reduction factors increase only very slowly, a fact indicating that in each of the following petri-dishes about the same amount of bacteria is being delivered with a merely slight tendency of decrease. On the skin surface the reservoir of test-bacteria that can potentially be released is thus very large. It is not too important how long the finger tips are rubbed in the petri-dish as only a slight increase of the reduction factors results from the prolonged procedure.

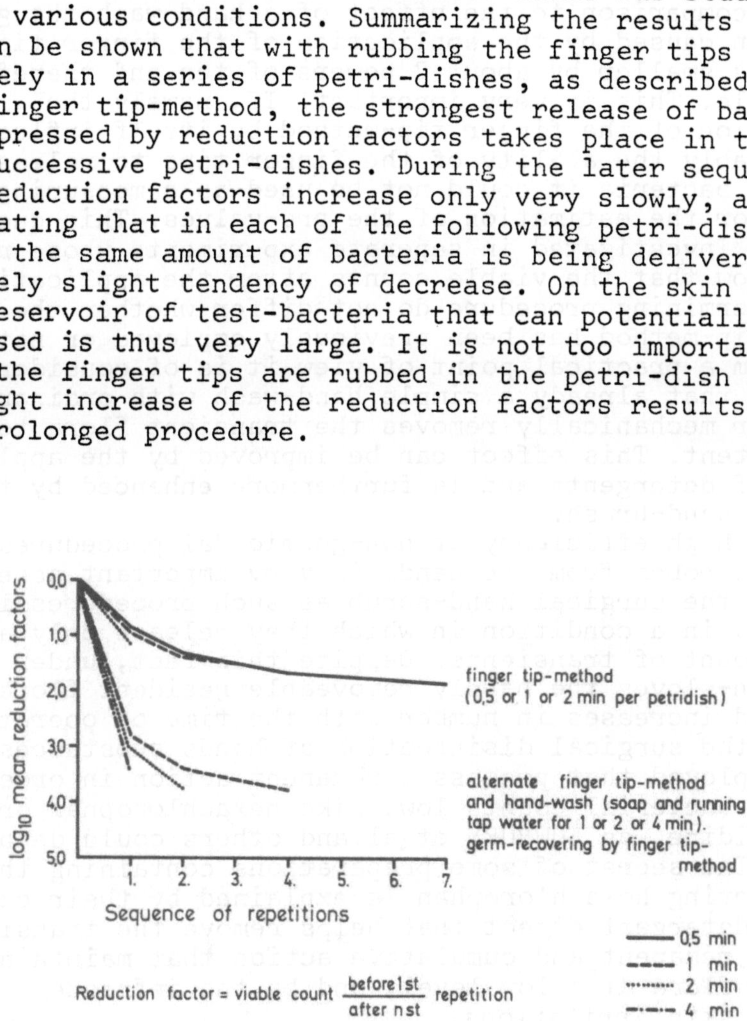

Figure 2. Kinetics of the release of testbacteria

If one interrupts the sequences of this proceeding by hand-washes with soap and running tap water after each "rubbing", the kinetics of the transient flora under the conditions of an ablution can be studied. In Fig.2 it is demonstrated that the effect of the first ablution-procedure is by far the greatest as subsequent hand-washes do not furthermore increase very much the germ-reduction already achieved. With both proceedings,namely finger tip-method alone and with alternate ablutions, there exists a tendency towards the fact that within a defined period of time the repetitive use of these procedures causes a reduction of viable counts greater than that achieveable by their single application.

In comparison to the effect of a hand-wash the germ-reduction caused by the application of the finger tip-method is smaller by about 2 powers of ten and therefore negligible. This is very important! If, namely the application of the finger tip-method by itself influenced considerably the ability of the finger tips to release the test bacteria it could not be used as a measuring method for the estimation of the pre-values. This question was also investigated in seperate experiments whose results show that the viable counts after the application of a degermining procedure do not differ whether the finger tip-method has been previously employed or not.

From a practical point of view it is of considerable interest that already a simple hand-wash with ordinary tap water mechanically removes the transient flora to a great extent. This effect can be improved by the application of detergents and is furthermore enhanced by the use of a hand-brush.

The high efficiency of non-germicidal procedures to remove microbes from the hands is very important aspect also for the surgical hand-scrub as such procedures leave the hands in a condition in which they release only a small amount of transients. Despite this fact, under the operation-gloves the hardly removeable resident flora remains and increases in number with the time of operation. So, for the surgical disinfection of hands substances have to be employed that possess a remanent action in order to keep the bacterial counts low, like hexachlorophan or chlorhexidine, as LOWBURY et al.and others could demonstrate. The secret of some preparations containing the slowly acting hexachlorophan is explained by their excellent detergent effect that helps remove the transients, by their remanent and cumulative action that maintain the resident flora at a low level, and by the infrequent occurence of skin irritations.

TOPICAL CHEMOTHERAPY OF SKIN DISEASE

Alan Lyell, Consultant Dermatologist

Royal Infirmary, Glasgow G4 0SF, U.K.

SUMMARY

There is a limited place for topical chemotherapy because few patients have disease (excluding warts) that are primarily due to infection. Impetigo contagiosa, tinea of the open skin, superficial candidal infection and scabies are within reach of and usually amenable to topical agents. Antiseptic skin cleansers are used in acne vulgaris, and to control the carriage of pathogenic staphylococci. The greatest actual use of topical chemotherapy, often in combination with corticosteroids, is made on vague indications, for example in eczema, where there is assumed to be an important infective element. The disadvantages include upsetting the ecology of the skin microflora, breeding resistant pathogens, staining or sensitizing the patient's skin and producing untoward effects by absorption. The potential sensitizers include the bases of medicaments. Attention is drawn particularly to the insidious clinical picture of sensitization to neomycin, and it is suggested that this antibiotic should be abandoned for topical use.

The skin may seem to be the ideal site to which to apply chemotherapy, since it is apparently so accessible, and the problem of absorbing sufficient drug from the alimentary tract to reach an effective tissue concentration ought not to arise. However, contrary to lay belief, few skin diseases are infectious, and their seeming accessibility is often negated by the effective barrier that the epidermis offers to the penetration of drugs - a barrier that can be overcome to some extent by the choice of vehicle.

TABLE 1

INCIDENCE OF INFECTIVE SKIN DISEASE IN HOSPITAL PRACTICE, EXPRESSED AS A PERCENTAGE OF TOTAL OUT-PATIENT ATTENDANCES

Warts	25
Fungal	2.5
Coccal	2
Scabies	2
Candidal	0.5

TABLE 2

PERCENTAGE OF PATIENTS ATTENDING CONTACT DERMATITIS CLINIC, SHOWING POSITIVE PATCH TEST REACTIONS TO TOPICAL MEDICAMENTS

Neomycin	7.6
Clioquinol	3.5
Chlorquinaldol	3.4
Benzocaine	1.8

(By courtesy of Dr. S.L. Husain, Contact Dermatitis Investigation Unit, Glasgow)

TABLE 3

PERCENTAGE OF PATIENTS ATTENDING CONTACT DERMATITIS CLINIC, SHOWING POSITIVE PATCH TEST REACTIONS TO BASES OF TOPICAL MEDICAMENTS

Wool alcobols	7.0
Parabens	3.0

(By courtesy of Dr. S.L. Husain, Contact Dermatitis Investigation Unit, Glasgow.

In practive only the most superficial infections and infestations are amenable to topical chemotherapy, and these comprise a mere 7% of the out-patients attending the Skin Department of the Glasgow Royal Infirmary (Table 1). On the other hand 25% of our patients come with warts. But the wart virus is difficult to reach with topical applications, being well protected by ketatin, and the most practical way of dealing with warts is by physical destruction. These figures for incidence apply to hospital practice: It is probable that superficial bacterial and fungal infections are commoner in general practice than these figures suggest, the hospital receiving only the failures and missed cases. By the same token the incidence of warts in general practice may well be lower, because all practitioners like to have a got at treating tinea and impetigo, but few make any determined effort to deal with warts.

Impetigo contagiosa is an example of an infection that responds well to topical chemotherapy. The causative organisms (staphylococci and/or streptococci) are superficial, and a high local concentration of antibiotic can be achieved, that may seem to contradict _in vitro_ laboratory tests of sensitivity. For example, 3% chlortetracycline hydrochloride ointment will deal with many cases of impetigo from which _Staphylococcus aureus_ resistant to this antibiotic _in vitro_ can be recovered. But the problem comes when staphylococci that are totally resistant to chlortetracycline are encountered. Here there is an important conflict between the aims of the dermatologist and of the microbiologist. The dermatologist wants preimarily to cure his patient, while the microbiologist is concerned to limit the development of strains of _Staphylococcus aureus_ that are resistant to the newer antibiotics. For although the recent epidemic of serious gram negative infections may seem to have eclipsed the importance of _Staphylococcus aureus_, in fact life-threatening staphylococcal infections continue to pose a serious problem. Consequently the microbiologist advises the dermatologist to avoid topical antibiotics that are useful in resistant systemic staphylococcal infections, such as fusidic acid, and recommends those that have a limited systemic use, such as neomycin. The dermatologist's objection is that neomycin has become a leading cause of contact dermatitis (Table 2). While on the subject of contact dermatitis from topical medicaments, it should be mentioned that the bases also play a part (Table 3), and it is now necessary for dermatologists to have details of these if they are to prescribe rationally.

The skin-sensitizing capacity of neomycin is perhaps new to you, and it is still not recognised by the profession at large. One reason for its having been overlooked is that the clinical course of neomycin sensitization tends to be insidious, whereas sensitization to many other topical agents, such as clioquinol, is usually acute, is therefore easily recognised, and the application is withdrawn. Another reason is that noemycin is often presented in a mixture with a corticosteroid, the corticosteroid moiety partially suppressing the dermatitis caused by neomycin. Clinical interpretation of the onset of neomycin dermatitis therefore tends to be that the originally helpful application has 'lost its effect'. A change to an alternative application is made, but since many such applications also contain neomycin, there is a considerable chance that neomycin will be continued. I have seen several patients whose allegedly psycho-somatic dermatosis was due to neomycin sensitivity, as it happened that all of the many topical applications used on them had contained this drug. Neomycin may be comparaitvely safe for use where the epidermal barrier is intact, for it is poorly absorbed in this circumstance, but since it is impossible thus to limits its prescription by non-dermatologists, it would seem that to discontinue its topical use would be a major step in reducing the increasing incidence of contact dermatitis. Chlortetracycline has been a popular application because it seldom causes dermatitis. Fusidic acid looks like being equally harmless in this respect, but if its topical use is to be discouraged to reserve it for treating life-threatening staphylococcal infections, it would seem preferable to risk manifest clioquinol dermatitis than occul sensitization of the patient to neomycin. A more rational procedure might be to use a combination of antibiotics, but only one of the eight combinations listed in a recent "MIMS' is free of neomycin.

The position in regard to the topical treatment of fungus infections is the reverse of that in coccal infections, because encouraging _in vitro_ tests of new anti-fungal agents have seldom been reflected in satisfactory _in vivo_ activity. With the possible exception of miconazole (Mandy and Garrott, 1974), which is still being evaluated, the most reliable topical applications remain Whitfield's ointment and Castellani's paint, the latter having an unwelcome colour. The biggest advance in the treatment of dermatophytosis was the introduction of oral griseofulvin, since it allowed fungi that were growing in places that in places that were inaccessible to topical agents to be reached. It is still not fully appreciated that griseofulvin is inactive against candidal infections.

Candida albicans is an opportunist pathogen, and the basis of its management is to consider why it has gained a foothold. Disturbance of the ecology of the intestinal flora by broad spectrum antibiotics is a common cause. Infections in diabetics respond poorly, if at all, until the diabetes has been controlled. Chronic paronychia depends heavily upon local conditions provided by wet occupations (housewives) and trauma (gardeners). Oral candidiasis, often misdiagnosed as a contact stomatitis from denture materials - an exceedingly uncommon occurrence - requires expert dental advice and a review of the patient's nutritional status, haemoglobin and serum iron levels. Provided that such factors are taken into account the topical treatment of candidal infection is usually fairly successful, but there are a few unfortunate patients suffering from an inherent inability to deal with Candida albicans, and some of these may be helped by the recently discovered transfer factor.

Dealing with scabies is largely a matter of technique. It is essential that the whole family should be treated simultaneously, irrespective of whether they are itching or not, advice that is made difficult if mother and the children are registered with one general practitioner, father with another, and grannie with a third. The whole body surface, except the head, must be treated, and it is surprising how many intelligent adults forget the soles of their feet. There is a vogue, sanctioned by Prescribers Notes, for using malathion, but I have reservations about this substance, which I believe to be a potential environmental poison. Sulphur ointment remains very effective, if somewhat messy, with gamma-benzene hexachloride, a cosmetically more acceptable alternative.

Antiseptic skin cleansers of the type used for surgical scrubbing-up have a use in acne vulgaris, in patients afflicted with crops of boils and in the care of the infant's skin. The aetiology of acne is complicated, but contrary to old belief Staphylococcus aureus is very unimportant. The organism most intimately concerned is the acne bacillus, which, by its lipolytic activity converts the non-irritant fatty acids present in the sebum into irritant ones (Marples et al, 1972). Therapy usually combines oral tetracycline with local skin cleansing. A possible untoward result of this regime is overgrowth of gram negative organisms on the skin, with a consequent gram negative folliculitis (Fulton et al, 1968), that can only be aggravated by persevering with this treatment. A mildly comedogenic effect of certain skin cleansers has also been described recently (Mills and Kligman, 1975). Boils, folliculitis and carbuncles reflect the carriage of 'pathogenic'staphylococci on the patient's skin, fed from a focus that is usually the nose or gut. Unknown host factors must be concerned, because 'healthy' carriers of apparently identical strains are commonplace. A logical way to tackle the problem, for the lesions themselves are not accessible to topical therapy, is routine washing of the skin with antiseptic cleansers, of which the most popular has been hexachlorophane, combined with topical antibiotics to the nostrils, to try and control skin carriage. Hexachlorophane has also been used widely as a skin cleanser in the nurseries of maternity hospitals, to control the troublesome staphylococcal skin infections that affect the babies - for infant skin is readily colonised by staphylococci, and the environment in which the babies find themselves is likely to abound in pathogenic strains. Since doubt was cast on the safety of hexachlorophane, due to serious, sometimes lethal effects attributed to its absorption, other cleansers have been tried, but often with less success.

Hexachlorophane has now been banned by the F.D.A., and an article directed against complacency in its use appeared in a recent issue of the Archives of Dermatology (Catalano, 1975). An alternative method of control has been to colonise the skin of the infants deliberately with a 'non-pathogenic'strain of *Staphylococcus aureus* (Light et al, 1967).

The greatest actual use of topical antibacterial agents is made on somewhat vague indications, as an anti-infective addition to topical corticosteroids. That such addition can be helpful clinically is true, but only in certain circumstances. Seborrhoeic eczema is a case in point. Atopic eczema in general does perfectly well with plain corticosteroid applications, but when heavily secondarily infected with *Staphylococcus aureus* it may help to combine the topical corticosteroid with an anti-staphylococcal agent. But any chronic superficial dermatosis becomes colonised by micro-organisms, and although it is tempting to attribute some harm to them, the evidence for them harming the patient is scanty. The regrettably low level of general dermatological knowledge gives the representative of the drug firm a field day in peddling his wares containing ever more potent corticosteroids combined with a wider spectrum of antibacterial activity. A great deal of this potency is wasted on eczemas that would respond satisfactorily to hydrocortisone, combined on occasion with clioquinol or chlortetracycline. As regards the harm that may result we are seeing an increasing number of patients with iatrogenic manifestations. Contact dermatitis in respect of the medicaments and their bases has been mentioned. We also see the red face induced by potent corticosteroids, peri-oral eczema, striae, skin atrophy and steroid acne. The potentially harmful results of disturbing the ecology of the skin microflora have not been explored. Occasionally the anti-infective spectrum is insufficiently broad to cover the particular infection present, for example candidal infection or tinea. The name *tinea incognito* (Ive and Marks, 1968) has been coined to describe the quiet by confident way in which a fungus infection flourishes under these circumstances. Not even scabies escapes this ritual anointing, and a colleague of mine scandalised the patient's practitioner, by saying that he was surprised that the *Acarus* that he had recovered and looked at under the microscope was not moon-faced.

I hope that this contribution does not strike you as having been too destructive in its criticisms. It was not intended to be so. The good that has resulted from topical chemotherapy of skin diseases speaks for itself, and we are grateful for the blessings that have been dispensed on our behalf. My object has been to try and achieve a sense of proportion by discussing some of the limitations and shortcomings of this apparently simple means of treatment, and to show that the simplicity is illusory. But that is a lession that has to be learnt painfully in every branch of medicine if there is to be real progress, and I trust that you will receive my remarks in this spirit.

REFERENCES

Catalano, P.M. (1975) "Hexachlorophane - not a cry of 'wolf'" Arch. Dermatol., 111, 250-251.

Fulton, J.E., McGinley, K., Leyden, J., Marples, R.R. (1968) Gram negative folliculitis in acne vulgaris. Arch. Dermatol., 97, 349-353.

Ive, F.A., Marks, R. (1968) Tinea incognito. Brit.Med.J., 3, 149.

Light, I.J., Walton, R.L., Sutherland, J.M., Shinefield, H.R., Brackvogel, V. (1967) Use of bacterial interference to control a staphylococcal nursery outbreak: Deliberate colonization of all infants with the 502A strain of Staphylococcus aureus. Amer.J.Dis.Child., 113, 291-300.

Mandy, S.J., Garrott, T.C. (1974) Miconazole treatment for severe dermatophytoses. J.Amer.med.Ass., 230, 72.

Marples, R.R., Downing, D.T., Kligman, A.M. (1972) Influence of Pityrosporum species in the generation of free fatty acids in human surface lipids. J.invest.Derm., 58, 155-159.

Mills, P.H., Kligman, A.M. (1975) Acne detergicans. Arch. Dermatol., 111, 250-251.

CONTAMINATION OF ANTISEPTICS AND USE OF PRESERVATIVES

D.A. Norton

School of Pharmacy and Pharmacology

University of Bath BA2 7AY

SUMMARY

Antiseptic substances such as benzalkonium chloride, chlorhexidine and organic mercurial compounds are also employed as antimicrobial preservatives in pharmaceutical preparations. Some of these substances have been implicated in accidental contamination involving loss of preservative efficiency and infection hazards particularly from organisms of Pseudomonas species.

The use of antimicrobial preservatives in topically administered ophthalmic solutions is described. Eye drops of the British Pharmaceutical Codex and commercial preparations of at least equivalent standard appear to be adequately preserved.

The growing employment of plastic contact lenses particularly those possessing hydrophilic properties and their requirements for cleansing and disinfecting solutions has inspired investigation into the antimicrobial efficiency of contact lens solutions. Appraisal is made of microbial "challenge" tests and the significance of the technique employed. Evidence from three groups of workers indicates that whilst it may be difficult to define an absolute standard for antimicrobial efficiency of contact lens solutions onus rests on the manufacturer to demonstrate by adequate quality control procedures that each product can efficiently combat accidental contamination by a limited range of pathogens.

The term "antiseptic" is generally used to describe substances which inhibit the growth or destroy micro-organisms and which can be applied to living tissues, as compared with "disinfectants" which are too toxic or corrosive to be so applied but which are suitable for application to inanimate objects. (Anon 1964).

Among the commonly used antiseptics recognized pharmaceutically as antimicrobial or preservative agents are benzalkonium, chlorhexidine (Hibitane) and phenylmercuric salts. Some of these have been incriminated in reports of incidence of infection in patients to whom the antiseptic solutions have been applied (e.g. Linton and George 1966, Spiller et al 1971).

However, since 1966 the British Pharmaceutical Codex has recommended the use of those antiseptics as antimicrobial preservatives in eye-drops. Aqueous eye-drops, unless in single-application form, are presented in a vehicle which is both bactericidal and fungicidal. Chlorhexidine acetate 0.01% w/v, benzalkonium chloride 0.01% w/v or phenyl-mercuric acetate or nitrate 0.002% may be used, the eye-drop solutions then being sterilised by an approved method viz. autoclaving, bacterial filtration or by heating with the stipulated bactericide at 98°C to 100°C for 30 minutes.

By examining residues of eye-drops issued to hospital out-patients Hugo and Wilson (1970) and the Department of Pharmaceutical Sciences of the Pharmaceutical Society of Great Britain (1969/70) have evaluated the "in-use" efficiency of these procedures. Their results taken together with evidence on sterilisation times following artificial "challenge" with Pseudomonal organisms (Table 1) albeit determined under different test conditions, give reasonable assurance of the effectiveness of benzalkonium and chlorhexidine as antimicrobial preservatives when used in the recommended concentration with compatible medicaments and adjuvants. Phenylmercuric nitrate, although effective, is slower in achieving sterilisation.

Contact lens solutions, which have varying functions, are usually formulated to contain lower concentrations of antimicrobial preservatives (Benzalkonium 0.004%, chlorhexidine 0.001% and Phenylmercuric nitrate 0.001%) because preservatives may be absorbed by the plastic contact lens material, the magnitude of uptake and subsequent release of preservative into the eye being greatest with the hydrophilic type lenses.

Recent work (Norton et al 1974) in which 34 commercially available contact lens solutions were examined for antimicrobial efficiency against four different organisms showed that of

TABLE 1 Anti-Pseudomonal activity of certain Bactericides

Workers	Substance & Concentration	Organism & Approximate Inoculum	Temperature	pH	Time to Sterilise
Richards & McBride (1971)	Benzalkonium chloride 0.1% w/v	Ps.aeruginosa 10^6 orgs/ml^{-1} (NCTC)	37°C	8.1	>15 <30 mins
	Phenylmercuric nitrate 0.002% w/v	-ditto-	37°C	8.1	>45 <60 mins
Hugo & Foster (1964)	Chlorhexidine acetate 0.05% w/v	Ps.aeruginosa 10^2 orgs/ml^{-1} (NCTC 7244)	18°C	7.2	15 mins
	-ditto- 0.005% w/v		18°C	7.2	30 mins
Brown (1968)	Phenylmercuric nitrate	Ps.aeruginosa (3 strains) 10^6 orgs/ml^{-1} (NCTC 6750) (NCTC 7244) (NCTC 8203)	22°C	8.6	5 hours

14 solutions used to soak and disinfect lenses only 4 inactivated all 4 test strains within 1 hour, 7 within 4 hours, while 6 solutions allowed growth of one or more test strains after 24 hours contact. McBride and McKie 1974, independently have produced similar results.

Richards (1975) reported differences in anti-pseudomonal activity in four of six preparations tested by both Norton et al and himself and found growth after 4 hours contact with 0.004 % benzalkonium whereas Norton et al found no growth after 15 minutes.

Richards suggested that the difference was due to harvesting techniques but repetition of the work did not confirm a difference in the efficiency of the antimicrobial substance explainable by variations in growth or harvesting conditions. This emphasises the need for standard procedures when assessing antimicrobial efficiency so that different laboratories may produce comparable results when testing identical products. The protocol of Kelsey and Maurer (1974) shows admirably the extent of detailed control which is necessary.

Davies and Norton (1975) have suggested parameters for microbial challenge tests. Variation in any of the conditions will markedly affect the results obtained and they suggest that for the guidance of manufacturers and the safety of users it would be sensible to base challenge tests on knowledge of the potential danger to the patient consequent upon the use of a contaminated solution. Unfortunately reliable information on the incidence of eye infections amongst contact lens wearers is not readily available.

In the absence of an absolute standard for antimicrobial efficiency of contact lens solutions onus rests upon manufacturers to demonstrate by adequate quality control procedures that their products can combat accidental contamination efficiently.

REFERENCES

1. Anon (1964) British Medical Journal (ii), 1513.

2. British Pharmaceutical Codex 1963, Supplement 1966 p.77. (The Pharmaceutical Press, London).

3. Brown, M.R.W. (1968). Journal of Pharmaceutical Sciences, 57 (3) 389-392.

4. Davies, D.J.G. and Norton, D.A. (1975). Journal of Pharmacy and Pharmacology, 27 (5), 383-4.

5. Department of Pharmaceutical Sciences, Pharmaceutical Society of Great Britain, Laboratory Reports P69/10, P69/14 and P70/5.

6. Hugo, W.B. and Foster, J.H.S. (1964). Journal of Pharmacy and Pharmacology 16 Supplement 124T - 126T.

7. Hugo, W.B. and Wilson, J.V. (1970). Pharmaceutical Journal, 204, 714.

8. Kelsey, J.C. and Maurer, Isobel M. (1974). Pharmaceutical Journal 213, 528-530.

9. Linton, K.B. and George, E. (1966), Lancet (i) 1353-55.

10. McBride, R.J. and Mackie, Mary A.L. (1974).
Journal of Pharmacy and Pharmacology, 26, 899-900.

11. Norton, D.A., Davies, D.J.G., Richardson, N.E., Meakin, B. J. and Keall, A. (1974).
Journal of Pharmacy and Pharmacology, 26 841-846.

12. Richards, R.M.E. (1975).
Journal of Pharmacy and Pharmacology, 27 (5), 381-2.

13. Richards, R.M.E. and McBride, R.J. (1971).
British Journal of Ophthalmology, 55, 734.

14. Speller, D.C.E., Stephens, M.E. and Viant, A.C. (1971).
(Letter to Editor) Lancet, (i) 798-9.

CHLORHEXIDINE IN THE CONTROL OF DENTAL PLAQUE

J. L. Honigman

Imperial Chemical Industries Limited (Pharmaceuticals Division)
Mereside, Alderley Park, Macclesfield, Cheshire

The establishment of bacterial plaque is essential for the development of dental caries and periodontal disease. The plaque which precedes caries forms by the adhesion of bacteria to the tooth pellicle which is further modified by other constituents in the buccal cavity derived from salivary secretions and food. A similar type of plaque precedes gingivitis which becomes increasingly important as a reason for tooth loss with age.

A number of agents have been tested in an attempt to eliminate the bacterial element in plaque and thereby prevent its formation (Figure 1). It would be undesirable to use antibiotic substances for fear of producing resistant strains which could unnecessarily complicate subsequent therapy should these give rise to systemic infection. Hexachlorophane has been found to be very weak as a plaque preventive. The quaternary ammonium compounds, although effective against salivary organisms, have such a relatively short life in the mouth, due to their speedy removal by the normal processes of salivation and mastication, that their usefulness is extremely limited. Victamine C is an organo-phosphorus compound which has been used to prevent crystal accretion which occurs when calculus forms as a consequence of negligent oral hygiene. Zinc salts have an astringent effect but there is little evidence to show that they are superior to placebo for plaque inhibition. Chlorhexidine, on the other hand, does not suffer the disadvantages of being used for systemic infections, is adsorbed on to the tooth surface and has been the subject of over one hundred papers which have confirmed its activity against the organisms concerned and its definite inhibitory effect against plaque formation.

Kanamycin	Penicillin
Erythromycin	Tetracycline
Chloramphenicol	Chlortetracycline
Vancomycin	Actinobolin
Polymyxin B	Spiramycin
Hexachlorophene	
Cetylpyridinium	Benzethonium
Dequalinium	Hexetidine
Victamine C	
Zinc	
Chlorhexidine	

Figure 1. Antibacterial Agents Tried for Plaque Prevention

Some of the factors favouring plaque formation are inattention to the minutiae of personal dental hygiene, the fact that some areas are not easily reached by the toothbrush, diet and hormonal status. Methods of assessing the degrees of plaque severity and the condition of the gums by graded scoring have been developed by Silness and Löe.

Agent	Medium / bacterial source / MLC %				
	Blood agar / saliva	Blood agar / oral Strept and Staph	Clark / saliva	Thioglycollate / saliva	P.I.
Chlorhexidine gluconate	0.1	0.003125	0.00625	0.025	0.23
Chlorhexidine acetate	0.025	0.003125	0.00625	0.025	0.19
Iodosan	25	12.5	6.25	50	1.95
Benzalkonium chloride	0.00625	0.0015625	0.00078125	0.003125	0.47
Aminoacridine HCl.	0.0125	nil	nil	nil	1.43
Proguanil HCl.	0.1	nil	0.2	0.2	1.50
H_2O_2 (3%)	nil	nil	1.5	nil	1.15
Ethanol (50%) w/w	nil	nil	nil	nil	1.92

Figure 2. MLC's of Antimicrobial Agents Used as Mouthrinses Against Salivary Bacteria

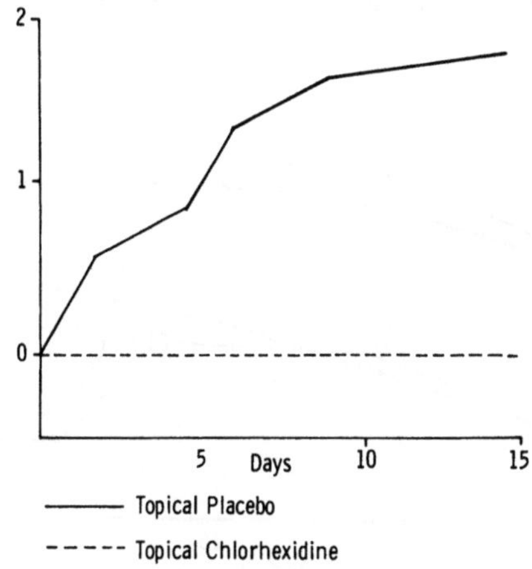

2% Topically once daily

Figure 3

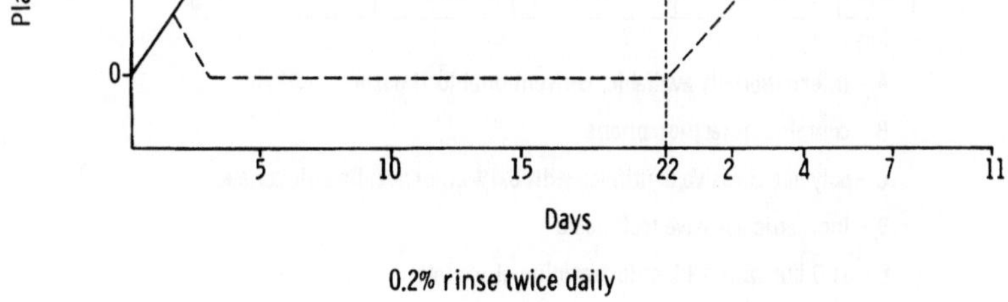

0.2% rinse twice daily

Figure 4

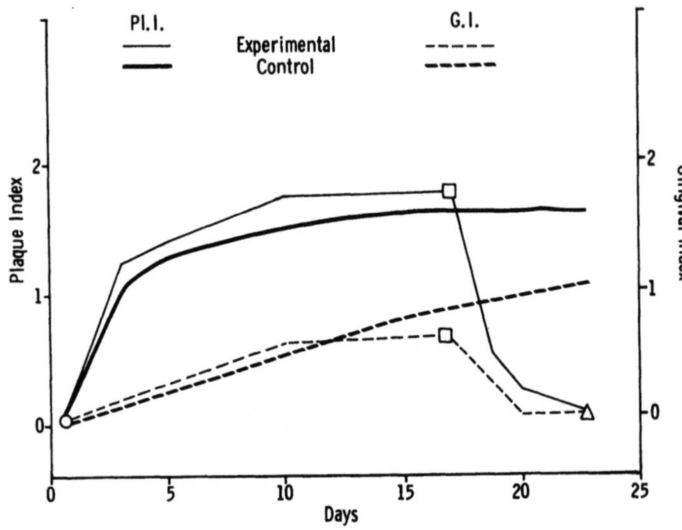

Control - 24 days no hygiene
Experimental - 17 days no hygiene

Figure 5

	P.I. values (Mean)	Antibacterial activity		
		Blood agar	Glucose	Thioglycollate
A	1.67	0.10	0.10	nil
B	1.51	0.10	0.50	0.50
C	0.88	1.00	1.00	0.50
D	1.85	nil	nil	nil
E	0.76	1.00	1.00	1.00

Key

A - internationally available, conventional toothpaste

B - contains hexachlorophane

C - polymer abrasive dentifrice with 0.6 % chlorhexidine gluconate

D - inorganic abrasive toothpaste

E - as D but with 0.8 % chlorhexidine gluconate

Figure 6

The relevance of antibacterial activity to the reduction of plaque has been shown by Gjermo, Baastad and Rolla, 1970 (Figure 2) in which a comparison between various antibacterial agents for potency against salivary bacteria and their effectiveness against plaque was made. The greater the activity against the organisms concerned; the lower the plaque index found in practice when these agents were used in mouth rinses. The lack of effect of quaternary ammonium compounds despite their high antibacterial potency is due to their lack of substantivity to the tooth surface. This limits the length of time for which they can act and, as plaque forms fairly rapidly, duration of activity is an important factor here. In fact, it would appear that the binding property of chlorhexidine to oral tissues contributes considerably to its success in inhibiting plaque formation.

I am indebted to the work of Löe and Rindom Schiott, 1970 for the next three figures (3-5). Plaque can be completely removed by routine scaling and polishing of the teeth. Plaque-free subjects were divided into two groups one of which used a chlorhexidine mouthrinse while the other was supplied with a placebo. The test group remained plaque-free for the 15-day period of the trial while the placebo group displayed increasing plaque (Figure 3). Allowing plaque to form for two days before instituting mouthrinsing, demonstrates the ability of chlorhexidine to eliminate plaque after it has begun to form. Withdrawal of the chlorhexidine rinse after 22 days, allowed a fairly rapid accumulation of plaque (Figure 4). Even after plaque had been allowed to form over a 17-day period, chlorhexidine produced a pronounced reduction in both plaque and gingival indices within a few days (Figure 5).

The chlorhexidine mouthrinses while most effective in reducing dental plaque did seem to have certain disadvantages. For example, the bitter taste was rather difficult to mask and a brown stain could be produced in certain individuals which appeared not only on the teeth but also on the dorsum of the tongue. Although various ingenious reasons were given for these idiosyncratic responses - they were particularly difficult to identify since there was great individual variation, it was felt that the introduction of a gel formulation would make it easier to cope with the problem of taste and at least limit any staining which might occur to the tooth surface. There had also been some reports of mucous desquamation and parotitis with the rinse which may well have been coincidental but, in any case, could be expected to be less likely occurrences if material was only applied directly to the tooth surface.

Gjermo and Rolla, 1970, compared a number of dentifrices (Figure 6) for their effect on plaque. The antibacterial effect against salivary organisms and the ability to inhibit plaque correlates in the same way as these did the various rinses described above.

Hull and Davies, 1973 (Figure 7), painted the teeth of beagle dogs with a 0.5% chlorhexidine gel. A placebo gel and untreated group of dogs showed no difference in their ability to form plaque but there was a highly significant reduction in plaque index between these groups and the test group. After a twelve week period in this trial, chlorhexidine was no longer applied to the test group who soon developed plaque to the same extent as the previous placebo and control dogs. Flotra, 1973 (Figure 8), showed that whether the gel was applied to the teeth by brushing or by cap splints, the plaque index would still be reduced by using a chlorhexidine gel.

1. 0.5% CHX - gel
2. Gel
3. Control

(2 and 3: No difference; 1 vs. 2 and 3: Highly significant difference)

12 weeks

1. Further 4 weeks without treatment

Figure 7. Beagle Dogs (Hull and Davies, 1972)

Brushing		P.I.
Experimental group	6 weeks	0.18 - 0.24
Control	6 weeks	0.4 - 0.7
Cap splint		
Initial		1.56
After 4 weeks		0.56

Figure 8. 0.8% CHX - epileptic children (Flotra, 1973)

1. Scale and polish
2. Toothpaste - 3 weeks
3. 1 % CHX - gel } 6 weeks with cross over
4. Placebo }

	Before	CHX	Placebo
Plaque	1.52	0.35	0.88

Figure 9. (Bassiouny and Grant, 1975)

Plastic applicators - three week periods

	After Placebo	After CHX
Mean Debris Index per tooth surface	1.39	0.58
	P = < 0.001	
Mean Gingival Index per tooth surface	1.04	0.78
	P = < 0.001	

Figure 10. (Usher, 1975)

More recently, Bassiouny and Grant, 1975, have reported the results of a cross-over trial, as shown (Figure 9). The results given for plaque indices have been bulked such that those for each group do not take account of whether the active gel was used before or after placebo. The figure denoted "Before" refers to the reading after stage 2, that is, after using a normal toothpaste for three weeks following the standard scale and polish. These differences were statistically significant. Usher, 1975, reported on the successful use of chlorhexidine gel in mentally retarded children using plastic applicators (Figure 10). This trial was also a cross-over design and the results have been bulked, as before, irrespective of the order of use of active and placebo gels. As can be seen, the results have high statistical significance.

It is certain that for those patients who have physical or mental disabilities which do not allow them to carry out an efficient dental toilet or, alternatively, who have already acquired periodontal disease such that the normal brushing process becomes distressingly painful, a means is now available from which they can derive immense benefit. By preventing plaque formation after various dental surgical procedures, the healing process might well be accelerated because of the reduced likelihood of infection causing further inflammation of the soft tissues of the periodontium.

References

Bassiouny, M.A. & Grant, A.A.,
I.A.D.R. Conference, London, 1975 Abst. L460
Davies, R.M. & Hull, P.S.
J.periodont.Res. 8 Suppl.12, 22-27, 1973
Flotra, L.,
J.periodont.Res. 8 Suppl.12, 41-44, 1973
Gjermo, P., Baastad, K.L. & Rolla, G.,
J.periodont.Res. 5 102-109, 1970
Gjermo, P. & Rolla, G.
Scand.J.dent.Res. 78 464-470, 1970
Löe, H. & Rindom Schiott, C.
J.periodont.Res. 5 79-83, 1970
Silness, J. & Löe, H.
Acta odont.Scand. 22 121-135, 1964
Usher, P.J.
Brit.dent.J. 138 217-221, 1975

SOFRAMYCIN TREATMENT OF THE NASAL CARRIER AFTER 14 YEARS

BRYAN C. STRATFORD AND SHIRLEY DIXSON

ST. VINCENT'S HOSPITAL

MELBOURNE, AUSTRALIA

SUMMARY This paper details the results of treatment with "Soframycin" of nasal carriers both of Staphylococcus aureus and Gram negative bacilli. There were three experiments. The first experiment was a failure in that the results of the treated wards were poor, but it was found that patients were being allowed both to swab and spray themselves! This experiment however, allowed us to determine baseline carriage rates in untreated Control Wards. Experiment 2, again of one month's duration but with more control excercised showed better results. The best results were in a short (10 day) experiment involving only 3 wards where S.D. both swabbed and treated the patients.

INTRODUCTION In 1960, nasal carriers of *Staph. aureus* were considered to be potent sources of hospital acquired infection. In addition both patients and staff with lesions or who carried the organism on their hands, skin, perineum etc. were implicated in infectious outbreaks.

In subsequent years Gram negative bacilli (resistant to many antibiotics) replaced *Staph. aureus* as the prime cause of post-operative wound infections. However, more recently *Staph. aureus* has again emerged as a serious cause of wound sepsis.

Although, in 1960, we found that in certain special circumstances we were able to clear 100 per cent of 85 nasal carriers of *Staph. aureus* in 24 hours using "Soframycin" nebulisers, it was decided to repeat the experiment looking at Gram negative bacilli as well as *Staph. aureus*. On this occasion we used the whole hospital (670 beds) as either Control or Treated Wards.

MATERIALS AND METHODS Swabs: "Trans-cul" swabs (Denver Chemical Mfg.Co) were employed because they allowed the swab immediately to be placed in a modified Stuart's Transport Medium.

Method of Swabbing: each Ward Sister was given printed instructions detailing the combined superficial and deep method of nasal sampling described by us, 1960 (Stratford et al.), together with an explanatory diagram, see Fig 1.

Methods of Identification: Swabs were plated out onto horse blood agar and incubated at 35–37°C for 48 hours. *Staph. aureus* was identified on colonial morphology and confirmed by coagulase testing. Gram negative organisms were identified according to the methods of Cowan & Steel (1965). Sensitivity or otherwise to "Soframycin" was determined by using a framycetin disc (100 mcg. Oxoid) on Mueller Hinton agar with 5 per cent defibrinated sheep red blood cells as described by Ericsson & Sherris (1971).

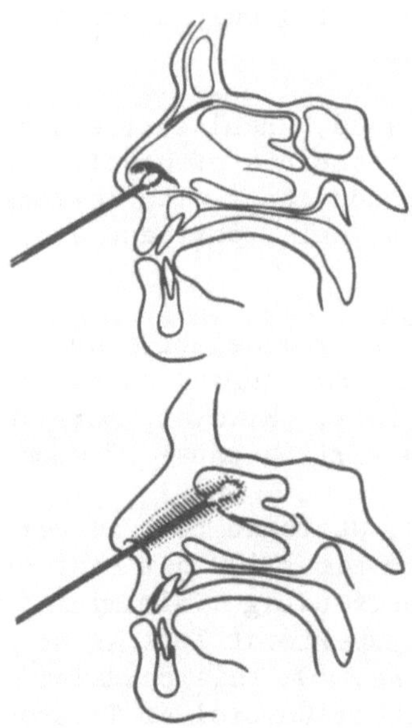

Figure 1. Method of Taking Deep Nasal Swab

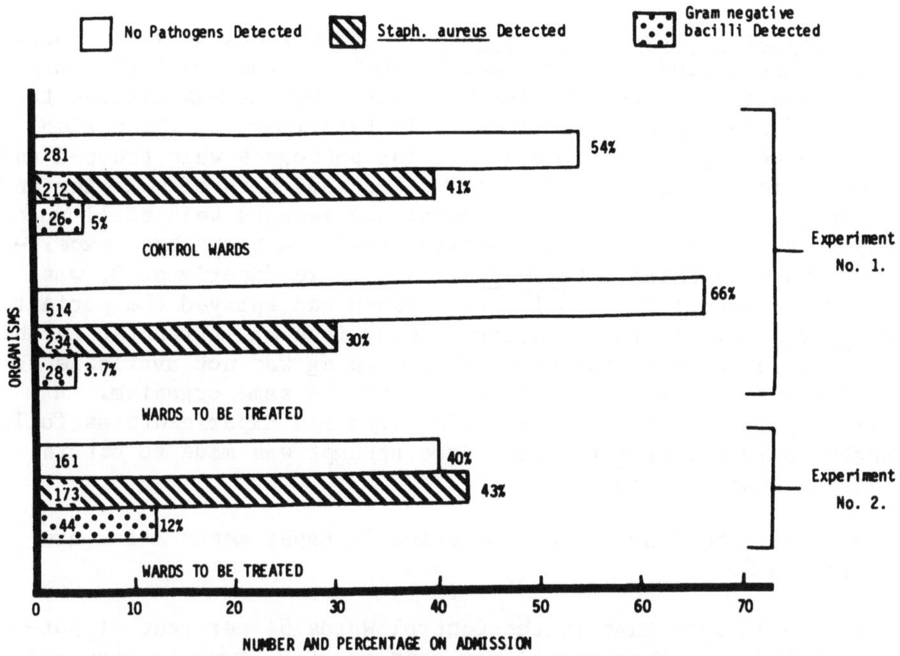

Figure 2. Findings on Admission.

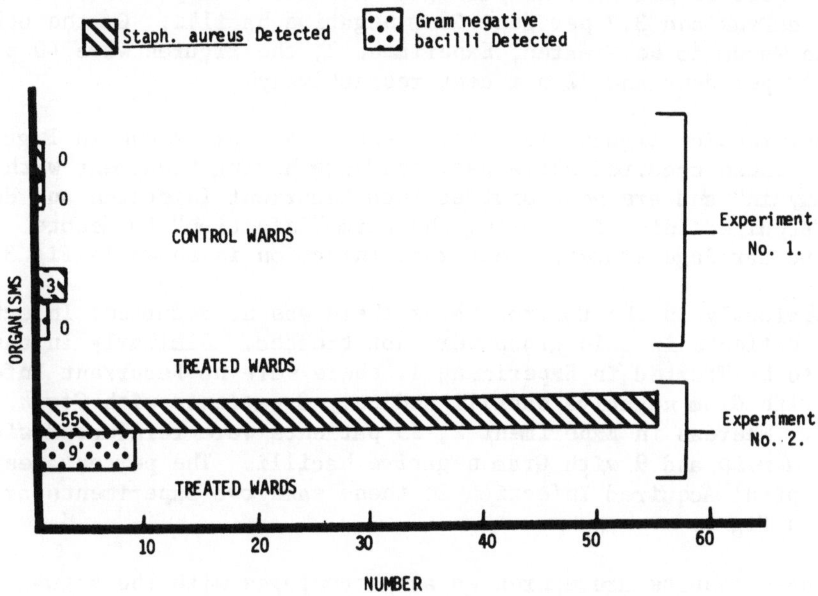

Figure 3. Number of Recurrent Infections.

Differences Between Experiments: in Experiment 1. which lasted one month and included Control and Treated Wards (medical, surgical and specialist) the results were such that it was decided to alter the design of the experiment. In Experiment 2, which also lasted one month, only patients carrying pathogens were treated and more emphasis was given to the correct methods both of swabbing and treatment. Despite this extra control the results were still much at variance with our original observations. In both these experiments swabs were taken twice weekly. Therefore Experiment 3, was designed and one of us (S.D.) both swabbed and sprayed the patients once daily. Correlation with wound infections was attempted in this last experiment. Unfortunately, phage-typing was not available so a similar antibiogram was taken to denote the same organism. A number of patients had to be excluded from all Experiments as follow-up swabs could not be obtained. Some attempt was made to obtain figures on staff carriage rates.

RESULTS. The findings On Admission in Experiments 1 & 2 are shown in Fig 2.

It can be seen that in the Control Wards 54 per cent of patients carried no pathogens, 41 per cent carried *Staph. aureus* and 5 per cent Gram negative bacilli. The actual numbers of patients are overprinted on the left of the bars of the histogram.

In the Wards to be Treated in Experiment 1. the corresponding figures were 66 per cent no pathogens detected, 30 per cent carried *Staph. aureus* and 3.7 per cent Gram negative bacilli. On the other hand in Wards to be Treated, Experiment 2, the figures were 40 per cent, 43 per cent and 12 per cent respectively.

Reinfection figures for Experiments 1 & 2 are shown in Figures 3 & 4. These occurred while patients were having treatment with "Soframycin" and are best divided into Recurrent Infection and Hospital Acquired Infection, using the term "Infection" to denote positive carriage states. Recurrent Infection is shown in Fig 3.

Obviously in the Control Wards there was no Recurrent Infection as the patients in this group were not treated. Similarly in the Wards to be Treated in Experiment 1. there were no Recurrent Infections with Gram negative bacilli and only 3 patients with *Staph. aureus*. Whereas in Experiment 2, 55 patients were reinfected with *Staph. aureus* and 9 with Gram negative bacilli. The percentages for Hospital Acquired Infection in these same two Experiments are shown in Fig 4.

These results are expressed as percentages with the actual numbers of patients involved overprinted on the left hand side of the bars of the histogram. In the Control (untreated) Wards, 67 per cent acquired *Staph. aureus* and 33 per cent Gram negative bacilli.

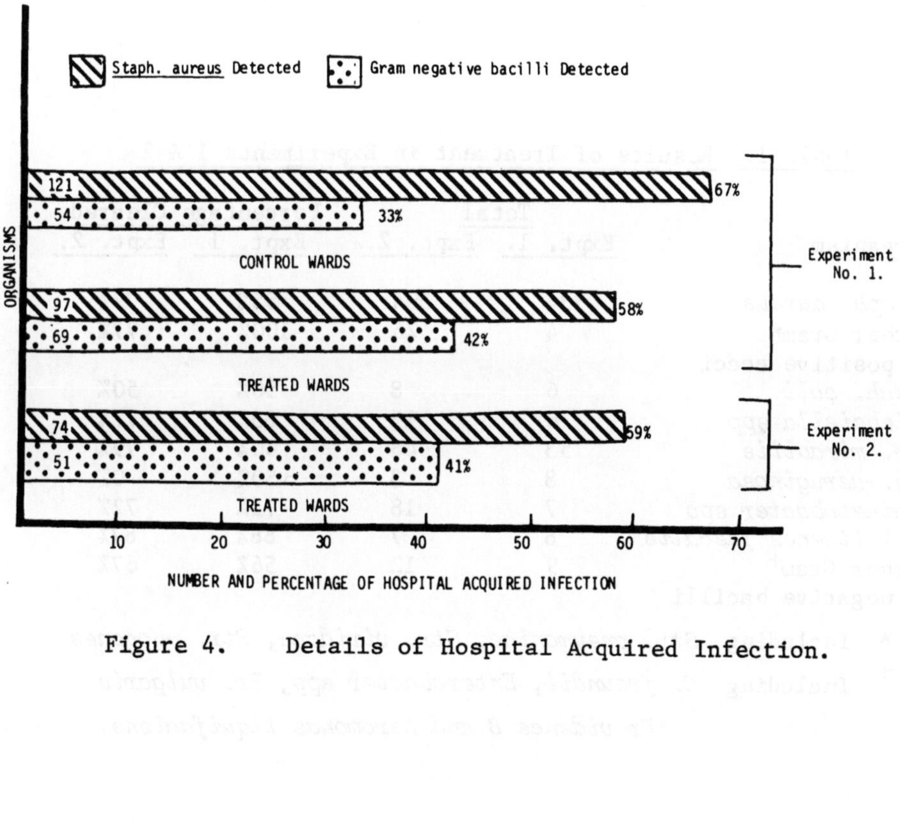

Figure 4. Details of Hospital Acquired Infection.

The corresponding figures for the Treated Wards in Experiment 1. were 58 per cent and 42 per cent. In Experiment 2, the figures were 59 per cent acquired *Staph. aureus* and 41 per cent Gram negative bacilli. The conclusion drawn at this stage is that Hospital Acquired Infection is not very different whether patients are being treated or not. But the important point is -"what was the effect of "Soframycin" treatment on all these carriers?" The question is answered in Table 1.

Table 1. Results of Treatment in Experiments 1 & 2

Organism	Total Expt. 1.	Total Expt. 2.	Percentage Cleared Expt. 1.	Percentage Cleared Expt. 2.
Staph. aureus	334	304	55%	77%
Other Gram* positive cocci	4	26	100%	77%
Esch. coli	6	8	50%	50%
Klebsiella spp	6	13	83%	77%
Pr. mirabilis	53	48	60%	79%
Ps. aeruginosa	8	3	50%	0%
Acinetobacter spp	7	18	71%	72%
Alkaligenes faecalis	8	7	88%	87%
Other Gram+ negative bacilli	9	12	56%	67%

* Including *Str. pneumoniae, Str. viridans, Str. pyogenes*

\+ Including *C. freundii, Enterobacter spp, Pr. vulgaris Providence B and Aeromonas liquifaciens.*

The "total" figures shown here refer to the sum of patients positive On Admission, plus those who experienced Recurrent Infections, and those who had Hospital Acquired Infections. On the left of the table are shown the causative organisms and on the right the percentage of those cleared with treatment. The two findings of importance are first, the percentage of *Staph. aureus* cleared, and second, the percentage of various Gram negative bacilli cleared.

The difference in results obtained in Experiment 1. compared to Experiment 2, requires explanation. When we found only 55 per cent clearance of *Staph. aureus* after one month in Experiment 1. we went to the wards and found that despite our instructions patients were allowed both to swab and treat themselves! This almost certainly accounted for the low figures obtained. The improved results in Experiment 2. reflect more control being exercised on these points.

The final results of Experiments 1 & 2 is shown in Table 2.

Table 2. Time for Clearance of 417 Carriers of Staph. aureus In Experiments 1 & 2

	≤ 3 days	≥ 4 days
Experiment 1.	109 (59%)	75 (41%)
Experiment 2.	170 (73%)	63 (27%)

This shows the time required for clearance of *Staph. aureus*, and illustrates that when more control of treatment is enforced then the rate with which the carriage state was lost increased substantially - from 59 to 73 per cent in 3 days or less.

Table 3 shows the results of Experiment 3 where all the daily swabbing and treatment was carried out by one of us, using the patients in 3 orthopaedic wards.

Table 3. Results of Experiment 3 (Treated Ward)

	Findings on Admission	Reinfection		No. Cleared	Time of Clearance	
		Recurrent	Hosp. Acq.		≤3	≥4
No Pathogens detected	17	NA	NA	NA	NA	NA
Staph. aureus	26	0	5	26/31	25	1
Gram negative bacilli	5+	0	1*	5/6	5	0

NA Not applicable + All Proteus mirabilis * Acinetobacter cloacae

The Experiment lasted only 10 days and involved 58 patients. Adverting to *Staph. aureus*, 26 carried on admission - or at the start of the Experiment - and 5 acquired it in hospital. Twenty six of these 31 were cleared by "Soframycin", ie. 84 per cent, and two isolates of *Streptococcus pneumoniae* were also cleared. Twenty five of these 26 cleared in less than 3 days (ie. 96 per cent). Of the Gram negative bacilli, there were 5 patients carrying *Proteus mirabilis* and all of these cleared within 24 hours with treatment. A single patient acquired *Acinetobacter cloacae* and failed to respond to treatment.

We were able to show that 3 patients' whose wounds became infected carried the same strain of *Staph. aureus* in their noses.

Another figure, not shown earlier, as it was not a truly representative sample was that 45 of 114 staff carried pathogens in their noses, - mainly *Staph. aureus*, ie. nearly 40 per cent.

DISCUSSION In 1960 we used a number of antibacterials in both spray and ointment form in an attempt to decide which was most effective, Stratford et al.(1960). Framycetin with gramicidin and phenylephrine "Soframycin" nebuliser was found to be the best. At that time in a series of 85 carriers of *Staph. aureus* 76 per cent were clear of the organism after 2 hours and 100 per cent after a second application at 24 hours. The present figures are not quite so impressive for *Staph. aureus* (84 per cent cleared), but of considerable interest is the efficiency of the spray against Gram negative bacilli.

A paper by Porter et al.(1963) gave results apparently significantly different from our own, but there were a number of variables. In 1963, Rubbo et al. repeated our original experiment using 157 patients and showed a very considerable reduction of *Staph. aureus* carriage, but not so great as in 1960. The findings presented in this paper show that with due care in both sampling and treatment, 84 per cent of *Staph. aureus* can be cleared, and also a very important finding viz. that the same comment applies to many Gram negative bacilli found in general hospitals.

Before proceeding any further one must ask the question, "is the nasal carriage of pathogens important?" If the answer is no, then the use of any topical antibacterial is unnecessary. However, most published reports answer the question in the affirmative, but the literature is too vast to be reviewed here. Some authors, eg. Gould & Cruickshank (1957) and Williams (1959) have suggested that acquired staphylococcal infections - in as many as 80 per cent according to Gould (1957)-may result from autogenous infections.

Williams et al.(1959) proved that patients who were or became carriers of *Staph. aureus* developed three times as much post-operative sepsis as did those who were never carriers and they further stated "that self-infection is important in the aetiology of the septic lesions." Our figures for a short experiment (No. 3) are marginally higher than this. In a chest unit, Weinstein (1957) showed that 37 per cent of nasal carriers developed surgical infections compared to 11 per cent of infections in patients who were not carriers.

The nasal carriage of *Staph. aureus* was shown to bear an important relationship to the occurrence of wound infections in some circumstances by auto-infection, Weinstein (1959), Williams et al. (1962), Rountree & Beard (1968) and in other circumstances by cross-infection to other patients by dispersal through the air, Stokes et al.(1965), and Williams et al.(1962). However, Henderson and Williams (1963) found only two of 6 patients acquired sepsis with the nasal strain amongst 64 carriers in 100 surgical patients - the other 4 acquiring "ward" strains. But these "ward" strains almost certainly came from other patients or staff, in that order. Davidson et al.(1971) noted a slight but significant increase in post-operative sepsis amongst nasal carriers, confirmed by our results in Experiment 3. Similar findings were reported by Lindbom (1964), and Lindbom et al.(1967) and Lindbom & Laurell (1967).

Since the early 1960's Gram negative bacilli have replaced *Staph. aureus* as the prime cause of hospital acquired infection and indeed many seriously ill patients carry such organisms in their noses and elsewhere, Stratford et al.(1968), Gallus et al. (1969). However, the findings presented in this present paper show that the ubiquitous staphylococcus is again becoming a problem, but that "Soframycin" nebuliser is the best treatment both for this and Gram negative organisms.

The conclusion reached is that the suppression of nasal carriage is a useful measure before elective surgery especially in patients admitted to hospital some days prior to operation. But the treatment of the nasal carrier per se will not necessarily reduce the incidence of hospital acquired infection, Gillespie et al.(1959), but can be considered as one of many measures for the environmental control of this disease.

The problem is further complicated by the fact that non-carriers can acquire the carriage state whilst in hospital; those that are already carriers may change their organism to a more virulent type; further, Gram positive organisms may be replaced by Gram negative ones. Other patients, probably intermittent carriers, as we have shown, lose their organisms without treatment, which confirms the finding of McNeill et al.(1961), who discussed these matters as they related to *Staph. aureus*. Jarvis & Wigley (1961) confirmed the efficacy of "Soframycin" treatment of the nasal carrier, but noted that the same phage-type re-emerged 12 days after ceasing treatment.

In 1961, Jacobs et al. found that minor nasal abnormalities in 178 nurses were associated with an increased nasal carriage rate of

Staph. aureus and confirmed that fact that a combined superficial (vestibular) and deep (middle turbinate) swab detected 17 per cent more carriers. The work of Atkins & Marks (1952) and Roodyn (1960 a & b) showed that the nose acted as a reservoir from which infection occurred.

Other workers such as Barber & Warren (1962) correctly stated that not all *Staph. aureus* are of equal virulence whether acquired in the operating theatre or the ward, and named phage-type 80/81 as the most important strain at that time. However, we contend it is easier to treat all patients as actual or potential carriers, rather than wait on the results of phage-typing which we consider of most importance in epidemic tracing.

Henderson & Williams (1961), using "Naseptin" cream concluded that this compound had no effect on the number of post-operative wound infections but found the infection rate to be higher in carriers than in non-carriers. In 1960, we found "Naseptin" cream to be a poor alternative to the "Soframycin" nebuliser, but the effects of the former were enhanced if the components were used as a spray. In 1964, White advised the use of gentamicin cream and quoted impressive results. We would not agree to the use of topical gentamicin within the hospital environment because of the risk of inducing resistant strains of organisms to a most important systemic antibiotic. Ruckley & Calder (1965) confirmed the efficacy of "Soframycin" and the requirement for taking a correct nasal swab for diagnosis.

The most recent study implicating the nasal carrier is that of Rebel et al. (1975) who concluded that infection of renal haemodialysis shunts was acquired principally from the nose.

With all the above facts and figures it appears necessary to reduce the ward load of microorganisms by whatever means available. One such is the treatment of the nasal carrier. Indeed, an economic case can be made out for treating all patients (and ? staff) as either actual or potential nasal carriers of pathogens. The cost saving to the laboratory would be considerable.

In conclusion, we learnt two lessons from these Experiments. First, the swab must be taken properly (see Fig 1.) and must be a combined superficial/deep swab. Second, the nebuliser must be used correctly as stated in our 1960 paper ie. the nebuliser should be employed so as to reach the anterior nares, then enough (0.2 ml.) of liquid jet should flood the deeper recesses of the nose so that the patient has to spit out any excess fluid. Once daily application is enough. Both these instructions should be taught to student nurses.

ACKNOWLEDGEMENTS Our thanks are due to the Honorary Medical Staff of St. Vincent's Hospital for their co-operation in allowing us to use their patients, and to Dr. W. M. C. Keane, Medical Superintendent for permission to publish these results. Roussel Pharmaceuticals Australia Pty. Ltd. generously supplied the "Soframycin" nebulisers and the "Trans-cul" swabs. All the Microbiology Staff particularly Miss B. Bell deserve our thanks for willingly undertaking the extra work involved in these experiments.

REFERENCES

1. Atkins, J.B., and Marks, J. (1952) Brit. J. industr. Med. 9, 296.
2. Barber, M., and Warren, S. (1962) Lancet, 2, 374.
3. Cowan, S.T., and Steele, K.J., (1965) "Manual for the Identification of Medical Bacteria" Cambridge University Press.
4. Davidson, A.I.G., Clark, C., and Smith, G. (1971) Brit. J. Surg. 58, 333.
5. Ericsson, H.M., and Sherris, J.C. (1971) Acta path. microbiol scand. Section B. Suppl. 217.
6. Gallus, A.S., Stratford, B.C., Matthiesson, A.S., and Dixson, S. (1968) Lancet, 1, 68.
7. Gillespie, W.A., Alder, V.G., Bradbeer, J.W., Ayliffe G.A., and Wypkema, W. (1959) Lancet, 2, 781.
8. Gould, J.C., (1957) Hospital Coccal Infections, P. 32, Association of Clinical Pathologists, Readings.
9. Gould, J.C., and Cruikshank, J.D. (1957) Lancet, 2, 1157.
10. Henderson, R.J., and Williams, R.E.O. (1961) Brit. med. J. 2, 330.
11. Henderson, R.J., and Williams, R.E.O. (1963) J. clin Path. 16, 452.
12. Jacobs, S.I., Williamson, G.M., and Willis, A.T. (1961) J. clin Path., 16, 519.
13. Jarvis, A.W., and Wigley, R.D., (1961) Lancet, 2, 1168.
14. Lindbom, G. (1964) Acta. chir. scand., 128, 421.
15. Lindbom, G., Laurell, G., and Grenvik, A., (1967) Acta. path. microbiol. scand., 69, 219.
16. Lindbom, G., and Laurell, G., (1967) Acta. path. microbiol. scand., 69, 246.
17. McNeill, I.F., Porter, I.A., and Green, C.A. (1961) Brit. med. J., 2, 798.
18. Porter, I.A., McNeill, I.F., Miller I.T., and Green, C.A. (1963) Brit. med. J., 1, 1515.
19. Rebel, M.H., Van Furth, R., Stevens, P.,Ősscher-Zonderman, L. and Noble, W.C., (1975) J. clin. Path., 28, 29.
20. Roodyn, L. (1960 a) J. Hyg., Camb., 58, 1.
21. Roodyn, L. (1960 b) J. Hyg., Camb., 58, 11.
22. Rountree, P.M., and Beard, M.A., (1968) Med. J. Aust., 1, 577.
23. Rubbo, S.D., Stratford, B.C., Christie, R., and Dixson, S. (1963) Brit. med. J., 2,252.

24. Ruckley, C.V. and Calder, M.A. (1965) Scot. med. J., 10, 235.
25. Stokes, E.J., Hall, B.M., Richards, J.D.M., and Riley, D.J. (1965) Lancet, 2, 197.
26. Stratford, B., Rubbo, S.D., Christie, R., and Dixson, S. (1960) Lancet, 2, 1125.
27. Stratford, B.C., Gallus, A.S., Matthiesson, A.S., and Dixson, S. (1968) Lancet, 1, 68.
28. Weinstein, H.J. (1959) New. Eng. J. Med., 260, 1303.
29. White, A., (1964) Am. J. of Med. Sci., 248, 52.
30. Williams, R.E.O., (1959) Lancet, 1, 190.
31. Williams, R.E.O., Jevons, M.P., Shooter, R.A., Hunter, C.J.W., Girling, J.A., Griffiths, J.D., and Taylor, G.W., (1959) Brit. med. J., 2, 658.
32. Williams, R.E.O., Noble, W.C., Jevons, M.P., Lidwell, O.M., Shooter, R.A., White, R.G., Thom, B.T., and Taylor, G.W., (1962) ibid. 2, 275.

THE EFFECT OF ANTIMICROBIAL AGENTS ON THE UMBILICAL CORD

R.H. GEORGE

Birmingham Maternity Hospital

Queen Elizabeth Medical Centre
Edgbaston, Birmingham B15 2TG

The umbilicus is often the primary site of colonization with Staphylococcus aureus in the newborn (Jellard 1959). Treatment of the cord with hexachlorophane has been shown to reduce colonization and infection (Gillespie et al. 1958), but it is reported that colonization and infection with Gram-negatives increases (Conn 1969). This paper reports studies of the umbilical flora in babies treated with a number of anti-bacterial talcs and the effect of some of them on separation of the cord.

MATERIALS AND METHODS

Babies of at least 38 weeks gestation and born by vaginal delivery were included in these studies. At birth the cord was severed and ligated with a latex band. Babies were washed with soap and water shortly after birth but were not bathed thereafter. Except for cord treatment the management of all babies was identical. Hexachlorophane was used routinely by the staff for handwashing.

The umbilicus of all babies was cleansed with spirit each morning and if soiling was observed at subsequent nappy changes. The control group received no other treatment. Talc containing either 0.33% hexachlorophane, 0.2% or 1% chlorhexidine hydrochloride or 0.2% chlorhexidine acetate was applied after the spirit to the other babies. Immediately prior to treatment on the second, fourth and sixth days the umbilicus was sampled by the author with moistened swabs. Culture was performed for 48 hours at 37°C after inoculation onto blood agar, MacConkey agar and letheen agar (Baltimore Biological Ltd.). Anaerobic cultures were also set up on blood agar. Growth was assessed in one of four grades:-

no growth, scanty (less than ten colonies per plate), moderate and heavy.

Coagulase positive staphylococci were identified as Staphylococcus aureus and coagulase negative as Staphylococcus albus. Other organisms were identified according to Cowan and Steel (1966).

The day on which the cord separated was studied in those babies receiving 1% chlorhexidine hydrochloride, 0.2% chlorhexidine acetate and a group treated with hexachlorophane and whose umbilicus was painted at birth and on day four with aqueous triple dye. Further studies were carried out later with 1% chlorhexidine hydrochloride talc to which 3% zinc oxide had been added.

RESULTS

The number of cultures which were sterile decreased progressively with postnatal age. In the control group the umbilicus of 48% was sterile after 24 hours, of 11% after 3 days and of 4% after 5 days. This was accompanied by a fall in the number of sample yielding a scanty growth. The bacteriological findings on the fourth and sixth days of life are shown in tables 1 and 2. Escherichia coli was the most frequently isolated Gram-negative organism. Proteus mirabilis, P. vulgaris and Klebsiella aerogenes were the only other Gram-negatives frequently isolated. Streptococcus faecalis was the most frequently isolated organism amongst a variety of 'others', which included members of the genus Bacillus, Clostridium, Corynebacterium and other streptococci.

Statistical analysis (Chi^2) was carried out on the results obtained on days four and six. Males and females were analysed separately, because males tended to be more frequently colonized. 1% chlorhexidine hydrochloride was significantly better in both sexes and on both days at preventing colonization with Gram-negatives than when used at a concentration of 0.2% and than hexachlorophane ($p<0.05$ to <0.01). It was significantly better than the control treatment in males but not females, nor compared with chlorhexidine acetate.

The number of sterile cultures obtained in each group was compared. 1% chlorhexidine hydrochloride was significantly better than 0.2% hydrochloride ($p<0.001$), the control group ($p<0.001$), and in females both chlorhexidine acetate ($p<0.01$) and hexachlorophane ($p<0.001$). In males the difference was not statistically significant with the last two agents. If comparison was made with a combined group of those yielding no growth and scanty growth,

TABLE 1

COLONIZATION OF UMBILICUS ON FOURTH DAY

	CONTROL	STERZAC	HIBITANE HCl 0.2%	HIBITANE ACETATE	HIBITANE HCl 1%
NO GROWTH	7 (10)	14 (18)	8 (10)	34 (29)	46 (53)
±	4 (6)	7 (9)	7 (9)	13 (11)	14 (16)
S.ALBUS	29 (43)	37 (47)	25(32)	53 (45)	16 (18)
S.AUREUS	17 (25)	15 (19)	28 (36)	13 (11)	8 (9)
G-VES	15 (22)	14 (18)	17 (22)	9 (8)	3 (3)
OTHERS	6 (9)	7 (9)	7 (9)	4 (3)	2 (2)
TOTAL	68	79	78	118	87

± = scanty growth   % in parenthesis

Sterzac = hexachlorophane. Hibitane = Chlorhexidine

1% chlorhexidine hydrochloride was significantly better than all other treatments on both days and in both sexes.

The results of cord separation are shown in table 3. Statistical analysis of the number of babies with the cord separated prior to day 9 showed that separation was significantly faster when zinc oxide was included in the talc ($p<0.001$).

TABLE 2

COLONIZATION OF UMBILICUS ON SIXTH DAY

	CONTROL	STERZAC	HIBITANE HCl 0.2%	HIBITANE ACETATE	HIBITANE HCl 1%
NO GROWTH	2 (4)	7 (11)	4 (6)	15 (17)	30 (44)
±	3 (6)	3 (4)	2 (3)	15 (17)	13 (19)
S.ALBUS	21 (41)	44 (67)	17 (28)	40 (46)	13 (19)
S.AUREUS	16 (31)	15 (23)	30 (49)	12 (14)	9 (13)
G - VES	10 (20)	20 (30)	20 (33)	8 (9)	3 (4)
OTHERS	5 (10)	9 (14)	4 (6)	3 (3)	0 (0)
TOTALS	51	66	61	86	68

± = scanty growth   % in parenthesis

Sterzac = hexachlorophane. Hibitane = Chlorhexidine

TABLE 3

TIME OF SEPARATION OF CORD

COMPOUND	NO. OF BABIES	DAY OF SEPARATION 3	4	5	6	7	8	9	10	11	12	13	14	15	>15
HEXACHLOROPHANE 0.3% WITH TRIPLE DYE	122	0	2	10	12	23	23	17	17	9	2	5	1	0	1
CHLORHEXIDINE ACETATE 0.2%	113	0	1	3	4	22	20	22	20	10	9	0	2	0	0
CHLORHEXIDINE HYDROCHLORIDE 1%	60	1	0	1	3	7	7	11	12	6	6	2	1	2	1
CHLORHEXIDINE HYDROCHLORIDE WITH 3% ZnO_2	54	1	10	9	11	7	7	4	3	1	1	0	0	0	0

DISCUSSION

Reports of hexachlorophane toxicity (Kimbrough and Gaines 1971) led to its withdrawal from many maternity hospitals. Epidemics of staphylococcal infection have been reported (Ayliffe et al. 1972; Dewar et al. 1972; Scopes et al. 1974) demonstrating the continuing need for an antistaphylococcal agent to prevent infection in the newborn. In these studies treatment was confined to the umbilicus. A number of babies with sterile umbilical cultures had staphylococcal skin lesions elsewhere, demonstrating the need for more widespread treatment if colonization of the baby is to be prevented.

Previous studies have compared the effect of treatment on the colonization rate with S.aureus. The author feels that this will vary over a period of time with the level of contamination of the environment by this organism. Because these studies were carried out over a period of 2 years the ability of the talcs to prevent colonization with any organism has been used as a measure of their activity.

Cord separation has been shown to depend on the time elapsing between birth and ligation of the cord (Bernstine et al. 1959) and the method of ligation (Laursen 1963). The role of Gram-negative organisms in delaying cord separation has been reported

(Ibister 1951) and the effect of antibacterial agents (Huntingford et al. 1961). In the present studies separation of the cord was more rapid in babies colonized with Gram-negatives except in the group treated with chlorhexidine talc containing zinc oxide. Gillespie et al. (1974) observed delayed separation using chlorhexidine talc without zinc oxide. In the present studies delayed separation was also observed, but this was overcome by the addition of zinc oxide, possibly associated with its astringent properties.

1% chlorhexidine hydrochloride talc would appear to be a suitable alternative to hexachlorophane for prevention of staphylococcal infection in the newborn, with the advantage of activity against Gram-negative organisms.

Ayliffe, G.A.J., Brightwell, K.M., Ball, P.M. and Derrington, M.M. (1972), Lancet, 2, 479.
Bernstine, J.B., Ludmir, A. and Fritz, M. (1959), American Journal of Obstetrics and Gynecology, 78, 69.
Conn, N.K. (1969), Scottish Medical Journal, 14, 23.
Cowan, S.T. and Steel, K.J. (1966), Manual for the Identification of Medical Bacteria. Cambridge University Press. London.
Dewar, J., Porter, I.A. and Smylie, H.G. (1972), Lancet, 2, 712.
Gillespie, W.A., Simpson, K. and Tozer, R.C. (1958), Lancet, 2, 1075.
Gillespie, W.A., Corner, B.D., Burman, D. and Alder, V.G. (1974), Journal of Hygiene, 73, 311.
Huntingford, P.J., Welch, G., Glass, U. and Wetherley-Main, G. (1961), Journal of Obstetrics and Gynaecology of the British Commonwealth, 68, 179.
Ibister, C. (1951), Medical Journal of Australia, 2, 386.
Jellard, J. (1959), The British Journal of Clinical Practice, 13, 43.
Kimbrough, R.D. and Gaines, R.D. (1971), Archives of Environmental Health, 23, 114.
Laursen, H. (1963), Acta Obstetricia at Gynecologica Scandinavica, 42, 43.
Scopes, J.W., Eykyn, S. and Phillips, I. (1974), Lancet, 2, 1392.

MECLOCYCLINE, AN ANTIBIOTIC FOR TOPICAL USE

Loris Jacopo Bononi

Chair of Chemotherapy Institute of Pharmacology

University of Turin

Meclocycline or 7-chloro-6-methylene-5-hydroxytetracycline belongs to the class of the 6-methylenetetracyclines (1). Meclocycline is one of the most active tetracyclines *in vitro*. Against strains of *Shigella* and *Salmonella* *in vitro* studies report meclocycline to be equal or superior to streptomycin and chloramphenicol (2). Several investigations have confirmed the *in vitro* broad spectrum activity of meclocycline (2, 4, 16, 19, 24, 25), and pointed out a marked antitreponema activity *in vitro* and an antiborrelia activity *in vivo* (3). The *in vivo* activity of meclocycline *per os* against *Staphylococcus aureus* infection has been negative. The *in vivo* activity of meclocycline parenterally against *Staphylococcus aureus* infection has been comparable to that of tetracycline (26). In rats, oral meclocycline is very active on aerobia, coliforms and (which is unusual for a tetracycline) also on mycetes (7). Meclocycline is exceedingly insoluble in water, poorly soluble in serum, very poorly absorbed from the gastrointestinal tract and not absorbed through the skin (4, 8, 9). Meclocycline in the chloroform/water system appears to be somewhat more lipophilic than other tetracyclines, except doxycycline (23). The oral absorption of meclocycline would expect to be better, in consequence of this fact, however, experiments in animals and in man show a very poor gastrointestinal absorption (6, 11, 26) and a possible explanation is offered by the very high mucin binding found *in vitro* (4). No blood levels of meclocycline have been found in five normal male subjects after 3, 6, 12 hours from a 25 mg/capsule orally administered of hydrochloride. No blood levels of meclocycline have been found in the same five subjects after 3 days of treatment with meclocycline hydrochloride (25 mg. q.i.d) after 3, 6, 12 hours from the last administration (26). Meclocycline also has a high affinity for tissues and serum proteins and complexes strongly with metal ions (23). Based on the data available, it seems that meclocycline should be effective especially in two sectors of chemotherapy:

(a) infections of the skin (10, 20, 21),

(b) infections of the alimentary tract (11).

Preliminary trails would also suggest the use of meclocycline in the treatment of trachoma (12, 13, 14).

As far as point (a) is concerned, meclocycline meets some very important requisites: "Antibacterial preparation for topical application to the skin should have a broad spectrum since many superficial infections have a mixed bacterial flora. The agent must be non-irritating and non toxic to leucocytes and other phagocytic cells and granulation tissue, and the antibacterial drugs liable to give rise to hypersensitivity should not be used. Antibiotics suitable for systemic administration should be avoided, so that if drug-resistance or skin hypersensitivity should occur, the patient is not thereby deprived of the benefits of a valuable drug for systemic treatment should this become necessary."(15) Meclocycline is a broad spectrum antibiotic which cannot be used by systemic route, is not absorbed through the skin and has shown neither local (22, 21, 9, 27, 20) nor general toxicity when administered for topical use (16). The U.V. irradiation has no influence on the chemotherapeutic activity of meclocycline (16). "Since the skin is the principal reacting organ in allergical reactions a substance with a low sensibilization rate, which is not employed for systemic therapy, is of particular importance for topical application. A group sensibilization cannot be excluded, but allergical reactions, especially of such a severe type, following the application of tetracyclines are rare" (16). As regards point (b), meclocycline appears to be a good antibiotic for the treatment of bacillary dyssentery, bacterial food poisoning, cholera, and other bacterial diarrheas. Preliminary trails have shown that meclocycline is an effective, safe and well tolerated antibiotic for localized lower tract intestinal infections (11, 17, 18).

SUMMARY

Meclocycline is a semisynthetic tetracycline belonging to the class of 6-methylenetetracyclines, having peculair characteristics. The use of meclocycline in the treatment of the infections of the skin and of the alimentary tract of bacterial origin, appears advisable.

Thanks to Istituto Chemioterapica Italiano S.p.A. for having supplied the pure substance of meclocycline.

BIBLIOGRAPHY

1) Blakwood,R.K., Beereboom,J.J., Renhard,H., Stephens,C.R., Shach Von Wittenau: Journal Am.Chem.Soc. 81, 2773, 1961
2) Bononi, L.J., Filadoro, F., Renzini,G.: Attività antibiotica di un nuovo derivato del gruppo delle tetracicline Antibiotica 2, 60, 1964
3) Berti,T., Bononi,L.J., Cantelli Forti,G.,Scuka,M., S.E. Abdullahi: Atti 6° Congress of Chemotherapy,Tokyo,Antimic. Antib. Chemoth., I° Vol., pag. 394, 1970, Tokyo
4) Bononi,L.J., Di Carlo,F., Scrollini,F.,: Meclociclina. VII Riunioni Medico-Chirurgiche Internazionali - Convegno di Chemioterapia - Minerva Medica - Torino, 1975
5) Arena,F., Bononi,L.J., Persico,D., Rausa, L. : Rapporto tra assorbimento dopo somministrazione orale ed influenza sullo sviluppo animale di due nuove tetracicline. Antibiotica 4, 230, 1966
6) Bernardi,F., Bononi,L.J., Di Carlo,F.: 7-cloro-6-metilene-5-ossitetraciclina - Giorn.Ital.Chemiot. 17, 276, 1970
7) Bononi,L.J., Minelli Bertazzoni,E., Benoni,G.; Attività antibatterica intestinale della meclociclina nel ratto. VII Riunioni Medico-Chirurgiche Internazionali - Convegno di Chemioterapia - Minerva Medica - Torino, 1975
8) Gattini,P., Renzini,G.: Hematic Levels of meclocycline in adults treated with meclocycline ointment. Antibiotica - Vol. 10, No. 1-2, 1972
9) Scotta,S., Ceccarelli,G., Renzini,G.: Absorption of meclocycline after its application on the skin in children VIII Intern. Congress Chemoth. Athens 8/14 Sept. 1973
10) Ciaffi,G., Renzini,G.: La meclociclina in dermatologia Prospettive di terapia (In corso di stampa)
11) Goffredo,V., Bay, F.: Terapia della diarrea infettiva-Diarrea del viaggiatore e del turista - con meclociclina. Clinica Europea Vol. XIII - No. 5 , 1974
12) Malik,S.R.K., Gupta,A.N., Deb,W.C., Sood,G.C.: Clinico-cytological study of trachoma and the effect of GS 2989
13) Neema,H.V., Wath,K., Bal,A., Shukla, B.R.: GS 2989 in trachoma - Am. J. Ophthal. 57, 747, 1964
14) Neema, H.V., Nath, K., Bal, A., Josmi, O.P., Shukla, B.R.: Comparative therapeutic field trials of GS 2989 and oxytetracycline in trachoma - Brit. J. Ophthalm.49, 330,1965 Bietti, G.B.,: Natural history and diagnosis of trachoma Israel Journ. Med. Scien. 8, 1101, 1972
15) Garrod, L.P., O'Grady, F.: Antibiotici e Chemioterapia Ed. Il pensiero scientifico - Roma 1973 pag. 257
16) Schoog, M., Weith, H., Dimmling, T., Schimpf, A.,Winkler, E.: Pharmacolgical studies with a new antimicrobial cream Arzneim. Forsch. 6, 1022, 1972
17) Abreu, L.M.: Evaluacion de erecto de la Clorometiloxitetraciclina (GS 2989) en el tratamiento de la diarrea in-

fecciosa aguda. Rev. de Invest. 4, 93, 1964.

18) Alvarez, M.R., Olerte, T., Galindo, E., Joachin, A.: Accion del compuesto GS 2989 sobre distintos grupos de bacterias enteropatogenas aisladas de los Hisopos rectales de ninos con diarrea en Mexico. Rev. De Invest. 4, 99, 1964

19) Cipriani, P., Filadoro, F., Liani, M.: Concentrazioni minime inibenti di 3 antibiotici tetraciclinici nei confronti di 60 ceppi di batteri Gram-positivi e Gram-negativi, Giornate Mediche di Fiuggi, 27-29 Giugno 1972.

20) Schimpf, A., Schoog, M., Weih, H.: Clinical Experience with meclocycline in dermatology - Arzneim.Forsch. 22,1019 1972

21) Vaccari, R.: Attività clinica di un preparato ad uso topico a base di 7-cloro-6-metilene-5-ossitetraciclina. Giorn. Ital. Dermat. Vol. 109, No. 9, 1974

22) Caramia, F.: Electron microscope study of the skin after application of fluprednilidene with or without meclocycline - VIII Int. Congr.of Chemoth. Athens, 1973

23) Genazzani, E.: (Istituto di Farmacologia dell'Università di Torino): Dati non pubblicati.

24) Cavallo, G.: Antibacterial spectrum of meclocycline - Antibiotica (accepted for publication).

25) Ciaffi, G.: Antibacterial spectrum <u>in vitro</u> and <u>in vivo</u>- Protection test with meclocycline. Antibiotica (accepted for publication).

26) Biological Research Laboratories Istituto Chemioterapico Italiano S.p.A. Milan - Data not yet published.

27) Domenichini, F., Bobbio-Pallavicini, F., Fischetti, M.: Ricerche controllate sulla efficacia ....e tollerabilità di un nuovo derivato tetraciclinico ... Rivista Gen. Ital. Chirurg. Vol. XIII, No. 1, 1972

THE EFFECTIVENESS OF POVIDONE-IODINE, SAVLON AND CHLORHEXIDINE AS PRE-OPERATIVE VAGINAL DISINFECTANTS

N.M. Duignan, J.D. Williams and P.A. Lowe
Dept. of Obstetrics and Gynaecology and Dept. of Microbiology,
Birmingham and Midland Hospital for Women and
Dudley Road Hospital, Birmingham, England

SUMMARY

The effectiveness of Povidone-iodine, Savlon and chlorhexidine as pre-operative vaginal disinfectants was assessed by both *in vivo* and *in vitro* studies. Povidone-iodine removed 92% of pathogens present in vaginal aspirates and Savlon removed 88%, aqueous chlorhexidine removed only 46% of organisms and this difference was highly significant ($p < 0.001$). *In vitro* killing of *Bacteroides fragilis* occurred rapidly in dilute solution of povidone-iodine and on overnight culture in 1/100,000 chlorhexidine and 1/10,000 Savlon; the greatest reduction was obtained by a 2min preparation with povidone-iodine.

INTRODUCTION

Anaerobic organisms are commonly found as commensals in the urogenital tract and infections with such organisms may occur following pelvic surgery. Although these bacteria often give rise to only mild infections they may, on occasion, cause severe sepsis with associated thrombophlebitis (Ledger *et al*., 1971).

In this paper, the effectiveness of povidone-iodine, Savlon and chlorhexidine as pre-operative vaginal disinfectants is assessed by both *in vivo* and *in vitro* studies.

MATERIALS AND METHODS

Clinical Methods: Pre-operative vaginal aspirates were collected from 84 patients. After introducing a sterile bivalve speculum into the vagina 0.5 ml sterile saline was placed in the posterior fornix; 0.1 ml was then aspirated into a sterile pipette and inserted in 9 9 ml thioglycollate broth. The vagina was next cleansed with the appropriate disinfectant which was left *in situ* for selected periods ranging from 1 to 3 min. before being removed. A second vaginal aspirate was then collected in the manner already described. The disinfectants used were:

1) Betadine surgical scrub diluted 1 in 10 containing 0.075% available iodine

2) Savlon diluted 1 in 100 containing chlorhexidine 0.015% and cetrimide 0.15%

3) Aqueous chlorhexidine 0.05%

Laboratory methods: 0.1 ml quantities of each thioglycollate broth were distributed on to blood agar and MacConkey plates for aerobic culture and on to a blood agar plate for anaerobic culture. The Gas-Pak system was used for the anaerobic cultures and plates were examined after 24 and 72 hours.

The *in vitro* bactericidal activity of each disinfectant was tested against 6 strains of *Bacteroides fragilis*. 0.5 ml broth suspensions of *Bacteroides fragilis* were inoculated into concentrations of povidone-iodine ranging from 0.1 to 1% dilutions of the clinical solutions and subcultured at intervals of between 15 s to 5 min. The *in vitro* activity of Savlon and chlorhexidine was tested by using a tube dilution technique in thioglycollate broth sealed with liquid paraffin.

RESULTS

The organisms isolated from the vaginal aspirates are shown in Table I. More than 10^5 per ml bacteroides were isolated from 6 of the 84 patients (7%) and anaerobic streptococci (more than 10^5 per ml) were isolated from 26 patients (30%). Povidone-iodine was found to remove 92% of pathogens present, Savlon 88% and aqueous chlorhexidine 46%; the difference between chlorhexidine and the other disinfectants was highly significant ($p < 0.001$).

In vitro killing of *Bacteroides fragilis* occurred rapidly in dilute solution of povidone-iodine and on overnight culture in 1/10,000 Savlon and 1/100,000 chlorhexidine solution.

DISCUSSION

Bacteroides have been isolated from the vagine and cervix of 5 to 18% of non-pregnant patients (Bollinger, 1964; Ansbacher et al., 1971; Neary et al, 1973; Duignan and Lowe, 1975). It is

TABLE 1

ORGANISMS (MORE THAN 10^5 PER ML) ISOLATED FROM VAGINAL ASPIRATED BEFORE AND AFTER TREATMENT WITH DISINFECTANT. THE POST-DISINFECTION RESULTS ARE SHOWN IN PARENTHESES

Disinfectant	No. of Patients	Bacteroides	Anaerobic streptococci	Gram negative bacilli	Staphylococcus pyogenes
Povidone-iodine	35	4 (0)	10 (1)	6 (0)	4 (1)
Savlon	29	1 (0)	10 (1)	8 (1)	8 (1)
Chlorhexidine	20	1 (1)	6 (6)	5 (2)	7 (1)

frequently difficult to decide which organism or organisms are responsible for infections occurring after pelvic surgery, and the vaginal flora may not accurately reflect the organisms present in the pelvic tissues. The role of bacteroides and anaerobic streptococci in post-operative pelvic infection has been well documented by the isolation of these organisms in pus drained from pelvic abscesses or in blood cultures obtained after pelvic surgery (Ledger et al., 1971). The present study suggests that povidone-iodine is the most effective vaginal disinfectant against anaerobic organisms though Savlon also reduces the number of potential pathogens in the vagina. Whether use of these disinfectants eliminates post-operative pelvic infection due to anaerobic organisms remains to be determined.

REFERENCES

Ansbacher, R., Boyson, W.A. and Morris, J.A. (1967) American Journal of Obstetrics and Gynaecology, 99, 394.

Bollinger, C.C. (1964) Obstetrics and Gynaecology, 23, 251.

Duignan, N.M. and Lowe, P.A. (1975) Journal of Antimicrobial Chemotherapy, 1, 117.

Ledger, J.W., Sweet, R.L. and Headington, J.T. (1971) Surgery, Gynecology and Obstetrics, 113 837.

Neary, M.P., Allen, J., Okubadejo, O.A.and Payne, D.J.H. (1973) Lancet, ii, 1291.

A CONTROLLED TRIAL OF POVIDONE IODINE IN THE PREVENTION OF POST OPERATIVE INFECTION IN ABDOMINAL WOUNDS

O. J. A. GILMORE and P. J. SANDERSON

St. Bartholomew's Hospital and North Middlesex Hospital

London

In 1960 the Public Health Laboratory Service[1] concluded from a national survey that some 10% of all surgical wounds became infected. As a consequence of such infections patients each spent on average one extra week in hospital. The annual cost of this extra bed occupancy in England and Wales was then estimated at £3.3 millions. According to DHSS data[2], the comparable cost in 1973 was £22.3 millions.

While asepsis is an ideal towards which surgeons must strive, it is nevertheless an accepted fact that the exclusion of all organisms from the wound is probably impossible, particularly in operations on the bowel or in the presence of peritonitis. It is therefore suggested that the best attainable standards of asepsis should be complemented by the use of an applied antibacterial.

Lowbury and Ayliffe[3] have stated that most, if not all, the independently active antibiotics have probably been discovered, and there is a strong desire amongst microbioloigsts that antibiotics be conserved and their use undergo constant review. A reappraisal of the value of antiseptics in the prevention of post operative wound infection is therefore indicated. There have been few clinical trials of these agents in wound infection. Chlorhexidine[4] and Noxythiolin[5,6,7], both failed to reduce infection when instilled into abdominal wounds prior to closure. Neither antiseptic however was applied by aerosol.

The antimicrobial activity of iodine has been long known[8], but because of its insolubility in water, chemical instability and irritating effect on tissues, it has not been widely used. On the other hand, povidone iodine, a complex of the polymer polyvinylpyrrolidone with iodine[9] enhances the bactericidal activity of elemental iodine whilst making it soluble in water, chemically stable and non-irritant.

Previous experience has demonstrated the efficacy of an aerosol formulation of povidone iodine (Disadine DP) following appendectomy[10,11]. This was the first controlled trial in which an antiseptic was shown to prevent wound infection. We now report a trial of the use of povidone iodine in all forms of abdominal surgery. We also investigated the incidence of bacterial contamination of the wound at the time of operation and ascertained the frequency and nature of post operative wound infection.

MATERIALS AND METHODS

156 consecutive patients admitted to the North Middlesex Hospital, London, under the care of one consultant and undergoing abdominal surgery were included in a controlled trial. 12 patients were withdrawn, 9 because they died within 2 weeks of operation, one because of uncontrollable diabetes mellitus, one because the drain was brought out through the main wound, and the last because he required re-operation within two weeks. Random allocation of patients to a group who received an aerosol of povidone iodine and to a group who received propellant alone (control group) was achieved by using a table of random numbers. The method of skin disinfection in both groups was identical and the surgeons involved limited to those of one firm. In both groups the aerosol was sprayed into the wound for a period of 10 secs. from a distance of 10 inches (25 cm) after the peritoneum was closed, but before the parietal layers of the wound had been sutured. The materials used for suturing were standard and drains when required were brought out through a separate stab incision.

All wounds were inspected by the clinical microbiologist who was unaware of the operation performed or of the nature of the aerosol used. In deciding the state of the wound post operatively the criteria of Ljungquist[12] were adopted. The wound was assessed as clean or infected. It was infected if at any time a purulent discharge occurred. If a serous discharge occurred the wound was swabbed and classified as infected if bacteria were cultured from it. All patients were seen 6 weeks after operation and any wound discharging pus after the patient had returned home was included in the infected group. Throughout each patient's stay in hospital a careful watch was kept on any evidence of reaction to either spray.

At every operation following closure of the peritoneum but before spraying, a swab tip was rolled along the length of both wound edges. The swab was sent to the laboratory in Stewart's transport medium, and innoculated onto two blood agar plates and a

McConkey plate and into Robertson's meat broth. One blood agar plate was incubated aerobically and the other anaerobically. If no bacterial growth occurred, the plates were reincubated for a further 24 hours. The cooked meat broth was subcultured if the direct plates did not yield organisms at 48 hours. A swab was taken from each subsequently infected wound and treated in the same way.

Standard methods of bacterial identification were used.[13] When similar bacterial strains were isolated from the operative wound and from a post operative wound infection, they were regarded as belonging to the same strain if the results of the reactions tested were identical and the response to antibiotics did not differ by more than one drug.

RESULTS

Swabs of the operative wound were obtained from 133 patients. Bacteria were isolated from 65, indicating an operative wound contamination rate of 49%. 83 of the total of 131 strains of bacteria isolated at operation belonged to species usually associated with the skin flora. Staphylococcus albus was the organism most frequently found, but 30 of the total 47 strains isolated were recovered only from the cooked meat enrichment medium. Of the organisms associated with the gut flora, Escherichia coli was the predominant species followed by Streptococcus faecalis. (Table 1).

TABLE (1) Organisms isolated. *organisms regarded as belonging to gut flora, including (not listed) Anaerobic streptococci (1), Enterobacter sp. (1), Pseudomonas sp. (1), Proteus sp. (1), Klensiella sp. (1), Lactobacillus sp. (1), Clostridium welchii (1).

Organism	No. isolated at operation	No. isolated from wound infections	
		Total	Similar strain at operation
Staphylococcus albus	47	3	0
*Escherichia coli	25	8	6
*Streptococcus faecalis	11	3	1
Streptococcus viridans	10	1	1
Staphylococcus aureus	7	4	1
Micrococcus spp.	5	0	0
Haemolytic streptococci (not Strep. faecalis)	4	0	0
*Bacteroides spp.	3	3	1
*Others	19	7	1
Total strains	131	29	11

TABLE (2) Operative procedure related to contamination and infection.

Operation	Total Cases	% Contaminated at operation	% of each group infected Control	Povidone Iodine
Biliary tract	16	60	0	0
Miscellaneous	27	30	8	0
Appendicectomy	47	32	16	5
Gastroduodenal	25	46	23	22
Intestinal	17	90	64	12
Peritonitis	12	80	80	16
Total	144			

The nature of the organisms isolated varied according to the operative procedure. 40 of the 76 isolates obtained from cases of appendicectomy, intestinal resection or peritonitis belonged to the gut flora as opposed to skin flora, compared to only 7 of the 57 isolates obtained from all other cases. Significantly more patients with peritonitis ($P < 0.01$) or undergoing intestinal resection ($P < 0.002$) had contaminated wounds compared to those in other categories. 27% of patients in the contaminated group had malignant disease compared to 14% in the non-contaminated group. (Table 2).

Swabs were obtained from all infected cases excepting six patients whose infection only became manifest after they had left hospital. In 11 of the 18 patients whose wounds discharged in hospital, organisms present at the time of wound closure were isolated from subsequently infected wounds, a correlation rate of 61%. 29 strains of bacteria were isolated from infected wounds and 18 of these belonged to gut flora. In 6 patients the correlating organism belonged to gut flora, in 3 to the skin flora and in 2 patients there was a mixture. Eschericia coli was the organism most frequently isolated from the infected wounds and 6 of the 8 strains recovered corresponded with those found at operation. 4 strains of Staphylococcus aureus were recovered but only one corellated with that found at operation.

The incidence of post operative infection mirrored the incidence of operative contamination except in biliary surgery. 26% of patients with contaminated wounds developed infection compared to 10% with non-contaminated operative wounds ($P < 0.01$).

24 of 144 patients studied developed post operative wound infections. Three quarters of infected patients came from the control group in which the infection rate was 24.3% compared to 8.6% in those receiving povidone iodine. A comparison of spraying

TABLE (3) Incidence of Wound Infection

Group	Patients	Infected	Significance
Control (Propellant alone)	74	18 (24.3%)	P 0.01
Povidone Iodine	70	6 (8.6%)	

povidone iodine against the propellant alone was statistically in favour of the povidone iodine ($P < 0.01$). (Table 3). Of the 68 patients with sterile operative swabs, only 3% of the povidone iodine group became infected compared to 17% in the control group.

Interparietal povidone iodine resulted in a reduced infection rate after all forms of abdominal surgery. The reduction in infection in patients undergoing intestinal resection, of whom 90% had contaminated wounds was significant at the 4% level, while that obtained in patients with peritonitis of whom 80% were contaminated, was significant at the 5% level.

The randomnization method used resulted in the even distribution of patients between the two groups according to age, sex, body build, pathology, operation, surgeon and the use of antibiotics. Ten patients in the control group and 13 in the povidone iodine group received antibiotics in hospital. Patients whose wounds healed by first intention had a mean post operative stay of 10 days compared to 2 weeks in those who developed wound infection ($P < 0.05$). Finally, no reaction, local or general, was seen to either aerosol throughout the whole trial.

DISCUSSION

Davidson et al[14] in a computer analysis of 14 factors involved in wound infection identified a positive operative wound culture to be more than three times as significant as any other single factor. The greatest risk of infection occurred in abdominal surgery and both these authors and Jepson[15] found a greater hazard from organisms of the gut flora compared to those of the skin flora. An earlier survey[16] showed five times higher incidence of infection in patients with contaminated wounds. In this study 49% of the operative wounds were contaminated and 8 of the 11 organisms found both at the time of operation and in infected wounds belonged to the gut flora.

It has been concluded[16,17] that wound infection is increased by prophylactic antibiotics, but there is evidence that ampicillin[18] kanamycin[19] and cephaloridine[20] reduce infection when instilled into the wound after abdominal surgery. Short term systemic prophylaxis with cephalgridine[21,22] and gentamicin and lincomycin in combination[23] have also been shown to be effective.

The incidence of antibiotic resistant gram negative bacteria, however, continues to increase and will only be reversed by holding some antibiotics in reserve. A povidone iodine aerosol has been demonstrated in this trial to be a valuable alternative to antibiotics in the prophylaxis of post operative abdominal wound infection.

REFERENCES

1. Public Health Laboratory Service (1960) Lancet 2 659
2. Department of Health and Social Security (1975), Private estimate based on Hospital In-Patient Enquiry and Hospital Costing Returns.
3. Lowbury E.J.L. and Ayliffe G.A.J. (1974) Drug Resistance in Antimicrobial Therapy. Springfield. Charles C. Thomas.
4. Crosfil M., Hall R., London D., (1969) Brit. J. Surg. 56 906.
5. Bird G.C., Bunch G.A., Hoffman D.C., Humphreys C.S., Rhind J., Rosenburg I.L., Whittaker M., Wilkinson A.R., Hall R. (1971) Brit. J. Surg. 58 477.
6. Stoker T.A.M. and Ellis H.(1972) Br. J. Surg. 59 184.
7. Frazer-Moodie A. (1974) J.R. Coll. Surg. Edinb. 19 121.
8. Davaine (1873) Dictionaire Encylopedie des Sciences Medical. Paris. Asselin P. and Masson G. Page 335.
9. Siggia S. (1957) J. Am. Pharm. Assoc. 46 201.
10. Gilmore O.J.A. (1973) Lancet 1 1134.
11. Gilmore O.J.A. and Martin T.D.M. (1974) Br. J. Surg. 61 281.
12. Ljungquist U. (1964) Lancet 1 1095.
13. Cowan S.T. and Steel K.J. (1975) Manual for the Identification of Medical Bacteria. Cambridge University Press.
14. Davidson A.I.G., Clark C., and Smith G. (1971) Br.J.Surg. 58 333.
15. Jepson O.B. (1973) Ann. Surg. 177 178.
16. National Research Council (1964) Ann. Surg. 160 Supplement.
17. Altemeier W.A., Culbertson W.R. and Hummell R.P. (1968) Surg. Clin. North Am. 48 227.
18. Nash A.G. and Hugh T.B. (1967) Br. Med. J. 1 471.
19. Moylan J.A. and Brockenbrough E.C. (1968) Surg. Forum 19 66.
20. Evans C., Pollock A.V. and Rosenberg I.L. (1974) Br.J.Surg.61 133.
21. Polk H.C. Jun. and Lopes Mayor J.F. (1969) Surgery 66 97.
22. Evans C. and Pollock A.V. (1973) Br. J. Surg. 60 434.
23. Stokes E.J., Waterworth P.M., Franks V., Watson B., and Clarke C.C. (1974) Br. J. Surg. 61 739.

BETADINE

P.R. Zellner and E. Metzger
Berufsgenossenschaftliche Unfallklinik
Ludwigshafen-Oggersheim, Abteilung für
Verbrennungen, plastische und Handchirurgie;
Chefarzt: Priv.Doz. Dr.Dr. Zellner

In the late 19th century, the problem of burn infection had already been recognized and a local topical treatment was started during the time of LISTER, however, it was only at the beginning of the second world war that it first became possible to drastically reduce the mortality rate during the first 48 hours by means of infusion therapy; this did not influence the overall mortality as significantly as expected, owing to the fact that many patients died as a result of septicaemia at a later date.

Even though it had proved possible to reduce this complication, up to the present day it remains one of the major problems in burns, and there is no doubt that in a high percentage of cases mortality occurs as a direct consequence of infection. It ist presumed that the main source of infection come from the environment and to a lesser extent from the patient himself.

Our own series of 26.000 swabs taken over the last four years have shown a steady increase in gramnegative bacteria, with a predominance of proteus and clebsiella.

According to a close examination of 930 patients we know that in 30 % of cases pseudomonas is already present on the skin or in the anal region on admission. Otherwise, the infection starts in 38 % during the first week, and in 20 % during the second week after the accident.

With the help of a serotyping which we performed on 9500 specimens, we ascertained that in our unit the most hazardous areas (i.e. those in which cross-infection is most likely to occur) are those which are common to all patients - the bath room and dressing room. There was no evidence, however, to support the theory that the water tap and sluice present in the patient's room provide sources of infection.

Important factors governing the onset of infection are

extent of the injury - depth of the injury - age of the patient.

The diagramm illustrated here is taken from the work by Soerensen & Thompson.

The danger of infection may be reduced in two ways - on the one hand on the part of the organism of the patient himself, by means of humoral and cellular defence, antiserum and antibiotics; and on the other hand by conservative and surgical procedures.

It is worthwhile to recognize that no great difference exists between the specific antibody response against pseudomonas of vaccinated and non-vaccinated burned patients, and up to the present time, it has not proved possible to stimulate the poor response of the defence mechanism by means of active immunisation. Only passive immunisation has shown positive results in reducing death by septicaemia, but since this treatment involves the human donor pool, its application is difficult to accomplish.

Antibiotics are applied; their relative merits are discussed, and what appears to be evident from recent studies is that it is important to check the sensitivity of a strain present on the patient's wound, individually, against a certain antibiotic; and to check the level of the antibiotic itself present in the blood and tissue in order to control its proper spplication.

Regarding the environmental measures, we have aseptic and surgical procedures at our disposal, however, we are limiting our discussion here to the antiseptic topical treatment.

A topical antiseptic substance should contain the following properties:

1 - it must be atoxic and should not bring about any changes in metabolism.

2 - it must have a broad bactericidal spectrum.

3 - it should be able to enter and penetrate the necrotic tissue.

4 - it must be inert to the surviving and reproducing tissues.

5 - it should not cause antigenicity.

6 - it should not cause any bacteriological resistance.

In recent years different agents have been used:

1. Sulfamylon
2. Silver-Nitrate
3. Gentamycin
4. SSD

But the fact that different topic creams are used in different burn units indicates that no single one is totally efficient in its action. Unfortunately, there is no standard method for evaluating the different agents and their activity i.e. their bacteria-killing property.

Due to the fact that, in spite of all eforts, most extensive burns become infected, a positive bacteriological result does not provide sufficient conclusive evidence. The proof of good treatment in relation to mortality can only be accepted when a large number of patients are treated in one burn unit, and it must be borne in mind that in many cases even the pathologist has difficulty in making a specific post-mortem diagnoses due to septicaemia. So it would appear necessary to test the agent and its bactericidal efficiency by a quantitation of bacteria either on the wound surface or deep in the tissue; only such a test, in combination with the antibody response, will give some indication of the patient's prognoses.

Adopting the open wound method of treatment together with an antiseptic cream, we applied BETADINE - this cream being known to have a bactericidal function on the burn wound. Betadine which is Iodine with PVP, was applied four times per day to 1oo patients who all possessed burns of over 2o %. When using the cream, attention was paid to the following points:

1. Laboratory results - We established that there was no obvious influence of Betadine in relation to abnormal blood values; no change of electrolyts; no change of ph, and no change in the kidney function.

2. Clinical observation of the wound surface - The clinical application of the cream is simple - but is important to note that the diagnoses must be made prior to application because the Iodine content results in a brownish staining of the eschar. On observing the wound surface it had a generally clean appearance; there was no suppuration at the margins of the eschar; there were only two cases in which secretion collected beneath the eschar; otherwise the necrotic area was a hardened texture and could be stripped off easily in the operating room, leaving a clean surface.

3. Bacteriological results - Besides using the routine swab method we also employed the quantitation of bacteria according to the method of Brentano. The following results were evaluated:

   1 - no. of sterile wounds,

   2 - time of onset of infection

   3 - sort of pathogenic bacteria

   4 - no. of pathogenic bacteria

   5 - relation between number of pathogenic bacteria and depth and extent of the burn

   6 - Comparison between Betadine and other topic treatments in relation to number of bacteria on the wound.

Results in relation to the number of bacteria are shown in this series.

In 1oo patients, we too, 725 specimens for bacteria counting; of these 725, 537 were sterile and did not show any pathogenic bacteria. With relation to the number of patients, 45 showed no growth in the quantitative count, but out of these, in 14 cases we found pathogenic bacteria after further cultivation in broth.

In 26 cases we counted 10^2
In 10 cases we counted 10^3
In 11 cases we counted 10^4
In 8 cases we counted 10^5.

No case was beyond this density, and it has to be mentioned that in 16 patients the number of bacteria was reduced.

Apart from the sterile wounds it was shown that in 49 patients the infection started during the first week, and in 20 patients during the second week.

In our trial no relationship could be established between the depth of the wound and number of bacteria. But a relationship was established between the extent of the burn and the quantitation of bacteria whereby there was less colonisation in smaller burns, when compared with the results of the more extensive ones.

What was apparent was a marked difference between Betadine and two other topical treatments all of which had been evaluated in the same way, i.e. according to Brentano. Patients were treated in the same unit, according to the same routine and by the same staff. We think that in this study Betadine compares favourably. - In comparison to the other topic treatment there were more sterile cases, and the density in bacteria never went above 10^5.

We are well aware that our examination of the wound surface provides insufficient evidence for us to make a definite statement regarding the bactericidal action of a cream, but we intend to carry out a quantitation of bacteria test in the tissue itself in the near future. Furthermore, definite proof of penetration can only be established by means of an absorption test and our initial trials with such a test are too premature to be presented here.

In conclusion - in treating the burn wound we have to consider that

1. 3o % of patients are harbouring pathogenic bacteria on admission and consequently aseptic procedures have a limited value.
2. the defence mechanism of the victim cannot be stimulated actively,
3. that an extensive burn will become infected in spite of the treatment applied.
4. that early excision of the eschar does not necessarily indicate a better survival rate.

Therefore, in the localised treatment of the burn wound it is of vital importance that an antiseptic topical treatment be carried out - and of all the topical treatments used in our unit until now Betadine has provided us with the most rewarding results.

List of Contributors

Alder, V.G.
Alexander, E.R.
Andrews, J.
Angel, J.H.

Bek, E.
Bismuth, R.
Blackman, E.
Blaha, H.
Blenk, H.
Bodunkova, L.E.
Bononi, L.J.
Boon, P.F.G.
Botzenhart, K.
Bruce, B.
Burgogne-Berezin, E.
Burley, D.M.
Burman, D.
Bywater, M.J.

Cartwright, R.Y.
Case, D.E.
Cavanagh, P.
Cho, K.Y.
Conway, J.
Corner, B.D.
Coutsogeorgopoulos, C.
Csonka, G.W.

Davis, K.Y.
Dixson, S.
Duignan, N.M.

Edsall, J.
Emmerson, M.
Erdei, J.
Espinosa, M.

Fanciulli, S.
Farrell, W.
Felton, C.
Fekety, F.R.
Fomina, I.P.
Franz, G.
Fujii, R.

Gabriel, Sister M.
Garcia, E.
Garcia, J.A.
George, R.H.
Geuther, R.
Gillespie, W.A.
Gilmore, O.S.A.
Girling, D.J.
Goto, J.
Granitzka, S.
Grosset, J.
Gunda, T.

Harris, W.
Harrison, W.O.
Haupt, I.
Hernadi, F.
Hobby, G.L.
Hofstetter, H.
Holmes, K.K.
Honigman, J.L.
Hooper, R.
Hori, M.
Hossack, G.M.

Inamatsu, T.

Jaszberenyi, P.

Kaether, M.
Kattan, S.
Keane, C.
Kensit, J.G.
Kim, K.S.
Koller, W.
Konno, M.
Korpal, K.
Kosakai, N.
Kosasin, F.
Krasemann, C.

Lassus, A.
Lebek, G.
Levrier, M.
Lindberg, R.B.
Little, J.
Lowbury, E.J.L.
Lowe, P.
Lyell, A.

Marcinia, J.
Martin, F.
Mason, A.D.
Matsumoto, F.
McAinsh, J.
Metzger, E.

Mitchison, D.A.
Mittermayer, H.
Modai, J.
Muller, W.

Nakauchi, J.
Havashin, S.M.
Norton, D.A.

Oguri, T.
Ohmori, M.
Okada, J.
Otaya, H.
Ozawa, A.

Pacaud, G.
Parsons, R.L.
Pellegrini, R.
Perez,Urena, M.T.
Pinto-Ribeiro, M.M.
Poh, S.C.
Pollock, A.V.
Portoles, A.
Prentice, M.J.
Prieto, J.
Pruitt, B.A.

Qureshi, S.H.

Radwanska, E.
Rangoonwala, R.
Reeves, D.S.
Reimann, R.
Renkonen, O.V.
Rhemrev, P.E.R.
Ridgway, G.L.
Rostila, T.
Rotter, M.
Rubio-Lotvin, B.
Ruden, H.
Rushton, A.

Saenz, M.C.
Salton, M.R.J.
Samoilova, L.N.
Sanderson, P.J.
Sarubbi, F.A.
Schuhmann, E.
Shadomy, S.
Shiba, K.
Shimada, K.
Soyka, E.
Sparling, P.F.
Sperenskaya, O.N.
Stratford, B.C.
Suzukake, K.
Swyer, G.I.M.
Sykes, R.B.
Szabo, G.
Szelagowicz, B.

Taylor-Robinson, D.
Thrum, H.
Truffaut, C.
Turrell, D.

Ubukata, K.
Ueda, Y.
Uehara, Y.
Umezawa, H.
Urbanczik, R.

Wagner, G.
Weissenbacher, E.R.
Wewalka, G.
Williams, J.D.
Winrow, M.J.
Wise, R.
Work, C.

Zellner, P.R.
Zierski, M.
Zueva, V.S.

MIX
Papier aus verantwortungsvollen Quellen
Paper from responsible sources
FSC® C105338

If you have any concerns about our products,
you can contact us on
ProductSafety@springernature.com

In case Publisher is established outside the EU,
the EU authorized representative is:
Springer Nature Customer Service Center GmbH
Europaplatz 3, 69115 Heidelberg, Germany

Printed by Libri Plureos GmbH
in Hamburg, Germany